POCKET COMPANION TO ACCOMPANY

Avery's Diseases of the Newborn,
7th Edition

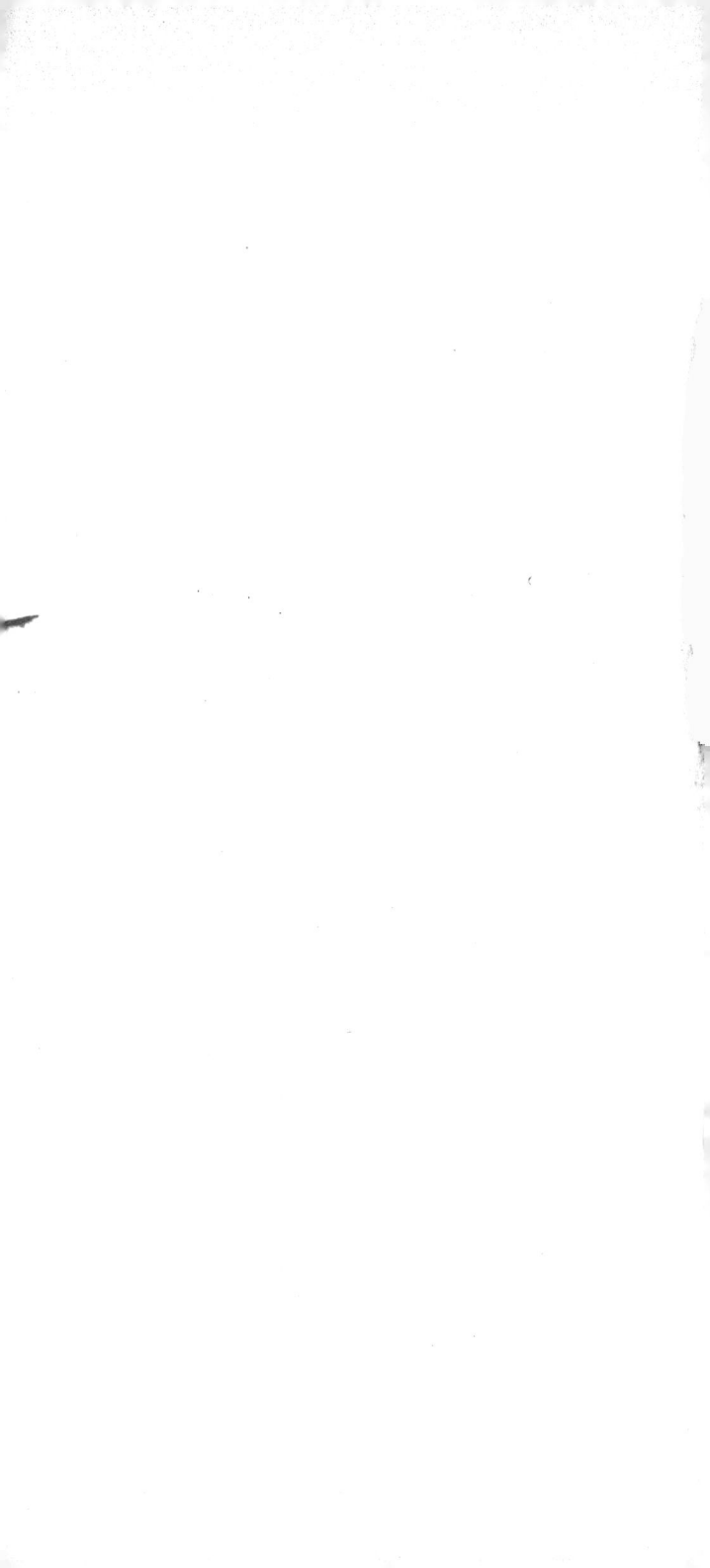

POCKET COMPANION TO ACCOMPANY
Avery's Diseases of the Newborn,
7th Edition

H. WILLIAM TAEUSCH, MD
Professor and Vice Chair of Pediatrics
University of California
Chief of Pediatrics
San Francisco General Hospital
San Francisco, CA

MARY ELLEN AVERY, MD
Thomas Morgan Rotch
Distinguished Professor of Pediatrics, emerita
Harvard Medical School
Department of Pediatrics
The Children's Hospital
Boston, MA

W.B. Saunders Company
A Division of Harcourt Brace & Company
Philadelphia   London   Toronto   Montreal   Sydney   Tokyo

W.B. SAUNDERS COMPANY
A Division of Harcourt Brace & Company

The Curtis Center
Independence Square West
Philadelphia, Pennsylvania 19106

Library of Congress Cataloging-in-Publication Data

Taeusch, H. William.
Pocket companion to accompany Avery's diseases of the newborn / H. William Taeusch, Mary Ellen Avery.—7th ed.

p. cm.

ISBN 0-7216-8146-8

1. Infants (Newborn)—Diseases, Handbooks, manuals, etc.
   I. Avery, Mary Ellen.   II. Title.   III. Title: Avery's diseases of the newborn.

RJ254.S3 2000   618.92'01—dc21

DNLM/DLC   99-24328

POCKET COMPANION TO ACCOMPANY AVERY'S
DISEASES OF THE NEWBORN,
7th Edition   ISBN 0-7216-8146-8

Copyright © 2000 by W.B. Saunders Company.

All rights reserved. No part of this publication may be reproduced or transmitted in any form or by any means, electronic or mechanical, including photocopy, recording, or any information storage and retrieval system, without permission in writing from the publisher.

Printed in the United States of America.

Last digit is the print number: 9 8 7 6 5 4 3 2 1

PREFACE

When I was in training a few decades ago, our peers, our professors, and a very few selected texts and journals were the sole sources of our educational input. Now, as we approach the next millennium, videos, the Internet, computer literature searches, CDs, audiotapes, and a multiplicity of journals are available to us in addition to texts. (One of our senior residents said that the TV show *ER* had contributed 25% of his medical knowledge.)

This volume, a synopsis of the seventh edition of *Avery's Diseases of the Newborn*, offers yet another way of providing just the right amount of information in just the right form. One of its virtues is that it is designed to fit in a pocket, to serve the student/practitioner when he or she does not have immediate access to a computer, a full text, or an all-wise teacher. We have attempted to give the essence of differential diagnosis and initial management but we have de-emphasized pathogenesis, alternative therapies, and prognosis. While our overall goal was to be concise, the authors of the chapters of the full text may be appalled at the extent to which their original contributions have been edited, and for this we apologize, suggesting only that the cut version may whet the appetite of many readers for the full text. We hope this synopsis will offer some direction when the physician caring for a newborn feels stuck. As always, we are interested in how this text serves your needs.

H. WILLIAM TAEUSCH
btaeusch@sfghpeds.uscf.edu

MARY ELLEN AVERY

CONTENTS

CHAPTER 1
Maternal-Fetal Medicine 1

PERINATAL SUBSTANCE ABUSE 1
NONIMMUNE HYDROPS 16
ANTEPARTUM FETAL ASSESSMENT 23
PRETERM LABOR AND BIRTH 29

CHAPTER 2
Genetics and Metabolism 34

GENETICS OF COMMON PROBLEMS PRESENTING IN THE NEWBORN 34
SPECIFIC GENETIC DISORDERS PRESENTING IN THE NEWBORN 49
INBORN ERRORS OF CARBOHYDRATE, AMMONIA, AMINO ACID, AND ORGANIC ACID METABOLISM 74
NEWBORN SCREENING 106

CHAPTER 3
Newborn Stabilization and Initial Evaluation 121

RESUSCITATION IN THE DELIVERY ROOM 121

CHAPTER 4
Newborn: General Principles of Care 138

TEMPERATURE REGULATION OF THE PREMATURE INFANT 138
ACID-BASE, FLUID, AND ELECTROLYTE MANAGEMENT 139

CHAPTER 5
Infections and Immunologic Defense Mechanisms 164

HUMAN IMMUNODEFICIENCY VIRUS INFECTION 164
VIRAL INFECTIONS 167

BACTERIAL INFECTIONS 184
FUNGAL INFECTIONS 222
PROTOZOAL INFECTIONS 224
SPIROCHETAL INFECTIONS 230

CHAPTER 6
Respiratory System 238

CONTROL OF BREATHING 238
RESPIRATORY DISTRESS IN THE NEWBORN 248
PNEUMOTHORAX AND OTHER AIR LEAK PROBLEMS 279
CHRONIC LUNG DISEASE 284

CHAPTER 7
Cardiovascular System 299

PATENT DUCTUS ARTERIOSUS IN THE PREMATURE INFANT 299
EVALUATION OF NEWBORNS WITH POSSIBLE CARDIAC PROBLEMS 305

CHAPTER 8
Nervous System 399

CENTRAL NERVOUS SYSTEM MALFORMATIONS 399
THE NEWBORN NERVOUS SYSTEM 413

CHAPTER 9
Gastrointestinal and Nutritional Conditions 436

DISORDERS OF THE INTESTINE AND PANCREAS 436
DISORDERS OF THE LIVER 444
PARENTERAL AND ENTERAL NUTRITION 450

CHAPTER 10
Bilirubin 463

PHYSIOLOGIC JAUNDICE 463
BILIRUBIN TOXICITY, ENCEPHALOPATHY, AND KERNICTERUS 467
UNCONJUGATED HYPERBILIRUBINEMIAS 470

CHAPTER 11
Hematologic System 479

HEMOSTATIC DISORDERS IN NEWBORNS 479

CHAPTER **12**
Renal and Genitourinary Systems **501**

   RENAL INSUFFICIENCY AND ACUTE RENAL FAILURE 501

CHAPTER **13**
Endocrine Disorders **508**

   DISORDERS OF CALCIUM AND PHOSPHORUS
     METABOLISM 508
   DISORDERS OF THE ADRENAL GLAND 518
   ABNORMALITIES OF SEXUAL DIFFERENTIATION 524
   DISORDERS OF THE THYROID GLAND 531
   DISORDERS OF CARBOHYDRATE METABOLISM 536

CHAPTER **14**
The Eye **544**

   RETINOPATHY OF PREMATURITY 544

Index **551**

NOTICE

Neonatology is an ever-changing field. Standard safety precautions must be followed, but as new research and clinical experience broaden our knowledge, changes in treatment and drug therapy become necessary or appropriate. Readers are advised to check the product information currently provided by the manufacturer of each drug to be administered to verify the recommended dose, the method and duration of administration, and the contraindications. It is the responsibility of the treating physician, relying on experience and knowledge of the patient, to determine dosages and the best treatment for the patient. Neither the publisher nor the editor assumes any responsibility for any injury and/or damage to persons or property.

THE PUBLISHER

CHAPTER 1

Maternal-Fetal Medicine

PERINATAL SUBSTANCE ABUSE

Substance abuse during pregnancy has been recognized for many decades. Awareness has also grown regarding the adverse impact of tobacco on pregnancy. The enhanced risk for various events in substance-abusing pregnant women is shown in Table 1-1.

OPIATES

Prevalence of opiate use among pregnant women is reported to range from 1% to 2% as high as 21% in a highly selected group of women. Rates for heroin use are higher in metropolitan areas and cities and are more concentrated in Northeast and West Coast cities. Opiate abuse is more common in groups of lower socioeconomic status.

Additionally, women who smoke during pregnancy are more likely to use opiates, alcohol, cocaine, amphetamines, and cannabis during pregnancy than nonsmoking women.

Of the opiate drugs known to be abused during pregnancy, heroin has been the most extensively studied. Heroin can be ingested by smoking or by the intranasal or intravenous routes. Intranasal use is common among women, especially in the western United States, whereas the intravenous route is more popular among users on the eastern seaboard. Reports from European countries suggest a trend away from intravenous injection of opiates. The use of noninjectable heroin may reduce the risk of human immunodeficiency virus (HIV) transmission; however, its wider use ensures the emergence of

TABLE 1–1
Enhanced Risk for Various Events After Substance Use During Pregnancy*

	Ethanol	Cigarettes	Cannabis	Opiates	Cocaine	Amphetamines	Barbiturates	PCP
Malformation	+	−	?	−	+	−	−	+
Abortion	−	+	?	?	+	+	−	+
IUGR	+	+	?	+	+	+	−	?
Prematurity	−	+	?	±	+	+	−	?
Withdrawal	±	−	−	+	−	+	−	−
Central nervous system sequelae	+	?	?	?	+	?	−	?
SIDS risk	+	+	?	+	+	?	−	?
Foster care	+	−	−	+	+	+	±	+

*Although risk is increased, the risk ratio ranges for the most part from 1 to 2 for these associations.
IUGR, intrauterine growth retardation; SIDS, sudden infant death syndrome; PCP, phencyclidine.

new groups of heroin users for whom intravenous use and risk is a major deterrent.

Many heroin-addicted pregnant women have poor general health with multiple medical problems associated with the drug abuse life-styles (Table 1–2). Intravenous use places the woman at risk for multiple infectious complications, including cellulitis, thrombophlebitis, hepatitis, endocarditis, syphilis, gonorrhea, and acquired immunodeficiency syndrome (AIDS).

Obstetric complications include higher incidence

TABLE 1–2

Drug Use, Alcohol Use, Smoking, and Other Issues for Child-Bearing Women

Suboptimal parenting
Physical, sexual, domestic violence
Poverty
Poor schooling, illiteracy, school dropout
Limited job skills, training
Limited jobs
Poor self-image, poor coping skills
Peer pressure
Ineffectual birth control, STD protection
Unplanned, unwanted pregnancy; teenage pregnancy
Poor nutrition and preconception health care
Poor access, receipt, and quality of prenatal care
Little family/father support
Stress
Psychological disorders, depression
Limited access to support services in community
Dependence/addiction
Pregnancy wastage
Increased risk of premature birth
Increased risk of fetal malformations
Fetal growth retardation
Fetal/neonatal death
Newborn to foster care
Attempts at rehabilitation
Increased risk of HIV, syphilis, hepatitis B or C, STDs
Incarceration
Recapitulation in next generation

STD, sexually transmitted disease; HIV, human immunodeficiency virus.

of spontaneous abortions, premature delivery and preterm labor, abruptio placentae, chorioamnionitis, increased risk for cesarean section associated with breech presentation, and fetal distress. Pregnant women who are opiate abusers have a 46% incidence of spontaneous abortions when using both methadone and cocaine and 16% when using methadone alone. These rates were significantly greater than nonsubstance abusers.

The classic neonatal withdrawal or abstinence syndrome includes a wide variety of central nervous system signs of irritability, gastrointestinal and feeding problems (diarrhea, hyperphagia), autonomic signs of dysfunction, and respiratory symptoms. The mortality rate in the past for infants with withdrawal syndrome has been estimated as high as 10% during the years of 1969 through 1979 in Amsterdam. Current estimates show marked improvement, with perinatal mortality rates currently less than 1%. Mortality is rarely associated with withdrawal alone but occurs as a consequence of prematurity, infection, and severe perinatal asphyxia.

There are a number of evaluation tools that are frequently used to assess the severity of opiate withdrawal after birth. The Neonatal Abstinence Score is a scale based on nursing observations of the severity signs of withdrawal. Others have introduced the Neonatal Narcotic Withdrawal Index as a rapid physician-based evaluation for neonatal signs of withdrawal. Using these scoring systems, the severity of the infant's withdrawal can thus be *quantified.*

Treatment includes soothing (swaddling, rocking, decreased environmental stimulation) as well as pharmacologic management. Medications most commonly used for opiate withdrawal include dilute tincture of opium, benzodiazepines, and phenobarbital.

The authors use starting doses of tincture of opium (0.4 mg/mL of morphine equivalent) of 0.1 mL/kg given orally. This dose can be increased by 0.05- to 0.1-mL increments until the symptoms are controlled. The usual dose for infants withdrawing at birth can range from 0.2 to 0.5 mL every 3 to 4 hours.

Sudden Infant Death Syndrome and Opiates

Numerous small studies and reports have suggested a link between maternal opiate use during pregnancy and an increased risk for sudden infant death syndrome (SIDS). A large 10-year study from New York showed that after controlling for known associated high-risk factors, the corrected risk ratio for SIDS among opiate exposed infants was two to four times greater than among infants not exposed to any perinatal drugs. The study found that differences in the rates of SIDS among ethnic groups disappear when women used drugs during their pregnancy. Whether the association between maternal opiate use and increased SIDS risk reflects pathology in the respiratory center of infants who eventually die from SIDS or whether this association is a reflection of other associated confounder(s) is still unclear. There are a number of maternal risk factors that may be associated with both opiate use and SIDS. Reports point to the strong association of maternal smoking in SIDS.

Because maternal withdrawal is believed to be associated with subsequent fetal withdrawal, fetal asphyxia, and spontaneous abortions, detoxification of a pregnant heroin user is infrequently attempted. Most women are treated with daily methadone maintenance throughout pregnancy.

Controversy continues over the most appropriate dose of methadone maintenance during pregnancy. Several investigators have not found that neonatal withdrawal symptoms, birth weight, length of pregnancy, and number of days infants require treatment for abstinence correlate with maternal methadone dosage. In contrast, others have reported significant correlation between the severity of neonatal withdrawal and maternal methadone dose. Investigators have found no correlation between neonatal serum levels of methadone and the maternal methadone dose at delivery, the maternal serum levels, or the severity of withdrawal symptoms in the neonates.

A number of studies have shown that opiate exposure in utero can have a prolonged effect on infant growth. Various investigators have shown that behavioral characteristics of infants are also affected by prenatal exposure to opiates. These infants showed significant differences in interactive behaviors, visual and auditory orientation, consolability, and state control.

Other significant developmental and learning deficits occur in both methadone-exposed and heroin-exposed children. Because opiate drug abusers use multiple drugs, including cigarettes, alcohol, cocaine, phencyclidine (PCP), and amphetamines, it is impossible to ascribe all adverse developmental effects to opiates alone. Additionally, maternal intelligence and maternal behaviors have significant effects on their children's performance on intelligence measures and social adaptive behaviors. Using regression analysis, one researcher showed that the amount of prenatal care obtained by the mother and the postnatal home environment were most predictive of the infant's future intellectual performance. Conversely the amount of maternal opiate use during pregnancy was not found to be predictive. Others have pointed to the adverse environmental effects of poverty and poor learning environment on the development of methadone-exposed children.

COCAINE

Cocaine is a highly psychoactive stimulant with a long history of abuse. Cocaine and other stimulants have become the drugs of choice for women in the United States, with estimates that up to 13% of women aged 18 to 25 use cocaine regularly. Women's use of cocaine as well as sexual activity to obtain drugs and maintain their habit has resulted in a marked increase nationwide in the birth of infants exposed to cocaine in utero.

The pharmacologic actions of cocaine include inhibition of postsynaptic reuptake of norepinephrine, dopamine, and serotonin neurotransmitters by sympathetic nerve terminals. Cocaine allows higher concentrations of neurotransmitters to interact with receptors. Higher levels of epinephrine and norepinephrine produce vasoconstriction, hypertension, and tachycardia. In adults, cocaine binds strongly to neuronal dopamine-reuptake transporters, thereby increasing postsynaptic dopamine at the mesolimbic and mesocortical levels and producing the addictive cycle of euphoria and dysphoria. Tryptophan uptake is similarly inhibited, altering serotonin pathways with resultant effects on sleep. Sodium ion permeability is blocked, producing the anesthetic effect of cocaine. The metabolites of cocaine are pharmacologically active and may themselves produce neurotoxicity in the pregnant woman or her fetus. Two forms of cocaine are commonly used, cocaine hydrochloride and cocaine base (either extracted by organic solvents or precipitated as crack using ammonia and baking soda). Crack, the most widely available form of freebase, is almost pure cocaine, and when it is smoked, it readily enters the bloodstream to produce levels similar to those occurring with intravenous use. Crack smoking appears to be particularly reinforcing and is associated with compulsive use, binges, and acceleration of the addictive process.

Many of the adverse perinatal outcomes with cocaine abuse are thought to be related to the effects of cocaine on uterine blood supply. An increase in maternal mean arterial blood pressure, a decrease in uterine blood flow, and a transient rise in fetal systemic blood pressure after an intravenous cocaine infusion have been found in fetal sheep. Additional animal studies demonstrated significant fetal hypoxemia associated with changes in uterine blood flow with cocaine infusion. Maternal hypertension and intermittent fetal hypoxia contribute to the increased risks for abruptio placentae, intrauterine growth retardation, and potentially the congenital anomalies seen in cocaine-exposed infants.

Cocaine and some of its metabolites readily cross the placenta and achieve pharmacologic fetal levels, although the exact mechanisms by which cocaine affects the fetus are not fully elucidated.

Women who use cocaine during pregnancy are at high risk for stillbirths, spontaneous abortions, abruptio placentae, intrauterine growth deficiency, anemia and malnutrition, and maternal death from intracerebral hemorrhage. Cocaine directly stimulates uterine contractions because of its alpha-adrenergic, prostaglandin, or dopaminergic effects, with resulting increased risk for fetal distress and premature deliveries. Abruptio placentae appears related to cocaine only when use occurs shortly before delivery. Other problems include evidence of fetal distress associated with abnormal fetal heart rate tracing and meconium staining (but not aspiration syndrome). These women are at high risk for premature labor, low-birth-weight infants, premature rupture of the membranes, and perinatal infections. The higher prevalence of sexually transmitted diseases has been associated with the trading of sex for drugs. A fourfold increased odds of cocaine exposure among infants with congenital syphilis has been documented; both injection and noninjection use of cocaine increases risks for HIV acquisition, with a 3.5-increased risk among women who trade sex for crack.

Diminished intrauterine growth and premature birth are the most common effects of gestational cocaine exposure, with effects on weight, height, and head circumference at birth. Head circumference among exposed infants is decreased, and it is postulated that fetal brain growth is impaired more than somatic growth.

Cocaine has been reported in association with a variety of congenital anomalies in animals, although the teratogenicity of cocaine has yet to be established in humans. Some of the fetal malformations could be explained by norepinephrine-mediated vasoconstrictive effects during organogenesis. Limb reduction deformities, intestinal atresia or infarction, and other vascular disruption sequences have been reported, although no increase was found in a population-based prevalence study. Central nervous system ischemic and hemorrhagic lesions have been reported inconsistently, both in term and in premature infants. The risk of genitourinary anomalies appears to be increased fourfold; these are the only anomalies well demonstrated in association with cocaine exposure.

Cocaine and Premature Delivery

Of all the problems attributed to cocaine use in the pregnant woman, the most common problem is that of premature delivery. Accordingly, infants born to these women may develop sequelae of prematurity: cerebral palsy, developmental delay, diminished intellectual capacity, and behavioral impairment. Several studies with sample sizes large enough to assess independent effects of cocaine on prematurity demonstrated this association. Another study showed no such association but was done in a woman receiving prenatal care, suggesting that in the absence of prenatal care, cocaine may bear an independent association with prematurity. Prematurity and intrauterine growth retardation also appear to be closely related to maternal life-style. In those populations studied in which the mother receives good prenatal care associated with drug treatment, the incidence of prematurity and intrauterine growth retardation is low.

Cocaine-exposed infants manifest a range of neurobehavioral abnormalities initially described as drug withdrawal, but these are more likely due to acute intoxication. Signs are present at birth or a few days thereafter, waning as cocaine and benzoylecgonine are cleared from plasma. The infants are hypertonic, irritable, and tremulous and may have abnormal crying, sleep, and feeding patterns, although controlled, blinded studies have demonstrated cocaine withdrawal signs in a lower proportion of cocaine-exposed infants than have unblinded studies. Tachycardia, tachypnea, and apnea have been noted with significant elevations in cardiac output, stroke volume, mean arterial blood pressure, and cerebral artery flow velocity resolving by day 2, consistent with an intoxicant effect of cocaine. Other early and late patterns of neurobehavioral abnormalities include a depressed state occurring immediately after birth and lasting 3 to 4 days (resembling the adult cocaine crash) and a late-emerging (onset 3 to 30 days) hyperirritable phase, which may be a manifestation of fetopathic effects of cocaine. Cocaine-exposed infants may have abnormal electroencephalograms or clinical seizures, perhaps the result of toxicity from benzoylecgonine, a major metabolite of cocaine.

Persisting behavioral, neurologic, and rearing problems are reported in these children. Significant impairment of orientation, motor, and state regulation among infants with documented cocaine exposure during only the first trimester has been reported. In contrast, one study noted no significant differences between a cocaine and polydrug group and a drug-negative group in mean developmental scores, although a significantly larger proportion of children in the drug-exposed groups had lower cognitive scores. Compromised motor performance in late infancy has been reported in exposed infants in a controlled longitudinal study. These motor abnormalities did not persist at 15 months, and both the exposed and the control group had motor scores significantly below norms for age. Variable outcomes of these studies may depend on the amounts and style of drug usage that vary with geographic area or on other covariates, such as nutritional status, poverty, and parental educational level. The neurodevelopmental problems among children exposed to cocaine may occur either from direct encephalopathic drug effects during gestation or from indirect effects of the social environment in which the developing infant is reared.

The incidence of SIDS may be greater in cocaine-exposed infants, although this increase appears less significant than those for methadone-exposed or heroin-exposed infants. Other studies demonstrate abnormal respiratory patterns and ventilatory control.

The pregnant woman with suspected or admitted gestational or intrapartum cocaine use should undergo urine toxicology screening after informed consent, recognizing that neither self-report nor urine screening are sensitive or specific tools for identifying intrapartum complications, neonatal morbidity, long-term outcome, or families at risk of child neglect or abuse. Identification offers the potential benefits of screening for sexually transmitted diseases, closer obstetric monitoring of maternal and fetal well-being, drug counseling, support and referrals for rehabilitation, and social service needs assessment.

The majority of infants, although at higher risk for medical complications, do not require intensive neonatal care; however, symptomatic infants often require more nursing care. Admission physical examination should document a maturational age examination, birth weight, head circumference, and length. Infants should be examined for any evidence of malformations (or anomalies related to concurrent alcohol exposure) or of complications of prematurity. Hypertonic, tremulous infants usually respond to swaddling, being held, decreases in ambient environmental stimuli (light and noise), pacifiers, and more frequent feedings. Studies such as electroencephalography, brain imaging, or renal sonography may add diagnostic or prognostic information when physical or neurologic abnormalities are noted, but these are not indicated for all exposed infants. Neurologic or ophthalmologic evaluation may document tone and ocular abnormalities in some otherwise asymptomatic infants, but it is not clear that all exposed infants should be referred for examination. Feedings in premature infants with cocaine exposure should be started with diluted formula with lower than usual volume increments because premature infants exposed to cocaine have been found to be at increased risk for both early-onset and late-onset necrotizing enterocolitis. Maternal cocaine use exposes infants to higher than expected problems with postasphyxial syndrome, and organ malfunction on this basis should be sought and treated.

AMPHETAMINES

The clinical effects of amphetamines are often indistinguishable from those of cocaine. Amphetamines also potentiate the action of norepinephrine, dopamine, and serotonin and are sympathomimetics similar to cocaine. Amphetamines may have some ability to block reuptake of released neurotransmitters. In contrast with cocaine, however, they appear to exert their central nervous system effects primarily by enhancing the release of neurotransmitters from presynaptic neurons. They may also exert a direct stimulatory action on postsynaptic catecholamine receptors.

The medical and obstetric complications of amphetamines are similar to those described for cocaine. Amphetamine toxicity has been described as more intense and prolonged than that seen with cocaine. Visual, auditory, and tactile hallucinations are common, and microvascular damage has been seen in the brains of chronic users. Amphetamine withdrawal is characterized by prolonged periods of hypersomnia, depression, and intense, often violent paranoid psychosis. Obstetric complications include an increased incidence of stillbirth. As in cocaine-using women, the pregnancies of amphetamine users are characterized by poor prenatal care, sexually transmitted diseases, and cardiovascular problems including abruptio placentae and postpartum hemorrhage.

Neonatal problems include prematurity and intrauterine growth retardation. Cardiovascular malformations have been described, but other studies have failed to show an increased risk. Neurodevelopmental abnormalities have been described both during the neonatal period and in long-term follow-up studies as late as 14 years. Intellectual capacity does not appear to be diminished among exposed infants. These children are described as exhibiting disturbed behavior, including hyperactivity, aggressiveness, and sleep disturbances. The neurobehavioral abnormalities appear to be associated with the extent and the duration of fetal exposure.

PHENCYCLIDINE

PCP, also known as angel dust, is a white crystalline powder soluble in water and alcohol. It can be inhaled, taken orally, or injected intravenously. Its popularity among young adults, especially women, however, relates to its low cost and its ability to be smoked. PCP is usually smoked sprinkled (dusted) on cigarettes (lovely) or marijuana (sherm). PCP increases epinephrine release, but its exact mechanism of action is not clearly understood.

There are limited data on the effects of PCP on pregnancy and the newborn. PCP readily crosses the placenta and has been documented in both the fetus and the newborn as well as in breast milk. The effects of PCP on the outcome of pregnancy appear to be dose related. In low doses, PCP has few side effects, although the anesthetic nature of the drug increases the frequency of precipitous deliveries at home, in ambulances, and in emergency departments. Other obstetric complications are not known to be increased. PCP is not associated with increased risks for prematurity, but 40% of PCP-exposed infants are small for gestational age.

A severe syndrome associated with PCP exposure in utero has been reported, with onset shortly after birth. The timing and severity of the symptoms, however, often present at birth, raise the question of whether the neurologic findings represent drug intoxication rather than drug withdrawal effects because PCP persists in the body, and especially in fetal brains, for prolonged periods. The neurologic findings in PCP-exposed infants were striking for the severity of the hypertonicity and hyperreflexia, often associated with spontaneous clonus and persisting for several weeks. Sudden episodes of agitation and fluctuating levels of consciousness have been described. Gastrointestinal symptoms, including abdominal distention, vomiting, and diarrhea, were also present in about 20% of the infants.

Congenital anomalies have been reported, but a clear causal association with PCP has not been verified.

ALCOHOL

The fetal alcohol syndrome (FAS) is an extensively documented teratogenic syndrome. FAS occurs in 1 to 2 per 1000 live births in most industrialized countries (as high as 20% of live births in a few reported subgroups of Native Americans), making it a major cause of mental retardation. FAS is estimated to occur in the infants of 30% to 40% of pregnant women who consume 3 or more ounces of absolute alcohol per day.

FAS is diagnosed by history and physical examination. There are no laboratory tests as yet that summate alcohol exposure during fetal life. The syndrome consists of prenatal and postnatal growth deficiency, microcephaly, and mental retardation associated with characteristic facies and diverse ocular defects. The microcephaly is a reflection of the damage to brain tissues that results from alcohol exposure. The facial features consist of short palpebral fissures, broad flat nasal bridge, short upturned nose, and long upper lip without distinct philtrum. Abnormal hand creases and cardiac anomalies have been described.

Women who are chronic alcoholics may also have a greater risk for abruptio placentae, spontaneous abortions, and stillbirths. Lesser degrees of alcohol consumption have been associated with fetal growth retardation, congenital anomalies, behavioral and neurologic abnormalities, and milder degrees of mental retardation—a condition termed by some *fetal alcohol effects* as compared with the more severe and clearly identifiable FAS.

The subsequent degree of mental retardation correlates with the degree of physical stigmata. The postnatal growth deficiency is prominent in infancy and persists into early childhood and may be associated with vomiting. Speech and language problems are common in older children. Behavioral problems, including severe hyperactivity and attention deficit disorders, contribute to the learning disabilities characteristically seen in these children.

CIGARETTES

Cigarettes are the drug most often used during pregnancy. Cigarette smoking has been associated with an increased risk of spontaneous abortion, stillbirth, fetal growth retardation, prematurity, and SIDS. The degree of intrauterine growth retardation is related to the number of cigarettes smoked. One pack (20 cigarettes) per day correlates with a 280-g weight decrement in term newborn infants. Maternal cotinine excretion is used as a marker to quantitate the degree of smoking. Studies have found a 1-g reduction in birth weight for every nanogram per milliliter of cotinine increase in maternal urine. The exact mechanism of the adverse effect on pregnancy is unknown. Cigarettes contain a number of potentially toxic compounds. Most theories involve the induction of fetal hypoxia either from carbon monoxide production or from nicotine-induced vasospasm; however, a direct cytotoxic effect has not been ruled out. Investigators have shown loss of neonatal hypoxia tolerance after prenatal nicotine exposure and suggested this as a causative factor in the increased risk of SIDS among offspring of mothers who smoke.

MARIJUANA

Marijuana is the illegal drug that is probably most frequently used during pregnancy. Marijuana is derived from the hemp plant *Cannabis,* with the most active ingredient being delta-9-tetrahydrocannabinol. Marijuana is associated with growth retardation. Neurologic abnormalities similar to a mild withdrawal syndrome with hypertonicity, irritability, and jitteriness have been seen in the newborn but without documented evidence of long-term sequelae. Marijuana is often used in combination with other drugs and potentiates the risk for prematurity and low birth weight. FAS may be more common among women who abuse alcohol with marijuana.

CAFFEINE

Caffeine exposure may occur in 75% of pregnancies in the United States. Caffeine is contained in coffee, tea, colas, and chocolate (100 mg/cup of coffee). Most studies detect increased risk of intrauterine growth retardation with intake in excess of 300 mg/day. That is to say, a detectable and significant increase of growth retardation occurs (relative risk about 1.5). Many studies also report increased risk of spontaneous abortion with caffeine exposure (e.g., risk of abortion increases by 1.017 for each cup of coffee/day in the first trimester). Most studies of caffeine, similar to those of other licit and illicit drugs, share problems of ascertainment; dose, duration, response, and confounding factors. For example, genetic differences may affect susceptibility to caffeine, caffeine may have fetotoxic additive effects with smoking, and drinks such as coffee may contain ingredients that have effects on pregnancy that are independent of caffeine. Granted these considerations, and to a greater degree than with other drugs discussed in this chapter, it is usually not possible to attribute growth retardation or spontaneous abortion in a specific case to caffeine.

BREAST-FEEDING

Psychotropic drugs are low molecular weight and lipophilic, which means that they are readily excreted in breast milk. Seizures and overdose symptoms have been reported in one infant whose mother used cocaine. Amphetamines appear in large quantities in breast milk. PCP has also been found to cross into breast milk readily. Because of the risk of toxicity, breast-feeding should be discouraged for known abusers of the previously mentioned drugs with the exception of those mothers in drug treatment programs in which their drug use is monitored closely.

NONIMMUNE HYDROPS

In 1943 Potter first distinguished between hydrops secondary to erythroblastosis fetalis and nonimmune hydrops in describing a group of infants with generalized body edema who did not have hepatosplenomegaly or abnormal erythropoiesis.

To understand the pathogenesis of hydrops, it is necessary to consider the forces underlying normal fluid homeostasis. Body water exists in two principal spaces: intracellular and extracellular. Intracellular volume is maintained largely by osmotic forces across the cell membrane and by the energy-dependent sodium transporter. In hydrops, the disorder is in the regulation of extracellular water such that fluid accumulates in the interstitium and body cavities.

The mechanisms in the pathogenesis of hydrops can ultimately be integrated through the Starling relationship. The Starling equation as applied to the balance of fluid across a capillary is as follows:

$$\text{Filtration} = K[(P_c - P_t) - R(O_p - O_t)]$$

where K = capillary filtration coefficient, P_c = hydrostatic pressure—capillary, P_t = hydrostatic pressure—tissue, R = reflection coefficient for solute, O_p = osmotic pressure—plasma, and O_t = osmotic pressure—tissue fluid.

Three possible mechanisms may be operative in infants with hydrops. These mechanisms include anemia, low colloid osmotic pressure with hypoproteinemia, and congestive heart failure with hypervolemia.

Infants with alloimmune hydrops (and several of the nonimmune hydrops conditions as well) have significant anemia. It has been proposed that anemia leads to congestive heart failure with increased hydrostatic pressure in the capillaries, causing vascular damage that results in edema. It is clear that a rapidly lowered hemoglobin concentration results in a need for greater cardiac output to maintain adequate oxygen delivery. This results in higher oxygen demands by the myocardium, which may be difficult to meet because of the anemia itself. The hypoxic myocardium may become less contractile and less compliant, with ventricular stiffness causing an increased afterload to the atria.

Infants who have erythroblastosis and hydrops seem to demonstrate a correlation between serum albumin concentration and the degree of hydrops. Initial therapy after birth, however, tends to raise the serum albumin toward normal rapidly, and with diuresis, these infants appear to have normal albumin concentrations. This suggests that their hypoalbuminemia may have been the result of dilution rather than the cause of the hydrops.

The most commonly diagnosed causes of nonimmune hydrops are cardiac disorders (about 40%).

Any state in which cardiac output is less than the rate of venous return results in an elevated central venous pressure (CVP). Increased CVP raises capillary filtration pressures and, if high enough, restricts lymphatic return. Both of these mechanisms may then contribute to interstitial fluid accumulation.

A fourth factor that contributes to hydrops is decreased lymph flow. If the rate of fluid filtration from plasma to tissues exceeds the rate of lymph return to the central venous system, edema and effusions form. Impairment of lymph flow may be caused by either a structural impedance or an increased CVP opposing lymphatic return.

Nonimmune hydrops has been described in association with a wide range of conditions (Table 1–3).

Prenatal ultrasound diagnosis of hydrops is made by observing generalized skin thickening of greater than 5 mm and two of the following: ascites, pleural effusions, pericardial effusion, or placental enlargement. Because the mortality and morbidity risk for hydrops is high, a rapid determination of the cause must be undertaken when the diagnosis is made so that appropriate intervention may preserve fetal well-being when possible. Ultrasound, in addition to revealing hydrops, may also yield information as to the cause. Cardiac defects and dysrhythmias are evident by fetal echocardiography and Doppler blood flow analysis. Fetal heart rate monitoring may be used to follow dysrhythmias. Other anomalies, including lesions such as teratomas and hemangiomas, which may create high-output failure states, may be visible as well.

Table 1–4 provides recommendations for the investigation of fetal hydrops.

NEONATAL EVALUATION

Table 1–5 presents the diagnostic evaluation recommended for newborn infants with nonimmune hydrops of unknown cause.

After successful resuscitation, including the intubation and administration of surfactant and placement of umbilical catheters, the clinical management can address both the cause and the complications of the hydrops.

TABLE 1-3

Conditions Associated with Hydrops Fetalis

Hemolytic anemias
    Alloimmune, Rh, Kell, c
    Alpha-chain hemoglobinopathies (homozygous alpha-thalassemia)
    Red blood cell enzyme deficiencies (glucose phosphate isomerase deficiency, glucose-6-phosphate dehydrogenase)
Other anemias
    Fetomaternal hemorrhage
    Twin–twin transfusion
Cardiac conditions
    Premature closure of foramen ovale
    Ebstein's anomaly
    Hypoplastic left or right heart
    Subaortic stenosis with fibroelastosis
    Cardiomyopathy, myocardial fibroelastosis
    Atrioventricular canal
    Myocarditis
    Right atrial hemangioma
    Intracardiac hamartoma or fibroma
    Tuberous sclerosis with cardiac rhabdomyoma
Cardiac arrhythmias
    Supraventricular tachycardia
    Atrial flutter
    Congenital heart block
Vascular malformations
    Hemangioma of liver
    Any large arteriovenous malformation
    Angiosteohypertrophy (Klippel-Trenaunay syndrome)
Vascular accidents
    Thrombosis of umbilical vein or inferior vena cava
    Recipient in twin–twin transfusion
Infections
    Cytomegalovirus, congenital hepatitis, human parvovirus, other viruses
    Toxoplasmosis, Chagas disease
    Coxsackie virus
    Syphilis
    Leptospirosis
Lymphatic abnormalities
    Lymphangiectasia
    Cystic hygroma
    Noonan syndrome
    Multiple pterygium syndrome
Nervous system lesions
    Absent corpus callosum
    Encephalocele
    Cerebral arteriovenous malformation
    Intracranial hemorrhage (massive)
    Holoprosencephaly
    Fetal akinesia sequence

Table continued on following page

TABLE 1-3

Conditions Associated with Hydrops Fetalis
Continued

Pulmonary conditions
   Cystic adenomatoid malformation of lung
   Mediastinal teratoma
   Diaphragmatic hernia
   Lung sequestration syndrome
   Lymphangiectasia
Renal conditions
   Urinary ascites
   Congenital nephrosis
   Renal vein thrombosis
Invasive and storage processes
   Tuberous sclerosis
   Gaucher disease
   Mucopolysaccharidosis
   Mucolipidosis
Chromosome abnormalities
   Trisomy 13, trisomy 18, trisomy 21
   Turner syndrome
   XX/XY
Bone diseases
   Osteogenesis imperfecta
   Achondroplasia
   Asphyxiating thoracic dystrophy
Gastrointestinal conditions
   Bowel obstruction with perforation and meconium peritonitis
   Small-bowel volvulus
   Other intestinal obstruction
   Prune-belly syndrome
Tumors
   Neuroblastoma
   Choriocarcinoma
   Sacrococcygeal teratoma
   Hemangioma of the liver
   Congenital leukemia
Maternal or placental conditions
   Maternal diabetes
   Maternal therapy with indomethacin
   Multiple gestation of parasitic fetus
   Chorioangioma of placenta, chorionic vessels, or umbilical vessels
   Toxemia
   Systemic lupus erythematosus
Miscellaneous
   Neu-Laxova syndrome
   Myotonic dystrophy
Idiopathic

TABLE 1–4

Investigation of Fetal Hydrops

Maternal

   Complete blood count and indices
   Hemoglobin electrophoresis
   Kleihauer-Betke stain of peripheral blood
   VDRL, rapid plasma reagin, and TORCH titers
   Anti-Ro, systemic lupus erythematosus preparation, sedimentation rate
   Parvovirus IgM, IgG
   Glucose-6-phosphate dehydrogenase, pyruvate kinase deficiency screening

Fetal

   Serial ultrasound evaluation
   Limb length, fetal movement
   Echocardiography

Amniocentesis

   Karyotype
   Alpha-fetoprotein
   Viral cultures; polymerase chain reaction for toxoplasmosis, parvovirus B19
   Establish culture for appropriate metabolic or DNA testing

Fetal Blood Sampling

   Karyotype
   Complete blood count
   Hemoglobin analysis
   IgM; specific cultures
   Albumin and total protein
   Measurement of umbilical venous pressure

From McGillivray BC, Hall JC: Nonimmune hydrops. Pediatr Rev 9:197, 1987. Reproduced by permission of Pediatrics.

Virtually all infants with hydrops require mechanical ventilation because of effusions, pulmonary hypoplasia, surfactant deficiency, pulmonary edema, poor chest wall compliance from edema, or, in some cases, persistent pulmonary hypertension of the newborn. The presence of persistent pleural effusions may necessitate the placing of chest tubes. Ascites may also compress the diaphragm and make lung expansion difficult.

TABLE 1–5

Diagnostic Evaluation of Newborns with Nonimmune Hydrops

System	Type of Evaluation
Cardiovascular	Echocardiogram, electrocardiogram
Pulmonary	Chest radiograph, pleural fluid examination
Hematologic	Complete blood cell count, differential platelet count, blood type and Coombs test, blood smear for morphology
Gastrointestinal	Abdominal radiograph, abdominal ultrasound, liver function tests, peritoneal fluid examination, total protein, albumin
Renal	Urinalysis, BUN, creatinine
Genetic	Chromosomal analysis, skeletal radiographs, genetic consultation
Congenital infections	Viral cultures or serology (including TORCH agents and parvovirus)
Pathologic	Complete autopsy, placental examination

Adapted from Carlton DP, McGillivray BC, Schreiber MD: Nonimmune hydrops fetalis: A multidisciplinary approach. Clin Perinatol 16:844, 1989.

A primary goal of fluid management is resolution of the hydrops itself. Maintenance fluids should be restricted, with volume boluses given only in response to clear signs of inadequate intravascular volume. The hydropic newborn has not only an excess of free extracellular water but also an excess of sodium. Volume given during resuscitation increases further the amount of water and sodium that must be removed. Initial maintenance fluids should not contain sodium. Serum and urine sodium levels, urine volume, and daily weights should be monitored carefully to guide fluid and electrolyte administration. Urinary sodium levels may help to differentiate between hyponatremia owing to hemodilution and urinary losses.

Shock may be a prominent feature in patients with hydrops. This may result from hypovolemia owing to capillary leakage, poor vascular tone and impaired myocardial contractility owing to hypoxia or infection, impaired venous return owing to shifting or compression of mediastinal structures, or pericardial effusion. Adequate intravascular volume must be maintained, and correctable causes of impaired venous return should be addressed. Peripheral perfusion, heart rate, blood pressure, and acid-base status should be monitored carefully.

ANTEPARTUM FETAL ASSESSMENT

Conditions in which fetal surveillance is traditionally considered mandatory are listed in Table 1–6.

Ultrasound has become an increasingly important tool in the evaluation of high-risk obstetric patients. In many obstetric practices, all pregnant women are offered an ultrasound evaluation of the fetus at some time. Although this practice is controversial, there are several well-recognized indications for sonography.

Accurate determination of pregnancy duration is a central goal of prenatal care. Although precise pregnancy dating is valuable in even uncomplicated pregnancies, this information is of critical importance in situations of marginal fetal viability and salvageability. A major additional benefit of routine sonographic scanning of pregnancies is the diagnosis of unexpected fetal anomalies.

TABLE 1–6

Indications for Fetal Surveillance

Threatened preterm delivery	Chronic maternal illness
Post-term pregnancy	Diabetes
Hypertensive disorders	Anemia
Intrauterine growth retardation	Hemoglobinopathies
	Cyanotic heart disease
Previous stillbirth	Collagen vascular disease
Decreased fetal movement	Renal impairment
Multiple gestation	

The use of maternally perceived fetal activity to identify fetuses at risk for distress or death has been proposed because of its relatively low cost, convenience, and applicability to a large population. A mean of 85 fetal movements in a 45-minute period occurred in a recent study (95% confidence limit of 14 to 232 movements).

The thesis that fetal movements decrease with hypoxia is central to understanding of the nonstress test (NST) and biophysical profile. A 1-hour observation period lacking 10 movements represented 3.5 standard deviations (99th percentile). Based on this and other observations, various methods of "kick counting" have been proposed. Perhaps the simplest of proven worth is that of Moore and Piacquadio, in which the patient records the time taken for 10 fetal movements to occur between 7 and 11 P.M. (the period of peak fetal activity). If the requisite 10 movements are not obtained after 1 hour of recording, further fetal evaluation is performed.

CONTRACTION STRESS TEST AND NONSTRESS TEST

The earliest fetal wellness test involving fetal heart rate monitoring was the contraction stress test (CST). This test assesses the response of the fetal heart rate to uterine contractions produced by administration of exogenous oxytocin or by nipple stimulation. In an oxygen-compromised fetus, contractions typically lead to late decelerations in the fetal heart rate. Although the CST remains a useful test, its disadvantages include significant time investment (45 to 60 minutes), the high frequency of uterine contraction hyperstimulation, and the need for close supervision.

Several observers noted that CSTs were rarely abnormal when fetal heart rate accelerations were present in association with movement. This clinical observation led to omission of the contractions, with simple monitoring for fetal heart rate accelerations. Because of its ease of use, universal applicability, and lack of contraindications, the nonstress test has replaced the CST as a first-line surveillance tool.

The NST is carried out with the patient supine with a lateral tilt. The fetal heart rate and uterine activity are recorded using an external transducer for up to 40 minutes. Usually uterine activity is monitored simultaneously, and the patient records perceived fetal movement with an event marker.

Criteria for a reassuring test are as follows:

- Observation period of 20 minutes.
- Baseline fetal heart rate between 110 and 160 beats/min.
- Short-term variability of ±5 beats/min.
- Two or more fetal heart rate accelerations of at least 15 beats/min lasting at least 15 seconds.
- No nonreassuring features (decelerations, tachycardia, bradycardia).

Abnormalities of amniotic fluid volume are associated with suboptimal pregnancy outcome. *Oligohydramnios* (inadequate fluid volume) is associated with increased frequency of fetal urinary obstruction, placental insufficiency, umbilical cord compression, fetal distress, meconium passage, and fetal asphyxia. Prolonged oligohydramnios interferes with normal lung growth, resulting in potentially lethal pulmonary hypoplasia. *Hydramnios* (excessive amniotic fluid volume) is associated with maternal diabetes, fetal esophageal obstruction, and duodenal atresia. Pregnancies complicated by hydramnios have increased rates of abnormal fetal lie, cesarean delivery, and abruptio placentae. The major diagnostic entities associated with abnormal amniotic fluid volume are listed in Tables 1–7 and 1–8.

BIOPHYSICAL PROFILE

Manning and associates developed the biophysical profile (BPP), which encompasses observations of fetal behavioral activity on ultrasound in addition to fetal heart rate reactivity. Prospective clinical studies have demonstrated generally good but varying predictive accuracies for each individual variable, but a combination of these measures improves the pre-

TABLE 1–7

Principal Diagnoses Associated with Oligohydramnios

Occult or overt premature rupture of membranes
Placental insufficiency
  Maternal hypertensive disease
  Autoimmune condition
  Chronic abruption
  Placental crowding in multifetal pregnancy
Urinary tract anomaly
  Renal agenesis
  Ureteral obstruction
  Urethral obstruction
  Polycystic or multicystic dysplastic kidneys

---

dictive accuracy substantially. The components of the BPP are listed in Table 1–9. A summary of possible scores and recommended actions is given in Table 1–10.

A positive finding in each of the BPP parameters is awarded a value of 2 to give a total score of 10. Outcomes in Manning's initial study were collected prospectively, and scores of 8 to 10 were found to correlate with good outcome.

Examination of amniotic fluid in late pregnancy for biochemical evidence of lung maturity may pre-

TABLE 1–8

Principal Diagnoses Associated with Polyhydramnios

Gastrointestinal obstruction
  Esophageal atresia
  Thoracic mass, pleural effusion
  Duodenal atresia
Central nervous system abnormalities
  Structural
  Chromosome
Cardiac anomalies
Fetal anemia
  Fetomaternal hemorrhage
  Blood group isoimmunization
  Parvovirus infection
Twin transfusion syndrome
Maternal diabetes
Constitutional macrosomia

TABLE 1-9
Elements of the Biophysical Profile

Nonstress test
  Reactive test = 2 points
Fetal breathing movements
  At least one episode of fetal breathing of 60-sec duration
    = 2 points
Gross fetal body movements
  At least three discrete episodes of fetal movement
    = 2 points
Fetal tone
  At least one episode of extension and return to flexion of
    extremities or spine or hand open/close = 2 points
Amniotic fluid volume
  At least one amniotic fluid pocket of at least 1 cm in depth
    = 2 points
Total available
  10 points

---

cede elective delivery or aid in timing of delivery in a compromised pregnancy. A variety of tests are available:

1. Lecithin-sphingomyelin ratio.
2. Phosphatidyl glycerol.
3. Phosphatidyl inositol.

In certain cases of apparent fetal compromise, it may be necessary to exclude potentially lethal chromosome anomalies before intervention and delivery. Amniocentesis for karyotyping or the more rapid fluorescent in-situ hybridization for identification of trisomies 13, 18, and 21 may thus be indicated.

Access to fetal blood provides the ultimate means of assessing fetal status—although not without significant procedural risk, carrying a fetal loss rate of 1%. Acid-base status and blood gases may be measured, although critical values for intervention have not been firmly established.

TABLE 1–10
Interpretation and Management of Biophysical Profile Score

Score	Comment	Perinatal Mortality Within 1 Wk Without Intervention	Management
10 of 10	Risk of fetal asphyxia extremely rare	<1/1000	Intervention only for obstetric and maternal factors
8 of 10 (normal fluid)	No indication for intervention for fetal disease		
8 of 8 (NST not done)	Equivalent to BPP = 10 with NST		
8 of 10 (abnormal fluid)	Probable chronic fetal compromise	89/1000	Determine that there is functioning renal tissue and intact membranes; if so, deliver for fetal indications
6 of 10 (normal fluid)	Equivocal test, possible fetal asphyxia	Variable	If the fetus is mature, deliver: In the immature fetus, repeat test within 24 h; if <6/10 deliver
6 of 10 (abnormal fluid)	Probable fetal asphyxia	89/1000	Deliver for fetal indications
4 of 10	High probability of fetal asphyxia	91/1000	Deliver for fetal indications
2 of 10	Fetal asphyxia almost certain	125/1000	Deliver for fetal indications
0 of 10	Fetal asphyxia certain	600/1000	Deliver for fetal indications

NST, nonstress test; BPP, biophysical profile.
From Manning FA, Morrison I, Harman CR, et al: Fetal assessment based on fetal biophysical profile scoring: Experience in 19,221 referred high-risk pregnancies. Am J Obstet Gynecol 157:880, 1987.

PRETERM LABOR AND BIRTH

Premature birth affects 11% of all pregnancies, resulting in 431,613 deliveries in the United States in 1994. Fewer than 1% of the deliveries were of infants less than 27 weeks' gestation, however.

Premature delivery is the delivery of any infant, of whatever cause, between 20 and 37 completed weeks of gestation. *Preterm premature rupture of the membranes* (PPROM) (sometimes called *preterm spontaneous rupture of the membranes*) is spontaneous rupture of the amniotic sac before the onset of labor (premature) before 37 completed weeks of gestation (preterm). It is distinguished from term premature rupture of the membranes (PROM) only by the gestational age of the pregnancy.

Premature delivery is strongly associated with social deprivation. Poverty, work away from home, teenage pregnancy, and single motherhood have all been identified as risk factors for preterm delivery. In the United States, race continues to be a major risk factor for prematurity, with blacks having a preterm birth rate of 18.1% compared with 9.6% in whites in 1994. Despite increasing access to health care, blacks continue to have a higher preterm delivery rate than their white counterparts regardless of economic status.

Smoking is strongly associated with premature delivery as well as other perinatal morbidities. Increased circulating carboxyhemoglobin, decreased oxygen delivery to the placenta and fetus, and nicotine have been postulated as reasons for the higher incidence of premature labor.

The use of recreational drugs, such as cocaine and crystal methamphetamine, is strongly associated with premature labor and delivery. Although associated comorbidities, such as sexually transmitted diseases, are undoubtedly important, these drugs have direct effects on the uterus and placenta. Cocaine especially is well known to result in maternal hypertension and placental abruption. There is some evidence that cocaine may also have a direct stimulatory effect on the myometrium resulting in contractions.

Up to 16% of women presenting with premature labor and intact membranes have microbiologic evidence of intra-amniotic infection on amniocentesis. Further work has demonstrated an even higher incidence of infection when markers such as intra-amniotic glucose and interleukin-6 are used.

Such evidence of overt and subclinical infection has led to much work on the use of antibiotics in premature labor. Related research has demonstrated that vaginal infection with anaerobic organisms, such as bacterial vaginosis, is a major risk factor for premature delivery. Early diagnosis and treatment of such infections has been shown to reduce the incidence of premature delivery. In addition, the presence of untreated urinary infections, including pyelonephritis, is associated with preterm labor and delivery.

As the number of fetuses per pregnancy increases, the mean gestational age at delivery decreases. Twins deliver at 35 weeks, on average; triplets, 33 weeks; quadruplets, 29 weeks; and so on.

The use of diethylstilbestrol (DES) in an attempt to salvage pregnancies at risk for spontaneous miscarriage was popular in the 1950s through the 1970s. It has become apparent that DES exposure in utero may result in genitourinary abnormalities in both male and female fetuses. Female congenital abnormalities include tubal, uterine, cervical, and vaginal conditions that result in infertility, spontaneous miscarriage, incompetent cervix, premature labor, and malpresentation. The abnormalities that result in premature delivery include cervical shortening and cervical matrix abnormalities that may result in painless cervical dilation or cervical incompetence.

As a result of the embryologic formation of the uterus by the uniting of bilaterally formed müllerian ducts, congenital abnormalities tend to be those of incomplete fusion. In general, the more incomplete the fusion, the greater the risk of premature delivery. The incidence of prematurity with bicornuate uterus is 16%, ranging to 8% in septate uterus.

Despite the importance of spontaneous preterm

labor, the vast majority of preterm infants are delivered for reasons of maternal necessity, such as severe preeclampsia, or fetal necessity, such as growth restriction. In all, only approximately 5% of premature deliveries are amenable to tocolytic therapy and potential prolongation of pregnancy.

TREATMENT

Bed rest, with or without sedation, is the most commonly used therapy for premature labor. Although there is evidence that strenuous activity may increase uterine activity, and walking is a commonly used method of encouraging early labor, there is no evidence that bed rest alone has any effect on the course of premature labor. Beyond its lack of proven efficacy, bed rest is difficult both to enforce and to comply with voluntarily.

The use of hydration to suppress premature labor is based on the premise that the inhibition of pituitary vasopressin also suppresses pituitary oxytocin production. The theory further posits that maternal pituitary oxytocin is the causal agent in premature labor. Randomized, controlled trials have shown no benefit of maternal hydration in the treatment of premature labor.

The use of benzodiazepines, barbiturates, and narcotics for the suppression of premature labor is common. There is no evidence that true premature labor can be halted by such measures, although the time that the patient spends sleeping may allow natural resolution of uterine irritability. The downside to the use of these drugs for this condition lies in the subsequent inability for the patient to be assessed for continuing symptoms.

The use of antibiotics to suppress premature labor has been proposed and tested but has not yet been shown to be of benefit.

When premature delivery seems inevitable or even likely, the only medical intervention that has been demonstrated to be beneficial is the administration of glucocorticoids, which are used not to inhibit preterm delivery but to mature various fetal organs more rapidly—particularly the lungs—in order to minimize immaturity. The glucocorticoid of choice is either betamethasone, 12 mg intramuscularly every 24 hours for two doses, or dexamethasone, 6 mg intramuscularly every 6 hours for four doses.

Antenatal glucocorticoids are maximally effective if delivery occurs between 48 hours and 7 days after first administration. Their use has been shown to result in a reduction in neonatal morbidity from respiratory distress, necrotizing enterocolitis, and intraventricular hemorrhage.

There are no contraindications to the use of corticosteroids in preterm labor except for imminent delivery (minutes away). Their use in PPROM has been demonstrated to be beneficial, with no increase in infection rate. Repeated courses of steroids in undelivered patients are controversial.

When a patient presents in active premature labor and there is no indication for delivery, tocolysis may be attempted. Tocolysis is the pharmacologic attempt to halt uterine contractions in an effort either to administer antenatal steroids or to improve maturity. All methods of tocolysis share common contraindications: cervical dilation greater than 4 cm, a contraindication to continued intrauterine existence for the fetus, and a contraindication to continued pregnancy for the mother.

Magnesium sulfate is the most commonly used tocolytic in the United States. Although its mechanism of action is not entirely determined, as a calcium antagonist it has a relaxant effect on both vascular smooth muscle and uterine muscle.

Terbutaline and ritodrine are the beta agonists used to suppress preterm uterine contractions. Their mechanism of action is the stimulation of beta-adrenergic receptors on smooth muscle cell walls, which results in smooth muscle relaxation. Stimulation of these receptors results in activation of adenylate cyclase and thus increases in intracellular cyclic adenosine monophosphate (cAMP). cAMP then activates protein kinase and phosphorylates intracellular proteins, decreasing intracellular calcium. In addition, myosin light chain kinase is phosphorylated, reducing its affinity for calmodulin.

These combined actions result in smooth muscle relaxation.

The inhibition of oxytocic prostaglandins $PGF_{2\alpha}$ and PGE_2 by indomethacin, ibuprofen, and sulindac is achieved via the inhibition of cyclooxygenase in the decidua. By blocking the free flow of calcium into and within smooth muscle cells, nifedipine and other calcium channel blockers relax vascular and uterine smooth muscle.

Oxytocin acts to cause uterine contractions through activation of a cell surface receptor on smooth muscles. Atosiban is a competitive inhibitor of the oxytocin receptor.

Currently investigational, nitric oxide donors such as glyceryl trinitrate show promise as tocolytics. The use of glyceryl trinitrate as a short-term uterine relaxant for breech version and breech extraction is described and appears safe.

Preterm Premature Rupture of the Membranes

PPROM is the most common precursor of preterm labor and delivery. It appears that many episodes of PPROM are the result of subclinical membrane infections or chorioamnionitis. Twenty-four percent of women suffering PPROM deliver within 24 hours, and of the remainder a proportion require induction within 24 hours for infection. The remaining pregnancies may remain undelivered for some time and are managed expectantly until the fetus is mature, the patient enters spontaneous labor, or chorioamnionitis ensues.

CHAPTER 2

Genetics and Metabolism

GENETICS OF COMMON PROBLEMS PRESENTING IN THE NEWBORN

TWINNING
Epidemiology

Monozygotic (MZ) twins account for approximately 30% of all twins, and dizygotic (DZ) twins account for about 70%. MZ twinning occurs sporadically, with no evidence of heritability. The incidence is approximately 1 in 260 births. The rate of DZ twinning, on the other hand, shows considerable racial and ethnic variation, being approximately 1 in 500 in Asians, 1 in 125 in whites, and as high as 1 in 20 in some African populations. There is a familial tendency to DZ twinning. The recurrence risk for a woman who has given birth to DZ twins is significantly greater than the general population risk. Other factors believed to influence the chance of DZ twinning are maternal age, parity, and availability of in vitro fertilization.

MZ twins, commonly referred to as "identical" twins, develop from a single fertilized ovum, carry identical genetic information, and are hence of the same sex. Approximately one half of MZ twin pairs are male, and one half are female. They result from splitting of the zygote sometime during the 14 days following fertilization. Placentation depends on when during this period the division takes place.

If separation is early, at the two-cell stage, two separate zygotes develop, each with its own placenta and amniotic sac (dichorionic-diamniotic; approximately 35% of MZ twins). The separate placentas may be fused or separate. More commonly, the inner cell mass splits within the same blastocyst cavity. These embryos share a placenta but have separate amniotic cavities (monochorionic, diamniotic; approximately 65% of MZ twins). Although the blood supply to each twin is usually well balanced, a variety of vascular anastomoses within the single placenta may occur.

Later separation of the embryo rarely occurs, resulting in the formation of twins with a single placenta and amnion sac (monochorionic, monoamniotic; <1% of MZ twins.) The splitting of the embryo during later stages of development may result in incomplete separation, giving rise to the formation of conjoined twins, an exceedingly rare phenomenon.

Congenital Malformations

An increased prevalence of anomalies at birth in twins, when compared with singletons, has been demonstrated in several large series. The structural defects seen fall into three categories. First, there are deformations imposed by the constraint of limited intrauterine space, which, as expected, are as common in MZ as DZ twins. Second, disruption of normal blood flow due to placental vascular communications in monochorionic (and hence MZ) twins can occur and give rise most commonly to anomalies of the central nervous, cardiovascular, and gastrointestinal systems. The most extreme example of this is the formation of an acardiac fetus, believed to result from artery-to-artery anastomoses between twin fetuses. Early in gestation the pressure in the artery of one twin exceeds that in the artery of the other. The circulation in the recipient twin is reversed, with blood entering the recipient through an umbilical artery and leaving through the umbilical vein, draining into vein-to-vein anastomoses. Severe structural defects in the recipient result, including acardia. The normal or "pump" twin must provide circulation for itself as well as its acardiac sibling and can develop cardiac hypertrophy, congestive heart failure, or hydrops fetalis. Vascular disruption lesions represent only a small portion of total malformations found in twins.

Structural malformations due to early defects of morphogenesis, the third category, are found more commonly in MZ twins. The etiology is believed to be closely related to the MZ twinning process itself. The factor responsible for zygotic separation may inflict further developmental damage during embryogenesis. Alternatively, embryos disrupted by splitting may be more vulnerable to teratogenic influences.

MZ twins are often discordant for congenital malformations, although less often than DZ twins, despite genetic equivalence. Determination of zygosity should not be based on phenotypic similarity or differences. For heritable abnormalities with known genetic etiologies, however, such as Down syndrome, concordance in MZ twins approaches 100%.

Zygosity Determination

Zygosity determination may be desired for any number of reasons, including for estimating the genetic prognosis in a twin of a patient with a genetic disease, for transplantation needs, for research purposes, or to gratify normal curiosity. From simple observations of sex and placentation, the zygosity of approximately half of all twins can be determined at birth: different-sex twins are dizygous (approximately 35%) and twins with a monochorionic placenta are monozygous (approximately 20%). Molecular diagnosis is the method of choice in the remainder, looking for differences in the large number of DNA markers available for testing. Twins who are not MZ are virtually certain to show different polymorphisms inherited from each parent. As discussed, determination of zygosity should not be based on phenotypic appearance.

CLEFT LIP AND PALATE

Of all cases of orofacial clefting (cleft lip with or without cleft palate [CL(P)]), about 50% involve both the lip and palate, 25% involve the lip only, and 25% involve the palate only. Cleft lip is unilateral in 80% of cases and bilateral in 20%. Associated cleft palate (CP) occurs in 70% of unilateral and 85% of bilateral cases of cleft lip. Other birth defects are present in about 7% to 13% of patients with cleft lip alone, 11% to 14% of patients with cleft lip and palate, and 35% to 50% of patients with CP. There are many multiple-malformation syndromes associated with cleft lip and CP. For this reason, a newborn with orofacial clefting requires a thorough evaluation to exclude a syndromic diagnosis and to provide accurate recurrence risk counseling. In some conditions, the other defects are obvious, but in others, such as van der Woude syndrome, the findings may be rather inconspicuous.

In van der Woude syndrome, an autosomal dominant condition, lower lip pits may be the only manifestation present in family members who carry the trait. Most cases of isolated CP and CL(P) conform to a multifactorial basis of inheritance in which genetic and environmental factors interact to cause clefting once a threshold effect is reached. Rare families with autosomal dominant clefting have also been reported. In genetic counseling, the empiric recurrence risks vary with the number of affected people in the family and their relationship to the offspring at risk.

CONGENITAL HEART DISEASE

Congenital heart disease (CHD) is the most common type of birth defect, occurring in about 1 in 140 newborns. CHD accounts for about 50% of children dying of birth defects, and approximately 15% of infantile deaths are due to CHD.

Cardiovascular embryology involves the expression of many genes for normal cardiovascular formation. Cardiac development is sensitive to genetic and environmental effects during the embryonic period, from the 2nd to the 8th week of gestation. Maldevelopment may occur from insults during this period or due to persistence of fetal structures. Many different anatomic types of CHD exist, reflecting the complexity of this process.

Approximately 20% to 45% of patients with

TABLE 2–1
Select Syndromes Associated with Congenital Heart Disease

Etiology	Cardiac Features
Chromosome	
Trisomy 21	AVC, VSD, ASD, ASCA
Trisomy 18	VSD, AVC, DORV, BAV, HLHS
Trisomy 13	ASD, VSD, PDA
Tetrasomy 22p (cat-eye syndrome)	TAPVR
Tetrasomy 12p (Pallister Killian syndrome)	VSD, CoA, ASD, PDA, AS
45,X (Turner syndrome)	CoA, HLHS, AS, ASD, VSD, MVP, BAV
Cri du chat (deletion 5p)	VSD, PDA, ASD
Wolf-Hirschhorn (deletion 4p)	ASD, VSD
Williams (deletion 7q/elastin)	SVAS, PPS
Alagille (deletion 20p)	PPS
DiGeorge (deletion 22q)	IAA, TOF, TArt
Velocardiofacial (deletion 22q)	TOF, VSD
Single Gene	
Adams-Oliver	VSD, PS, TOF, CoA
Apert	PS, VSD
Ellis–van Creveld	ASD, AVC, SA
FG	VSD, PS, HLHS
Holt-Oram	ASD, VSD, AVC
Kartagener	Dextrocardia
Marfan	Aortic dilatation, valve incompetence
Noonan	Valvular PS, CM
Neurofibromatosis type 1	PS, neurofibromata
Osteogenesis imperfecta	MVP, AR
Smith-Lemli-Opitz type 1	ASD, AVC, TOF, CoA
Thanatophoric dysplasia	ASD, PDA
Treacher Collins	VSD, PDA, ASD
Tuberous sclerosis	Rhabdomyomata, angiomata
Zellweger	PDA, VSD

CHD have one or more other congenital anomalies, and about 10% of patients with CHD have a syndromic diagnosis. Newborns with CHD should be carefully examined for evidence of dysmorphic features or other birth defects. If present, a chromo-

TABLE 2-1
Select Syndromes Associated with Congenital Heart Disease *Continued*

Etiology	Cardiac Features
Environmental	
Hydantoin	PS, AS, CoA, PDA
Maternal diabetes mellitus	VSD, CoA, TGA
Maternal SLE	Complete heart block
Maternal alcohol abuse	VSD, ASD, PDA, TOF
Maternal PKU	TOF, VSD, PDA, HLHS
Congenital CMV	MS, PS, ASD
Congenital rubella	PDA, PPS, ASD, VSD
Lithium	Ebstein anomaly, TA, ASD
Retinoic acid	IAA, TOF, TArt, VSD
Trimethadione	TGA, TOF, HLHS
Vitamin A	TArt, TGA, ASD, VSD, TOF
Unknown	
Laterality sequence (asplenia/polysplenia)	DC, TGA, TAPVR, TArt, AVC
CHARGE association	VSD, AVC, TOF
Goldenhar	VSD, TOF, ASD
Klippel-Feil	ASD, VSD
VACTERL association	VSD, various defects

AR, aortic regurgitation; AS, aortic stenosis; ASCA, aberrant subclavian artery; ASD, atrial septal defect; AVC, atrioventricular canal; BAV, bicuspid aortic valve; CoA, coarctation of the aorta; CM, cardiomyopathy; DC, dextrocardia; DORV, double-outlet right ventricle; HLHS, hypoplastic left heart syndrome; IAA, interrupted aortic arch; MVP, mitral valve prolapse; MS, mitral stenosis; PDA, patent ductus arteriosus; PS, pulmonic stenosis; PPS, peripheral pulmonic stenosis; SA, common atrium; SVAS, supravalvular aortic stenosis; TA, tricuspid atresia; TArt, truncus arteriosus; TAPVR, total anomalous pulmonary venous return; TGA, transposition of great arteries; TOF, tetralogy of Fallot; VSD, ventricular septal defect.

some analysis is indicated, and additional studies such as fluorescence in situ hybridization (FISH), DNA analysis, and metabolic testing may be required.

Specific types of CHD result from a myriad of chromosome, monogenic, environmental, and multifactorial effects on cardiac embryologic development (Table 2–1). The underlying basis of CHD is attributable to chromosome abnormalities in 5% to 6% of cases, single gene disorders in 3% to 5%, and environmental factors in 2%. The remaining 85% to 90% of cases of CHD have no definable cause and are usually considered multifactorial in origin.

Recently a deletion of chromosome 22q11 has been shown to be associated with three conditions associated with CHD: DiGeorge syndrome, velocardiofacial syndrome, and conotruncal anomaly face syndrome. FISH studies reveal a 22q11 deletion in about 90% of patients with DiGeorge syndrome and 75% of patients with velocardiofacial syndrome. The acronym *CATCH 22* has been termed to denote the phenotype associated with this deletion: *C*ardiac defect, *A*bnormal facies, *T*-cell defect, *C*left palate, *H*ypocalcemia. Even among patients with nonsyndromic conotruncal anomalies, approximately 20% to 30% have demonstrable 22q11 deletions. For this reason 22q11 FISH analysis is indicated for patients with tetralogy of Fallot, truncus arteriosus, aortic arch anomalies, or phenotypic features of DiGeorge or velocardiofacial syndromes.

Isolated nonsyndromic cardiac malformations are generally considered multifactorial, unless the family history indicates a specific mendelian pattern of inheritance. After one affected child with isolated nonsyndromic CHD, the recurrence risk for a sibling is 2% to 3%. The risk to the offspring is twofold to threefold greater if the mother has CHD than if the father has CHD. Recurrence risks are based on empiric data for isolated nonsyndromic CHD.

HYPOTONIA

Genetic diseases causing neonatal hypotonia can be found with all modes of inheritance (Table 2–2). Chromosome aberrations that can be associated with a floppy baby include trisomy 21, in which hypotonia is present in 95%, Miller-Dieker syndrome due to microdeletion at chromosome 17p13.3, and Prader-Willi syndrome due to absence of paternal chromosome 15q11. These infants are dysmorphic. Infants with Down syndrome have a well-known facial appearance with midface hypopla-

TABLE 2–2
Heritable Disorders Associated with Neonatal Hypotonia

Autosomal Dominant Transmission

Achondroplasia
Central core myopathy
Congenital fiber-type disproportion
Congenital hypomyelinating neuropathy
Congenital myotonic dystrophy
Ehlers-Danlos syndrome (I, II, III, IV, VII, VIII)
Hereditary motor-sensory neuropathy
Marfan syndrome
Minicore myopathy
Myotubular myopathy
Nemaline myopathy

Autosomal Recessive Transmission

Acid maltase deficiency (Pompe disease)
Amino acid dysmetabolism
Carnitine deficiency
Congenital fiber-type disproportion
Central core myopathy
Congenital muscular dystrophy
Congenital myasthenia syndrome
Ehlers-Danlos syndrome (VI)
Lissencephaly
Myophosphorylase deficiency (McArdle disease)
Myotubular myopathy
Nemaline myopathy
Organic acid dysmetabolism
Peroxisomal disorders
Phosphofructokinase deficiency
Pyruvate dysmetabolism (Leigh disease)
Spinal muscular atrophy (Werdnig-Hoffmann disease)

X-Linked Transmission

Cerebro-oculo-renal syndrome (Lowe syndrome)
Ehlers-Danlos syndrome (V)
Kinky hair disease (Menkes disease)
Mucopolysaccharidosis (Hunter syndrome)
Myotubular myopathy

Nonmendelian Transmission

Chromosome aberrations
Down syndrome (trisomy 21)
Miller-Dieker syndrome (17 deletion)
Prader-Willi syndrome (15q deletion)
Cytoplasmic DNA abnormalities
Mitochondrial myopathies

Adapted from DiMario FJ: Genetic diseases in the etiology of the floppy infant. Rhode Island Med J 72:357–359, 1989.

sia; epicanthal folds; and small, posteriorly rotated ears, among other findings. Infants with Miller-Dieker syndrome are microcephalic but are less obviously dysmorphic. They have forehead furrowing, a small nose with anteverted nostrils, upslanting palpebral fissures, and a thin upper lip. Computed tomographic (CT) imaging reveals the lissencephaly that makes this diagnosis. Patients with Prader-Willi syndrome may appear only slightly dysmorphic and can be missed if the diagnosis is not considered during the evaluation of hypotonia. Karyotype analysis and pertinent FISH studies should be performed on all hypotonic infants with a dysmorphic appearance.

The most well-known and most serious autosomal recessive disease giving rise to neonatal hypotonia is spinal muscular atrophy (SMA), or Werdnig-Hoffman disease. In its most fulminant form, newborns are profoundly weak and floppy, sometimes prenatally. The history of decreased fetal activity can sometimes be elicited. Tendon reflexes are weak or absent. The infants, however, are alert and sociable. Tongue fasciculations and tremors may be present. The carrier frequency for this disease is high, 1 in 80; therefore, although family history should be searched for consanguinity, it need not be present. SMA occurs in 1 in 20,000 to 25,000 newborns. The gene for SMA has been mapped to chromosome 5q11.2-13.3, and DNA diagnosis is available.

Inborn errors of metabolism are frequently associated with neonatal hypotonia. The presence of acidosis or hepatomegaly, or both, should alert the clinician to this diagnostic possibility in a hypotonic infant. Many heritable metabolic disorders have autosomal recessive inheritance, and some, such as carnitine deficiency, are treatable.

About 15% of babies born to mothers with myasthenia gravis are born with transient myasthenia gravis of the newborn, demonstrating severe hypotonia and weakness, facial diplegia, and pooling of oral secretions. These are manifestations of the mother's disease and treatment and are usually gone within 6 weeks. Some infants benefit from treatment with anticholinesterase drugs while symptomatic.

CONGENITAL DISLOCATION OF THE HIP

Congenital dislocation of the hip (CDH) is a common birth defect inherited as an isolated multifactorial trait or as a feature of a multiple-malformation syndrome. As an isolated condition, its incidence varies widely among different ethnic populations, ranging from about 1 in 1000 whites to 1 in 5000 blacks to 1 in 26 Native Americans in the southwestern United States. The highest frequency occurs among ethnic groups who "swaddle" their infants, such as Laplanders and Native Americans.

Other associated risk factors include breech presentation, firstborn status, and female sex. The fourfold to sixfold female-to-male predilection is believed to occur due to hormone-induced joint laxity. Other genetic factors include ligamentous laxity and shallowness of the acetabulum.

Many syndromes have been described in which CDH is a common feature, including connective tissue disorders such as skeletal dysplasias, Marfan syndrome, Ehlers-Danlos syndrome, and Larsen syndrome, as well as neuromuscular disorders such as Pena-Shokeir syndrome type I, congenital muscular dystrophies, and neural tube defects.

Isolated CDH shows aggregation among first-degree relatives in families, demonstrating multifactorial inheritance. MZ twins display about a 50% concordance rate compared with 5% among DZ twins.

PIERRE ROBIN SEQUENCE AND MICROGNATHIA

Descriptions of infants born with the triad of micrognathia, cleft palate, and respiratory obstruction were published as early as 1822. In 1923, however, French stomatologist Pierre Robin introduced the term *glossoptosis* to describe the tendency for the tongue to fall back into the airway, causing pharyngeal obstruction. He did not mention cleft palate as a problem in children with micrognathia until his second report in 1934. Pierre Robin sequence is now a well-recognized congenital condition involving a combination of micrognathia and/or retrognathia and glossoptosis causing upper airway obstruction, with or without a typically U-shaped CP. The designation *sequence* signifies the theory that the mandibular abnormality gives rise to the secondary problems of CP and airway obstruction. It is hypothesized that abnormal embryologic development of the mandible occurs between 7 and 11 weeks' postconception, resulting in a high tongue position in the nasopharynx that interferes with the medial growth of the lateral palatal shelves toward midline fusion. A U-shaped palatal cleft is created, and the upper airway becomes obstructed because of glossoptosis.

Possible mechanisms that may lead to the arrest of mandibular development include positional deformation from intrauterine constriction, intrinsic mandibular hypoplasia, and neurologic abnormalities that inhibit normal fetal mandibular movements such as swallowing. As such, the mechanisms that lead to the occurrence of Robin sequence are variable. In a study of 100 consecutive cases referred with the triad of findings associated with Robin sequence, only 17% were considered nonsyndromic. Eighty percent of children had other anomalies, and many had associated syndromes. The most common were Stickler syndrome in 34%, velocardiofacial syndrome in 11%, and fetal alcohol syndrome in 10%. The importance of making the underlying syndrome diagnosis cannot be overemphasized. Patients with Stickler syndrome have normal intellect but may have severe ocular abnormalities. Stickler syndrome is an autosomal dominant disorder. Patients with velocardiofacial syndrome usually have cognitive impairment and heart malformations, and they may develop psychiatric illness. Affected patients have a deletion of chromosome 22 and transmit the disease in an autosomal dominant fashion. Isolated Robin sequence appears to be sporadic, but when part of another syndrome it follows the inheritance pattern of the associated disorder.

Elliott and associates retrospectively reviewed 55 patients with confirmed Pierre Robin sequence to determine the associated presence of pediatric conditions such as respiratory distress, feeding difficulties, and middle ear pathology. Respiratory problems, often from airway obstruction, were present in 55% of patients. Respiratory difficulties may not be apparent immediately after birth but may develop sometime during the first week. Various treatment strategies are employed, including positioning, glossopexy, and tracheostomy placement. Fifty-five percent of patients had feeding difficulties, related more often to the airway obstruction and respiratory difficulties than to the palatal clefts. Many infants in this study needed feeding assistance to support nutrition until they were able to maintain sufficient caloric intake with oral feeds. Most (90%) of the patients reviewed had recurrent otitis media, most eventually requiring myringotomy tube placement. Careful monitoring for middle ear disease is crucial to prevent hearing loss and speech delay. The presence of an associated syndrome did not alter the prevalence of these medical problems.

In addition to the Robin sequence, there are more than 70 syndromes or conditions in which micrognathia is a prominent feature. The increasing recognition of micrognathia as an important marker for fetal genetic abnormality has prompted some investigators to establish fetal mandible measurement standards. One commonly accepted standard does not yet exist. Nonetheless, the currently available data indicate that the presence of micrognathia should prompt the search for other abnormalities, both in utero and after birth, and consideration of karyotype examination. Genetic counseling should be offered when fetal micrognathia and other sonographic findings are found.

ARTHROGRYPOSIS

Arthrogryposis refers to multiple congenital joint contractures that are nonprogressive and involve more than one area of the body. Arthrogryposis is found in a large heterogeneous group of disorders; more than 150 different syndromic conditions have been reported.

Multiple joint contractures occur at birth following any cause of limitation of movement in utero (Table 2–3). There are five etiologic causes: (1) neuropathy, either central or peripheral; (2) myopathy; (3) abnormal connective tissue involving joints; (4) in utero restraint; and (5) maternal illness. Neuropathies account for 90% to 95% of cases and myopathies for 5% to 10%.

Amyoplasia is considered the most common condition causing arthrogryposis, accounting for about one third of cases. In amyoplasia, all limbs are usually affected and muscle is replaced with fatty tissue and fibrous bands. The major joints are fusiform or cylindrical and firmly fixed. Sensation and cognitive development are normal. Abdominal wall defects occur in about 10% of patients, and 5% have evidence of amniotic bands with digital defects. Early physical therapy is essential to improve range of motion, and orthopedic surgery is often necessary. This condition is sporadic and most likely occurs from vascular compromise during midpregnancy.

TABLE 2–3

Examples of Different Causes of Arthrogryposis

Neuropathy

Trisomy 18
Fetal alcohol syndrome
Fryns syndrome
Smith-Lemli-Opitz syndrome
Zellweger syndrome
Congenital myasthenia gravis
Miller-Dieker syndrome

Myopathy

Amyoplasia
Nemaline myopathy
Schwartz-Jampel syndrome

Abnormal Connective Tissue

Larsen syndrome
Diastrophic dysplasia
Kniest dysplasia
Multiple pterygium syndrome
Freeman-Sheldon syndrome
Neonatal Marfan syndrome

In Utero Constraint

Twins
Amniotic band sequence
Oligohydramnios

Maternal Illness

Hyperthermia
Myasthenia gravis
Myotonic dystrophy
Multiple sclerosis

POLYDACTYLY

Postaxial polydactyly is common and occurs 10 times more frequently in blacks than in whites. It may occur in 3 to 4 in 1000 births, and much higher frequencies have been published in some countries, such as 17 to 27 in 1000 in Nigeria. When isolated, postaxial polydactyly is an autosomal dominant trait. It may be associated with genetic syndromes, however, in which case it follows the inheritance pattern of the syndrome. Postaxial polydactyly is a frequent finding in trisomy 13, and in Meckel syndrome, an autosomal recessive disorder characterized by encephalocele and cystic dysplastic kidneys. Other syndromes that feature postaxial polydactyly include oral-facial-digital syndrome type II (Mohr), Pallister-Hall syndrome, and short rib polydactyly syndrome.

Preaxial polydactyly may occur as infrequently as 8 in 100,000 births and is much more likely to be present as part of a syndrome. It is more often unilateral. It is two to four times more frequent in the Native American population than in whites or blacks. Thumb polydactyly, type I, may be as subtle as broadening of the distal phalanx, as seen in Rubinstein-Taybi syndrome, or it may be a full duplication.

Numerous homeobox genes are known to be expressed in various cell groups of the developing limb, guiding the developmental processes. Cells in the limb bud receive positional information, which allows them to differentiate into specific cell types and structures with anteroposterior and dorsoventral axes. Positional information is believed to be gained from chemical gradients set up by morphogen diffusion from specific groups of cells. Retinoids are probably important morphogens in limb bud development. It is likely that mutations involving *HOX* genes, growth factors, and morphogen receptors give rise to abnormalities of limb development. Candidate genes have been identified, and study of the molecular genetics of limb anomalies is ongoing.

AURICULAR TAGS AND SINUSES

Auricular tags and sinuses are relatively common mild malformations, each occurring in about 1% of newborns. More than 90% of cases are isolated and are usually unilateral. The birth prevalence of ear sinuses is somewhat greater for Asians and blacks than for whites. As isolated anomalies, ear tags and sinuses do segregate independently as autosomal dominant traits in some families.

Auricular tags are skin-covered nodules or appendages that often contain cartilage and represent remnants of the hillock of His. They are typically located anterior to the pinna but may be present anywhere along an arclike line from the temple to just below the tragus, conforming to the junction between the first and second branchial arches. They may also be situated anterior to the tragus down to the angle of the mouth, corresponding embryologically to the fusion of the mandibular and maxillary portions of the first branchial arch.

Ear tags may exist as a part of a multiple malformation condition, such as the oculo-auriculo-vertebral spectrum (Goldenhar syndrome), Towne-Brocks syndrome, Treacher Collins syndrome, cat-eye syndrome, Wolf-Hirschhorn (4p-) syndrome, and cri du chat (5p-) syndrome.

Auricular sinuses are usually shallow dimples, pits, or depressions of 1 to 3 mm in diameter, most commonly located on the anterior margin of the ascending helix or, less commonly, in the preauricular region. The rarest location is posterior to the auricle at the site of its attachment. Auricular sinuses are twice as common in females as males. Although ear sinuses are usually isolated anomalies, they are associated with several multiple malformation syndromes, including oculo-auriculo-vertebral spectrum, Beckwith-Wiedemann syndrome, branchio-oto-renal (Melnick-Fraser) syndrome, Peters-plus syndrome, and various chromosome aberrations.

Preauricular pits and ear tags may coexist in a number of syndromes, including oculo-auriculo-vertebral spectrum (Goldenhar syndrome), cervico-oculo-acoustic (Wildervanck) syndrome, and mandibulofacial dysostosis (Treacher Collins syndrome).

Hearing loss is associated with both ear tags and sinuses. In approximately 13% of isolated cases of ear tags, mild to moderate sensorineural hearing loss is present. Conductive and sensorineural hearing loss has also been described with ear sinuses. Hearing screening tests are warranted for patients presenting with either of these anomalies.

SPECIFIC GENETIC DISORDERS PRESENTING IN THE NEWBORN

TRISOMY 21 (DOWN SYNDROME)

Down syndrome is the most common autosomal trisomy compatible with live birth, occurring in about 1 in 700 to 800 newborns. Trisomy 21 due to meiotic nondisjunction provides the underlying basis in 92% to 95% of liveborns with Down syndrome, and translocation Down syndrome with 46 chromosomes accounts for 3% to 5% of cases. In most cases of translocation Down syndrome, one parent has a balanced robertsonian translocation between chromosome 21 and another acrocentric chromosome, most commonly chromosome 14. In approximately 3% of Down syndrome, mitotic nondisjunction occurs leading to trisomy 21 mosaicism.

Many fetuses with Down syndrome are now diagnosed by prenatal karyotyping initiated because of advanced maternal age or abnormal maternal serum analyte screening (triple test) or fetal ultrasonographic findings. Many prenatal ultrasound findings are associated with Down syndrome, including atrioventricular canal defect, the "double-bubble" sign of duodenal atresia, short femur or humerus lengths, nuchal thickening or translucency, echogenic small bowel, choroid plexus cysts, cerebral ventriculomegaly, hydronephrosis, nonimmune hydrops, fifth-finger clinodactyly, and cholecystomegaly.

If not prenatally diagnosed, most patients with Down syndrome are usually recognized at birth owing to the constellation of physical findings. Although no one physical feature is pathognomonic, a number of clinical signs are usually present in affected babies, allowing the nurse or midwife to frequently suspect the diagnosis first. Common neonatal features include a rounded head, third fontanel, brachycephaly, upslanted palpebral fissures, epicanthal folds, Brushfield spots, midfacial hypoplasia, flattened nasal root, small dysplastic pinnae, a large tongue in a small mouth, short neck, transverse palmar creases, brachydactyly, fifth-finger clinodactyly, a wide gap between the first and second toe, and hypotonia.

Diagnostic scoring systems have been devised. In Table 2–4, six or more out of 10 signs are considered virtually diagnostic in the newborn. In some cases, the diagnosis may be difficult because the features may be subtle or confounded by other factors such as prematurity and ethnic background.

Whenever the diagnosis is suspected, an immediate karyotype is indicated to definitively confirm or rule out the condition. The parents should be informed of the level of clinical suspicion and the need for a confirmatory cytogenetic study.

Numerous birth defects have been described in association with Down syndrome. Congenital heart disease comprises the common major malformation

TABLE 2–4

Ten Cardinal Signs of Down Syndrome in a Newborn

Sign	Frequency (%) in Affected Newborn
Poor Moro reflex	85
Hypotonia	80
Flat facial profile	90
Upslanted palpebral fissures	80
Morphologically simple, small, round ears	60
Redundant loose neck skin	80
Transverse palmar crease	45
Hyperextensible large joints	80
Abnormal pelvic radiograph	70
Fifth-finger clinodactyly	60

Adapted from Hall B: Mongolism in newborns. Clin Pediatr (Phila) 5:4, 1966.

in Down syndrome, occurring in about 45% of babies. The most frequently observed cardiac lesion is the atrioventricular canal defect; other lesions include ventricular septal defect (VSD), atrial septal defect (ASD), patent ductus arteriosus (PDA), and tetralogy of Fallot. An echocardiogram is indicated for all patients with Down syndrome, since the diagnosis of congenital heart disease may be missed by routine diagnostic means. The medical and surgical treatment of the heart lesions are the same as for chromosomally normal infants.

Gastrointestinal malformations also occur more commonly in Down syndrome. Approximately 2% to 5% of patients have duodenal atresia, and 2% have Hirschsprung disease. Other rarer associated anomalies include tracheoesophageal fistula, esophageal atresia, omphalocele, annular pancreas, duodenal web, distal small bowel atresia, microcolon, and anorectal anomalies.

Hearing loss of heterogeneous origin may be present to some degree in 40% to 75% of patients with Down syndrome. Middle ear disease is the most common cause of hearing problems.

Strabismus, myopia, cataracts, and glaucoma occur more frequently in Down syndrome, with 61% of patients requiring ongoing ophthalmologic care. A pediatric eye evaluation at 6 months or less and annually thereafter is recommended.

Atlantoaxial subluxation is an infrequent but serious complication of Down syndrome; cord compression and neurologic symptoms may result. Generalized ligamentous laxity is considered the basis for the atlantoaxial instability. The radiographic signs of instability (gap >4 mm) have poor predictive value and generally do not merit treatment. Flexion-extension radiographs are recommended prior to anesthesia and the initiation of high-risk sports.

Growth problems occur in virtually all patients with Down syndrome. At birth, the mean weight, length, and head circumference range between 10% to 15%. After infancy the growth velocity falls off so that linear growth retardation is the norm by 3 years of age. Growth curves for Down syndrome children have been published. Growth hormone has been used to treat short stature in some patients who do not have growth hormone deficiency. This controversial treatment has shown some favorable short-term results. As adults, obesity is a common problem, occurring in 96% of females and 71% of males.

Approximately 5% of patients with Down syndrome develop hypothyroidism; almost one third of patients have demonstrable thyroid autoantibodies. The thyroid dysfunction may occur at any age, and newborn screening followed by regular thyroid screening is indicated.

Approximately 1 in 150 children with Down syndrome develop acute lymphoblastic leukemia. Transient myeloproliferative disorder associated with splenomegaly and hepatic fibrosis may occur at birth and usually resolves spontaneously in the first year of life. Neonatal thrombocytopenia is also associated with Down syndrome.

Children with Down syndrome show a great deal of developmental variability. Language and motor delay become more pronounced during the second year of life. The degree of central hypotonia is correlated to some degree with later cognitive and motor development. I.Q. testing has revealed an extremely wide range, from 20 to 85. Most children attain the learning ability of a 6- to 8-year-old child, but some patients may exceed this level. The popular Down syndrome stereotype of a happy, affectionate, pleasant, music-loving person with moderate intellectual handicaps does not accurately reflect the great variety of personalities, including behavioral and psychological problems, in these patients. Epilepsy occurs in 5% to 10% of patients with Down syndrome, with peak onsets in infancy and late adulthood.

If a child with Down syndrome survives the infancy period, the prognosis for long-term survival is generally good; however, a shortened life span is still likely. About 44% of patients survive to 60 years of age and about 14% to 68 years. Beyond 40 years of age, virtually all patients display neuropathologic features of Alzheimer disease, but most patients do not develop frank dementia.

For complete or mosaic trisomy 21, it is unnecessary to obtain parental chromosome analyses since in virtually all cases their karyotypes will be normal. After a child with trisomy 21 is born to a mother, her risk of recurrence for Down syndrome at the time of amniocentesis is about 1% greater than her age-specific risk. For younger mothers, this increase over the age-specific risk is significant, whereas for older mothers, the increased risk is only incremental.

For de novo Down syndrome translocation, the recurrence risk is less than 1%. In the case of a mother carrying a familial robertsonian translocation, the risk for translocation Down syndrome is about 15% at amniocentesis and 10% at birth. For male translocation carriers, the recurrence risk is small, at about 1%.

TRISOMY 18 (EDWARDS SYNDROME)

Trisomy 18 occurs in about 1 in 6000 live births, with a 3:1 female:male preponderance. It carries a high intrauterine mortality rate. It is estimated that only 5% of trisomy 18 conceptuses survive to live birth, and 30% of fetuses diagnosed by mid-trimester amniocentesis succumb during the rest of the pregnancy.

Prenatal ultrasonography may provide important clues to the diagnosis of trisomy 18. Reported findings include growth retardation, oligohydramnios or polyhydramnios, heart defects, exomphalos, myelomeningocele, clenched fists, and radial limb anomalies. The combination of intrauterine growth retardation with any major birth defect should raise suspicion for trisomy 18. Maternal serum analyte screening has also been shown to be useful for the detection of trisomy 18; alpha-fetoprotein, uE3, and total human chorionic gonadotropin all demonstrate lower values than the normal population. The mid-trimester triple test can detect 66% of cases of trisomy 18 with a 0.4% false-positive rate.

At birth, physical findings are usually diagnostic of trisomy 18. Common features include intrauterine growth retardation (1500 to 2500 g near term); small, narrow cranium; prominent occiput; open metopic suture; low-set, posteriorly rotated, primitive pinnae; small mouth; micrognathia; short sternum; characteristic overlapping digits; hypoplastic fingernails; short, dorsiflexed great toes; and prominent heels with convex soles, termed *rocker-bottom feet*.

Many different major malformations are associated with trisomy 18. More common defects include congenital heart disease (ASD, VSD, PDA, pulmonic stenosis, coarctation), cleft palate, talipes equinovarus, omphalocele, colonic malrotation, renal anomalies, myelomeningocele, brain anomalies, choanal atresia, eye anomalies, vertebral anomalies, radial ray defects, hypospadias, and cryptorchidism.

Approximately 90% or more of babies with trisomy 18 die by 6 months of age, and about 5% are alive at 1 year. Female survivors significantly outnumber males. The major causes of death include central apnea, infection, and congestive heart failure. In the newborn period poor feeding is almost universal, so that gavage tube feeding is generally required.

Once the diagnosis is cytogenetically confirmed, the extremely poor prognosis should be fully explained to the parents. The caregivers should discuss the inappropriateness of aggressive life-sustaining therapies, which may inflict discomfort on the patient. Given the significantly shortened life span of such patients, most parents and providers jointly decide to forego heroic medical and surgical interventions. Arrangements to care for the baby at home may be considered if adequate medical, social, and emotional supports exist.

Rare long-term survivors with trisomy 18 have been described; profound somatic growth and mental retardation are the rule. In some patients, cardiac surgery has been performed, but this intervention has not been shown to improve outcome. Overall development does not progress much beyond that of a 6-month-old infant. Malignant tumors, such as Wilms tumor, hepatoblastoma, and neurogenetic tumors, have been described in some survivors.

There are rare anecdotal reports of recurrences of trisomy 18, as well as the occurrence of other autosomal trisomies following trisomy 18. In relatively small series of trisomy 18 index cases, this phenomenon appears extremely uncommon. Nonetheless, it is postulated that some women have a general predisposition to aneuploidy. In the case of young mothers, it is common practice to add a 1% risk to the maternal age–specific risk when estimating the recurrence risk of a viable autosomal trisomy.

TRISOMY 13 (PATAU SYNDROME)

Trisomy 13 has a birth frequency of 1 in 12,500 to 21,000 newborns, and it is estimated that only 2.5% of trisomy 13 conceptuses survive to birth.

Approximately 50% of cases of trisomy 13 can be diagnosed prenatally by using maternal age, maternal serum screening, and routine fetal ultrasonography. Prenatal ultrasound has the potential to visualize many of the major associated malformations, including holoprosencephaly, anophthalmia, facial clefting, nasal deformities, congenital heart disease, renal anomalies, omphalocele, and polydactyly.

In the newborn, the diagnosis is suggested by the presence of postaxial polydactyly, microcephaly, eye anomalies, cleft lip and palate, scalp defects, congenital heart disease, and renal anomalies.

Varying degrees of holoprosencephaly are present in 60% of patients, and seizures are quite common. Microcephaly is quite common, and the sutures are usually split with large fontanels. Microphthalmia, colobomas of the iris, abnormal ears, capillary hemangiomata, and cleft lip and/or palate are common facial findings. Localized scalp defects (cutis aplasia) in the parieto-occipital area are present in about 50% of cases. Approximately 80% of patients have some form of congenital heart disease, most commonly VSD, ASD, PDA, and dextocardia. Typical limb findings are transverse palmar creases, postaxial polydactyly, camptylodactyly, and hyperconvex narrow fingernails.

Survival is extremely limited with 80% of babies dying in the neonatal period and 3% surviving to 6 months of age. Physical and mental development is severely delayed. Patients are often blind and deaf, experience refractory epilepsy, and have feeding difficulties.

In the newborn period, management issues are similar to those of trisomy 18, in that decisions must be mutually reached regarding the goals of medical interventions. The dismal prognosis dictates that focus should be directed toward comfort measures and quality-of-life issues.

As in trisomy 18, the data on recurrences after having one child with trisomy 13 are incomplete, but available data suggest that recurrences are extremely rare. Nonetheless, a maternal age–related risk plus 1% is usually offered for the recurrence risk of any viable autosomal trisomy.

TURNER SYNDROME (45,X)

The cardinal signs of Turner syndrome include short stature, mild craniofacial abnormalities (epicanthal folds, high-arched palate), strabismus, auditory defects, a webbed or short neck, shield chest, renal anomalies, pigmented nevi, lymphedema of hand and feet, nail hypoplasia, primary amenorrhea, and congenital heart disease. The types of heart defects seen in Turner syndrome include bicuspid aortic valve, coarctation of the aorta, valvar aortic stenosis, and mitral valve prolapse. There is wide phenotypic variation in patients with Turner syndrome. The ultimate adult height in Turner syndrome is 135 to 150 cm. Delayed secondary sexual characteristics result from primary ovarian failure with lack of estrogen production.

Mental retardation is not a feature of Turner syndrome. Perceptual and spatial thinking may be impaired, however, leading to somewhat lower mean performance I.Q. Language as well as fine and gross motor skills may be delayed. Personality traits may be characterized by lack of aggressiveness, immaturity, shyness, and compliance.

Other medical problems later in life include a higher risk for autoimmune thyroiditis, hypothyroidism, hypertension, obesity, intestinal telangiectasia, non–insulin-dependent diabetes, osteoporosis, deafness, and aortic aneurysms.

Growth hormone therapy is commonly now used to treat short stature beginning at age 4 to 6 years. Cyclic hormonal therapy with estrogens and progesterone is usually initiated at puberty for the development of secondary sex characteristics, menses, and the prevention of osteoporosis. Infertility is highly likely secondary to primary ovarian failure (streak gonads), but assisted reproduction with in vitro fertilization of donated oocytes in hormonally treated patients has been successfully performed.

47,XXX

With a birth prevalence of 1 in 1200 female newborns, the 47,XXX syndrome has no specific phenotype in the newborn period. There is a higher rate of minor anomalies, such as clinodactyly, ear anomalies, and epicanthal folds. Many display taller stature with disproportionate leg lengths relative to trunk height. The average I.Q. is normal in the 85 to 90 range, with wide variations. Speech delay, neuromotor incoordination, and learning disabilities are more common. Although about 60% of 47,XXX females require special education in high school, some attended college and are highly competent adults. Personality traits such as shyness, immaturity, passivity, mild depression, and conduct disorders are also more commonly reported. Most patients undergo normal puberty, have normal reproductive capacity, and cope well as adults.

47,XXY

Klinefelter syndrome occurs in about 1 in 600 male newborns and is the most common cause of hypogonadism in males. Maternal and paternal meiotic nondisjunction contribute equally as the underlying mechanism. In the newborn there is no significant dysmorphic pattern, although fifth-finger clinodactyly occurs in about 25% of patients. The major features noted later include tall stature, hypogonadism, infertility, light facial hair, and an increased risk for developmental problems. Gynecomastia occurs in 15% to 30% of patients. The mean I.Q. is

85 to 90, with most patients falling in the normal range. Learning disabilities, especially those involving reading, expressive language, and auditory processing, are common. Behavioral problems may also exist, including immaturity, shyness, unassertiveness, low frustration tolerance, and poor peer relations. The onset of puberty is normal and the sexual orientation is generally heterosexual. Testosterone therapy in adolescence is indicated to promote secondary sexual characteristics.

47,XYY

The 47,XYY karyotype occurs in about 1 in 1000 male newborns and there is no recognizable physical phenotype. The 47,XYY syndrome originates from paternal nondisjunction in meiosis II. Although preliminary reports invoked the supernumerary Y chromosome as the basis for criminal behavior in some mentally retarded persons, prospective studies have not shown an increased risk of frank mental retardation or severe behavioral problems. There is an increased risk of hyperactivity, low impulse control, distractibility, and expressive and receptive language problems. Boys with 47,XYY have accelerated linear growth, becoming taller adults. Reproductive ability is not affected.

TRIPLOIDY

Triploidy occurs when the karyotype contains three copies of each chromosome: 69,XXX or 69,XXY. Approximately 15% of cytogenetically abnormal abortuses are triploid. Cytogenetic mechanisms include fertilization of one egg by two sperm (dispermy) and complete failure of nondisjunction in maternal meiosis. Most triploid conceptuses are spontaneously aborted, and of those liveborn, death in infancy is the rule. Patients with diploid-triploid mosaicism, known as *mixoploidy*, may survive with varying degrees of severity. A number of birth defects are associated with triploidy, including a large cystic placenta, low birth weight, hydrocephalus, neural tube defects, microphthalmia, colobomata, malformed ears, 2-3 syndactyly, cardiac septal defects, and ambiguous genitalia.

DELETION/CONTIGUOUS GENE SYNDROMES
Cri du Chat (5p−)

Partial deletion of 5p results in the cri du chat syndrome, named for the distinctive cry of a mewing cat in affected infants. The birth incidence is approximately 1 in 50,000 newborns. In the newborn period, patients present with the characteristic cry, low birth weight, microcephaly, craniofacial dysmorphism (round face, hypertelorism, downward-slanted palpebral fissures, epicanthal folds, and broad nasal bridge), and hypotonia. Approximately one third of patients have variable types of congenital heart disease, including ASD, VSD, and tetralogy of Fallot.

Over the first year of life, the catlike cry disappears and development progresses slowly. Mental retardation is generally severe, with reported I.Q. levels below 50 in infancy and below 20 in adulthood. Special education has been reported to be beneficial, with some adult patients reaching the developmental level of a normal 5- to 6-year-old child. Failure to thrive commonly occurs, and most patients survive to adulthood.

The cri du chat phenotype results from a deletion of the critical region of 5p15.2-p15.3. De novo deletions account for 85% to 90% of cases; 10% to 15% occur due to malsegregation of parental balanced translocations. Fine molecular mapping of the critical region is now in progress to determine which of the estimated 100 genes in the critical region are responsible for specific phenotypic features.

Lissencephaly/Miller-Dieker Syndrome (17p−)

The distal deletion of chromosome 17p leads to Miller-Dieker syndrome, characterized by facial dysmorphism and a severe neuronal migrational defect. Moreover, patients with isolated lissencephaly may also have deletions in the same region.

In Miller-Dieker syndrome, Type I lissencephaly is present, in which the surface of the brain is smooth without gyri. The craniofacial features include bitemporal hollowness, midfacial hypoplasia, a short nose with anteverted nostrils, micrognathia, and a protuberant upper lip with a thin vermilion border. Polyhydramnios is common during pregnancy owing to poor fetal swallowing. Postnatal growth retardation, seizures, profound mental retardation, and spasticity occur in most patients. The disorder carries a significant mortality rate in childhood.

A microdeletion of the critical region, band 17p13.3, results in Miller-Dieker syndrome and will be visible by high-resolution methods in only about 50% of cases. Using cytogenetic and molecular techniques, 17p13 deletions are detectable in about 90% of patients with Miller-Dieker syndrome and 15% of patients with isolated lissencephaly. A brain morphogenesis gene *LIS1* has been isolated from this region and is deleted in patients with Miller-Dieker syndrome and isolated lissencephaly. The diagnosis may be confirmed by either fluorescent in situ hybridization (FISH) analysis, polymorphic DNA markers, or direct *LIS1* mutational analysis. FISH probes for the 17p13 region are commercially available; most cytogenetic laboratories routinely offer specific testing for this condition.

Parental balanced translocations or pericentric inversions can account for recurrences in families, which previously were erroneously assumed to be due to an autosomal recessive trait.

DiGeorge/Velocardiofacial Syndromes (22q−)

The DiGeorge and the velocardiofacial (Sprintzen) syndrome (VCFS) were previously regarded as separate entities but have since shown phenotypic overlap when it was discovered that they contain deletions in the same 22q region.

In classic DiGeorge syndrome there is aplasia or

hypoplasia of the thymus and parathyroid glands, congenital heart disease, and dysmorphic facies. Hypoparathyroidism leads to neonatal hypocalcemia and possibly seizures. Thymic hypoplasia results in a T-cell deficiency, with increased susceptibility to infections. The congenital heart defects are predominantly conotruncal, including tetralogy of Fallot, truncus arteriosus, interrupted aortic arch, right-sided aortic arch, and septal defects. The craniofacial findings include low-set ears, micrognathia, cleft palate, bifid uvula, and hypertelorism with short palpebral fissures.

VCFS is considered to be an autosomal dominant condition with cleft palate, cardiac defects, speech and language difficulties, and typical facies. Some patients with VCFS have additional features found in DiGeorge syndrome, namely neonatal hypocalcemia and lymphoid hypoplasia. Twenty percent of patients with VCFS demonstrate cytogenetic deletions of chromosome 22q by high-resolution techniques. Using FISH analysis, more than 80% of patients with VCFS have deletions. About 90% of cases of 22q deletions are de novo.

Approximately 15% to 20% of patients with DiGeorge syndrome have chromosome abnormalities, mainly involving chromosome 22. Additionally, FISH or DNA dosage studies now demonstrate 22q deletions in about 90% of patients with DiGeorge.

DiGeorge syndrome and VCFS are now considered different manifestations of the same disorder, a loss of contiguous genes in the same region. The range of phenotype is quite wide and subtle dysmorphic features may be overlooked. In familial cases one parent may show features of predominantly VCFS but have a child with classic DiGeorge phenotype. The basis for the apparent autosomal dominant inheritance in VCFS has been shown to be due to the inheritance of a chromosome deletion from one of the parents.

WOLF-HIRSCHHORN SYNDROME, 4p(−)

Infants with the Wolf-Hirschhorn syndrome, due to distal deletion of the short arm of chromosome 4, have dysmorphic features evident at birth. Prenatal ultrasound findings can also suggest the diagnosis. This clinical entity was first delineated in 1965 when Hirschhorn and Cooper cited a case with midline fusion defects and a deletion of a group B chromosome, and Wolf and colleagues described a similar case and were able to show that the deletion was of chromosome 4.

Hallmarks of this syndrome include growth restriction of prenatal onset, typical craniofacial malformations, microcephaly, and midline closure defects, including scalp defects, cleft lip and/or palate, cardiac septal defects, and hypospadias. The facial features, described as the "Greek helmet facies," consist of ocular hypertelorism with epicanthal folds; high forehead with prominent glabella; and a long, straight, beaked nose with broad nasal bridge. The ears are simple, large, and low set. Hypotonia is common, as is the history of poor fetal movement.

Approximately a third of infants with Wolf-Hirschhorn syndrome die in the first year, but some have lived to adulthood. Severe growth and mental retardation are invariable, and those that survive usually develop seizures.

WILMS TUMOR–ANIRIDIA (WAGR)

Although it accounts for approximately 8% of all childhood malignancies, the diagnosis of Wilms tumor in the newborn is rare. When found, it is usually as a unilateral, asymptomatic abdominal mass. Hypertension, microscopic hematuria, and, rarely, gross hematuria can be found.

WILLIAMS SYNDROME

The most characteristic findings are distinctive facial features, growth and mental deficiency, cardiovascular anomalies, and infantile hypercalcemia in some cases. Williams syndrome usually occurs sporadically, but it can be inherited as an autosomal dominant disorder. The estimated incidence is 1 in 20,000 to 50,000 live births.

Many infants with Williams syndrome are born small for gestational age with mild microcephaly. The typical facial features of flat midface with depressed nasal bridge; anteverted nostrils; long philtrum; thick lips; a large, open mouth; and a stellate or lacy iris pattern may not be obvious at birth but become more striking with age. Most infants have a cardiovascular abnormality. Supravalvular aortic stenosis is the most common and is present in more than 50% of cases. Pulmonary artery stenoses are also characteristic, and other defects can be found. Hypercalcemia is present in only 5% to 10% of cases but can be severe, symptomatic, and persist into late infancy. Umbilical or inguinal hernias are more common than in the general population.

Feeding and growth are problematic during infancy, and these babies tend to be irritable and colicky. With age, Williams syndrome patients are more likely to develop strabismus, a hoarse voice, hypertension, and joint limitations. Most are mildly to moderately mentally retarded, but language skills are often disproportionately advanced and can mask the extent of the retardation. A characteristic, gregarious, "cocktail party personality" is described in these children. Although gross motor development is preserved, visual-motor integration is particularly impaired. Learning disabilities, most notably attention deficit disorders, are common.

Isolated supravalvular aortic stenosis (SVAS) also exists as a distinct, autosomal dominant trait. Linkage between this trait and *ELN*, which had been mapped to 7q11.23 in 1991, was identified in 1993. This led to the hypothesis that *ELN* was involved in the pathogenesis of Williams syndrome. When studied, it was found that most Williams syndrome patients are missing one copy (hemizygous) of *ELN*. Deletions in both the maternally and the paternally derived chromosome 7 have been found with no apparent predominance. In Williams syndrome, the microdeletion (submicroscopic, i.e., not visible by even high-resolution cytogenetic techniques) appears to be of the entire gene plus flanking DNA. SVAS mutations that have been defined involve only part of the gene.

EXTRA STRUCTURALLY ABNORMAL CHROMOSOME

Marker chromosomes, or extra structurally abnormal chromosomes (ESACs), are small 47th chromosomes occurring with an estimated birth prevalence of 0.60%. By definition, these chromosomes cannot be characterized by standard cytogenetic analysis owing to the paucity of bands represented. ESACs are heterogeneous in size and origin. An ESAC may or may not exert phenotypic effects, depending on whether critical coding regions are contained in the marker. Further definition of an ESAC is performed by FISH with chromosome-specific probes.

Inverted duplicated chromosome 15, denoted as *inv dup (15)*, accounts for about 40% of ESACs. These chromosomes are dicentric and bisatellited and contain two copies of the p arm, centromere, and proximal long arm. They have been described in normal and mentally retarded patients, who may have epilepsy, autistic features, and mild physical abnormalities.

Once an ESAC is identified in a patient, it is important to determine if its origin is de novo or familial. De novo markers carry a higher risk for phenotypic abnormalities than familial markers. Likewise the chromosome origin of the ESAC also is correlated with the likelihood of a phenotypic effect.

BECKWITH-WIEDEMANN SYNDROME

Genomic imprinting affects the inheritance pattern of Beckwith-Wiedemann syndrome, a common overgrowth syndrome that usually presents in the neonatal period. It is estimated to occur in one in approximately 14,000 births, but underdiagnosis is possible, because the severity of findings is variable and the diagnosis is more difficult to make at ages beyond childhood. The characteristic triad of findings in infants with Beckwith-Wiedemann syndrome include macrosomia, abdominal wall defect, and macroglossia.

Most infants are large for gestational age with weight appropriate for length, unlike infants of diabetic mothers who are more likely to be overweight for their length. They then grow along their growth curve usually at or above the 95th percentile. Advanced bone age is usually present. In a few patients, overgrowth may be asymmetric, resulting in hemihypertrophy. Visceromegaly is a frequent manifestation of overgrowth in affected patients. Histologically, cytomegaly of the various tissues of the adrenal gland, pancreas, kidney, liver, and spleen can be found.

The most distinctive facial feature of Beckwith-Wiedemann syndrome is macroglossia, which nearly all described patients exhibit. Slitlike linear creases of the earlobe and indentations of the posterior helix are characteristic ear findings. Facial nevus flammeus and prominent eyes with infraorbital creases are often seen.

Hypoglycemia, often severe and recalcitrant, is a neonatal problem in at least one third of cases. Prompt recognition and testing is important in infants manifesting other findings suggestive of Beckwith-Wiedemann syndrome to minimize the short- and long-term sequelae of this complication. Hypoglycemia responds to therapy but may persist for months, spontaneously resolving during infancy.

Abdominal wall defects are common and may vary from an omphalocele to umbilical hernia or simple diastasis recti. Early visceromegaly of abdominal organs is postulated to disrupt return of the intestine to the abdominal organs is postulated to disrupt return of the intestine to the abdominal cavity in early embryogenesis, giving rise to abdominal wall abnormalities. Prune belly, inguinal hernia, and diaphragmatic eventration have also been described in patients with Beckwith-Wiedemann syndrome.

SINGLE GENE DISORDERS
Cystic Fibrosis

Cystic fibrosis is an autosomal recessive disease caused by mutations of a gene located on the long arm of chromosome 7. Although it is often not clinically symptomatic in newborns, a variety of circumstances arise for which cystic fibrosis testing is desired or indicated in the perinatal period. An understanding of the genetic mechanisms of disease, the testing available, and the implications of results are vital to accurate diagnosis and counseling.

The clinical manifestations of cystic fibrosis are related to the build-up of abnormal, viscous mucus in a variety of organ systems. Principally affected are the lungs, pancreas, intestine, and reproductive tract. Most of the morbidity and mortality of the disease are from pulmonary manifestations of chronic bronchiectasis and infection.

Meconium ileus is the most common manifestation in the newborn infant and is present in 10% to 15% of patients with cystic fibrosis. They present with signs of small bowel obstruction within 24 to 48 hours, with failure to pass meconium, abdominal distention, and vomiting. Associated intestinal atresias may or may not be present. Occasionally meconium ileus is complicated by prenatal bowel perforation, in which case newborns may present with symptoms of an acute abdomen and peritonitis. Nonsurgical treatment of simple meconium ileus with a hypertonic contrast enema is often successful in liberating the abnormal meconium and meconium plugs. Although there are other causes, a high percentage of patients with meconium plugs, when tested, will be identified as having cystic fibrosis and should be tested. Furthermore, prenatal sonographic findings suggestive of intestinal obstruction or peritonitis or of echogenic-appearing fetal bowel should prompt consideration of cystic fibrosis testing.

Genotyping is now an important, powerful diagnostic tool for cystic fibrosis. Mutation analysis of patients already known to have cystic fibrosis may provide information that will allow risk assessment for family members. Genotyping can detect asymptomatic carriers. It has provided the possibility of prenatal testing for at-risk families. It can be performed on infants for whom sweat testing is not possible, such as premature or critically ill infants. In some cases, genotype analysis may be helpful in predicting phenotype. Furthermore, DNA needed for testing can be easily prepared from blood, buccal samples, or amniocytes.

MARFAN SYNDROME

Marfan syndrome is a hereditary disorder of connective tissue with the predominant clinical effects seen in the skeletal, ocular, and cardiovascular systems. Clinical findings in the skeletal system are long, slender fingers and toes, out of proportion to the length of the hands and feet (arachnodactyly); long, slender limbs relative to the body (dolichostenomelia); and anterior chest deformities of either pectus excavatum or pectus carinatum. Dolichocephaly, a high-arched palate, joint laxity, and flexion contractures can be seen. There is also a tendency toward development of kyphoscoliosis.

The cardinal ocular feature is ectopia lentis, with the lens usually anteriorly dislocated. Myopia is also common, and abnormalities of the cornea or iris can be present. Ectopia lentis has not been reported in a newborn with Marfan syndrome.

Involvement of the cardiovascular system is responsible for 90% of deaths related to Marfan syndrome. Progressive widening of the aortic root and mitral annulus can lead to mitral valve prolapse, often with regurgitation, aortic valve incompetence, and/or aneurysms or dissections of the ascending aorta. In infants with Marfan syndrome, the cardiac abnormalities are frequently found in the neonatal period.

Other systems can be involved as well. Spontaneous pneumothoraces due to pulmonary blebs, striae distensiae (stretch marks) without obvious cause, hernias, and dural ectasia (which is very specific to this disorder and therefore diagnostically important) are seen in older children and adults with Marfan syndrome.

Infants with Marfan syndrome have been described to have a characteristic facies with large, deep-set eyes; malar hypoplasia; megalocornea; and frontal bossing. Some authors have described the appearance as a "worried" or "old man" look. They may also have large, floppy ears and micrognathia.

MECKEL SYNDROME

The classic combination of congenital anomalies in patients with Meckel syndrome is occipital encephalocele, polydactyly, and polycystic kidneys. Gruber named this syndrome *dysencephalia splanchnocystica*. The much earlier description of the syndrome by Meckel was publicized years later by Opitz and Howe, leading to the current designation of Meckel syndrome. Other prominent features include hepatic fibrosis with bile duct proliferation, cleft lip and/or palate, and genitourinary abnormalities. The syndrome is lethal in the perinatal period and has an autosomal recessive pattern of inheritance. It can frequently be confused with trisomy 13 before karyotype results become available.

Other central nervous system abnormalities may be hydrocephalus, absence of olfactory lobes, or Dandy-Walker malformation. Microcephaly with marked sloping of the forehead is common. The polydactyly is usually postaxial (ulnar) and usually bilateral. Hands are more often affected than feet, but all four limbs may be abnormal. Nearly all males have hypoplastic penis and cryptorchidism.

NOONAN SYNDROME

The clinical findings of Noonan syndrome were described in 1963. The incidence has been estimated to be 1 in 1000 to 2500 live births. The typical appearance changes with age. In the newborn period, findings may be more subtle but may include a broad, sloping forehead; ocular hypertelorism; antimongoloid slant of the palpebral fissures; and a deeply grooved philtrum. The ears are thick, low-set, and posteriorly angulated. Mild retrognathia may be present. There is frequently a prenatal history of cystic hygroma, polyhydramnios, or hydrops fetalis, and the infant may be born edematous or hydropic. Excess nuchal skin or even webbing may be present, similar to Turner syndrome. Later in infancy, the eyes, still hyperteloric, appear prominent with thick, hooded eyelids, epicanthal folds, and ptosis. The nasal bridge is wide and depressed. Anterior chest deformities, pectus excavatum or carinatum, may be present. In childhood, the face is triangularly shaped, and the eyes are less prominent but neck webbing may become more prominent.

Other system involvement is common. Infants with Noonan syndrome may have early feeding problems, or even failure to thrive, which resolve. Although weight and length are usually normal at birth, short stature develops in the majority.

About half of patients have a cardiac problem. Pulmonary valve stenosis is the most characteristic, but hypertrophic cardiomyopathy is also seen, and many other structural defects can be found. Anterior chest deformities are common, and scoliosis develops in some. Many males with Noonan syndrome have unilateral or bilateral cryptorchidism, which is likely the reason for increased male infertility among patients. Females with Noonan syndrome have normal genitalia and usually normal fertility. A variety of neurologic problems have been reported, including seizures, hearing deficit, peripheral neuropathy, and schwannomas. Hair may be abnormally sparse or curly, and skin may have nevi, freckles, or café au lait spots, which may be difficult to distinguish from other neurocutaneous disorders. Bleeding problems have been found. When present, developmental delay, both motor and cognitive, are mild, and many children with Noonan syndrome have normal development.

The diagnosis of Noonan syndrome is currently based on clinical presentation. The karyotype is normal. Turner syndrome must be ruled out in females, and other syndromes in the differential, depending on the features of the individual case, may include fetal alcohol syndrome, Aarskog syndrome, neurofibromatosis type 1, LEOPARD* syndrome, Watson syndrome, or Williams syndrome.

SURFACTANT PROTEIN B DEFICIENCY

Surfactant protein B (SP-B) deficiency is an inherited disease of full-term newborn infants that leads

---

*LEOPARD = *l*entigines, *e*lectrocardiogram abnormalities, *o*cular hypertelorism, *p*ulmonary stenosis, *a*bnormal genitalia, *r*etardation of growth, and *d*eafness.

to lethal respiratory failure within the first year of life. It is refractory to mechanical ventilation, exogenous surfactant therapy, glucocorticoid induction of SP-B production, and extracorporeal membrane oxygenation. Lung transplantation has been effective in some infants.

This inborn error of surfactant metabolism causes what has been known as *congenital alveolar proteinosis,* an uncommon cause of respiratory failure in full-term newborns who have chest radiographs similar to that of the premature infant with surfactant deficiency but a severely progressive course ultimately leading to death. A family history of similar disease in siblings is frequently found. In 1993, the absence of SP-B protein was demonstrated in the lung of three infants (in a family) who died of congenital alveolar proteinosis.

RUBINSTEIN-TAYBI SYNDROME

First described in 1963, Rubinstein-Taybi syndrome is characterized by dysmorphic facies, broad thumbs and great toes, growth retardation, and mental deficiency. Only recently has the genetic basis for Rubinstein-Taybi syndrome been elucidated. Prevalence in the general population is roughly estimated to range from 1 in 300,000 to 700,000.

When typical features are present, newborns with Rubinstein-Taybi syndrome can be readily recognized. The facial features change with age, in fact, and diagnosis can be more difficult later in infancy. Classic craniofacial appearance includes puffiness; down-slanting palpebral features; epicanthal folds; a prominent and/or beaked nose with nasal septum sometimes extending below the alae; and a narrow, high-arched palate. Patients can have a grimacing smile. They are frequently microcephalic. The ears are low set and often malformed. There is abundant dark hair with low anterior and posterior hairlines. Eyebrows are heavy and eyelashes are long.

Broad thumbs and/or halluces are present in almost all reported cases. Angulation deformities of thumbs may be found as well. The terminal phalanges of other fingers can also be broad, but less so. Significant dermatoglyphic findings are excess dermal ridge patterning in the thenar and first interdigital areas of the palm. There is a tendency toward keloid formation. Most of the males have cryptorchidism. Congenital heart defects, including PDA, VSD, and pulmonic stenosis, have been reported in about a third of the patients.

All patients have mental retardation, most of the time severe, with expressive speech most prominently delayed. Seizures and absence of the corpus callosum have been reported.

DISORDERS OF UNKNOWN ETIOLOGY
CHARGE Association

First defined by Pagon, the CHARGE association is a constellation of nonrandomly associated malformations that occur together in varying combinations. The malformations include coloboma, heart disease, atresia choanae, retarded growth and development and/or central nervous system (CNS) anomalies, genital anomalies, and ear anomalies and/or deafness. Criteria used "arbitrarily" by Pagon for diagnosis were the presence of either choanal atresia or ocular coloboma or both, and a total of at least four of the seven most common findings, with retardation and CNS anomalies considered separately. As the diagnosis of an association serves to alert clinicians to look for other, perhaps occult, associated anomalies, attempts to further delineate minimal diagnostic criteria have not been reported.

The coloboma may be unilateral or bilateral and of the iris, retina, or disc, and degree of visual impairment depends on the defect. The most common heart defect is tetralogy of Fallot, and other conotruncal defects are seen. ASD is also common. Choanal atresia may be bony or membranous, unilateral or bilateral. Growth deficiency is postnatal, and mental retardation is extremely likely, although variable in severity. CNS anomalies have included arrhinencephaly, holoprosencephaly, Dandy-Walker malformation, and agenesis of the corpus callosum. Males usually have genital hypoplasia that may respond to androgen therapy. Typical ears are low set and posteriorly rotated and have abnormal pinnae. Deafness, ranging from mild to profound, is common.

Many other anomalies have been reported in patients with CHARGE association. Phenotypic overlap exists with several known malformation syndromes, most notably cat-eye syndrome, trisomy 13 and 18, and 4p− syndrome. In addition, the VACTERL association (see following section) needs to be considered in the differential. Choanal and coloboma abnormalities are less common in VACTERL, and skeletal anomalies are less common in CHARGE.

VACTERL ASSOCIATION

The nonrandom tendency for five types of birth defects to associate together was described in 1972. VATER is the acronym that was used to delineate these defects: *v*ertebral defects, *a*nal atresia, *tra*cheoesophageal fistula with *e*sophageal atresia, *r*enal defects, and radial limb dysplasia. The association was subsequently expanded to include congenital cardiac disease and other limb defects and is now more commonly referred to as the *VACTERL association*. Although each of these defects may occur as isolated anomalies, they frequently occur in varying combination. The probability of the simultaneous occurrence of any three of these defects in the same person, based on their individual incidences, is so unlikely that it suggests a nonrandom association. Patients exhibiting any three or more of these defects, when other chromosome, single-gene, or recognized syndrome disorders are ruled out, are considered VACTERL cases.

This combination of anomalies is not believed to represent a discrete single etiologic syndrome. Rather, a common type of defect in differentiating mesoderm involved in the early development of these separate tissues is suggested as the basis for the association. The proposed defect would occur prior to the 35th day of gestation, because all of the involved mesodermal processes are near completion by that time. Although teratogenic influences have been speculated, no recognized teratogen has been proven. Nearly all cases have been sporadic, and no chromosome abnormalities have been found. The incidence of VACTERL has been estimated at 1.6 in 10,000 live births in one large series.

The most common vertebral anomaly is hemivertebrae, but other anomalies can be seen. Most, but not all, patients with tracheoesophageal fistula also have esophageal atresia. Although the association was first described as having specifically radial limb anomalies, patients with VACTERL have been reported with a variety of upper limb anomalies, including preaxial polydactyly, a proximally placed thumb, and even humeral hypoplasia. The renal malformation is most commonly renal agenesis, either unilateral or bilateral, but combinations of other renal anomalies can be seen. A cardiac anomaly is the least specific of the findings, VSD being the most common. In fact, it has been recently suggested that the association of cardiac defects with other VACTERL components is not more frequent than with any other birth defects. A variety of anomalies not considered components of the VACTERL association have been reported in patients with VACTERL, including single umbilical artery, inguinal hernia, hydrocephalus secondary to aqueductal stenosis, urogenital malformation, other gastrointestinal atresias, cleft lip and/or palate, and choanal atresia.

GOLDENHAR SYNDROME

Goldenhar syndrome is a complex, heterogeneous combination of abnormalities most classically involving the face, ears, and eyes that is also referred to as oculo-auriculo-vertebral spectrum and hemifacial microsomia. The hallmark features are unilateral deformity of the external ear and hypoplasia of the ipsilateral half of the face. Epibulbar dermoids and vertebral anomalies were present in Goldenhar's original description. Coloboma of the upper eyelid is common. There is an extremely wide variety of anomalies included in this diagnosis, and more than one disorder may be found to account for this het-

TABLE 2-5
Inborn Errors of Carbohydrate Metabolism

Hereditary galactosemia
Glycogen storage diseases
Hereditary fructose intolerance
Fructose-1,6-bisphosphatase deficiency

---

erogeneity. Most cases are sporadic, but families demonstrating apparent autosomal dominant transmission have been reported. Most reported monozygotic twins are discordantly affected. The best estimates of incidence are between 1 in 3500 and 1 in 5000 live births with a slight (3:2) male predilection. Family recurrence risk is estimated to be 1% to 2%. Many chromosome aberrations have been described in association with this syndrome, but the genetic etiology remains unknown.

INBORN ERRORS OF CARBOHYDRATE, AMMONIA, AMINO ACID, AND ORGANIC ACID METABOLISM

The disorders that comprise the inborn errors of carbohydrate, ammonia, amino acid, and organic acid metabolism, respectively, are outlined in Tables 2–5 to 2–8.

TABLE 2-6
Inborn Errors of Ammonia Metabolism

Ornithine transcarbamylase deficiency
Argininosuccinicaciduria
Citrullinemia
Carbamylphosphate synthetase deficiency
Transient hyperammonemia of the newborn

TABLE 2-7
Inborn Errors of Amino Acid Metabolism

Maple syrup urine disease
Hereditary tyrosinemia type 1
Nonketotic hyperglycinemia
Methionine synthetase deficiency
Phenylketonuria

TABLE 2-8
Inborn Errors of Organic Acid Metabolism

Methylmalonic acidemia
Propionic acidemia
Isovaleric acidemia
Multiple carboxylase deficiency
Glutaric acidemia type 1

Fatty acid oxidation disorders
  Glutaric acidemia type 2
  Very-long-chain acyl CoA dehydrogenase deficiency
  Medium-chain acyl-CoA dehydrogenase deficiency
  Short-chain acyl-CoA dehydrogenase deficiency
  Long-chain 3-hydroxy acyl-CoA dehydrogenase deficiency
  Carnitine transporter defect
  Carnitine palmitoyltransferase type I deficiency
  Carnitine palmitoyltransferase type II deficiency
  Acylcarnitine translocase deficiency

Defects in ketone metabolism
  Ketothiolase deficiency
  Succinyl-CoA: 3-ketoacid-CoA transferase deficiency
  3-Hydroxy-3-methylglutaryl-CoA lyase deficiency

Primary lactic acidoses
  Pyruvate dehydrogenase complex deficiency
  Pyruvate carboxylase deficiency
  Phosphoenolpyruvate carboxykinase deficiency
  Mitochondrial respiratory/electron transport chain defects
    Barth syndrome
    Pearson syndrome
    Leigh disease

CoA, coenzyme A.

INBORN ERRORS OF CARBOHYDRATE METABOLISM

Hereditary Galactosemia

Galactose-1-Phosphate-Uridyltransferase (GALT) Deficiency

Galactose-1-Phosphate + Uridine Diphosphate (UDP) Glucose (UDPglucose) $\xrightarrow{\text{GALT}}$ UDPgalactose + Glucose-1-Phosphate

> Enzyme: Homodimer
> Gene Location: Chromosome 9p13
> Frequency: 1/35,000–60,000

The three enzymes of the galactose metabolic pathway that are responsible for the rapid hepatic conversion of galactose to glucose following ingestion of dietary lactose are erythrocyte galactokinase (GALK), GALT, and UDP galactose-4-epimerase. GALT deficiency is the most common of these disorders. The most frequent initial clinical sign is poor growth; vomiting and poor feeding also occur in most of the patients. Jaundice may be present in the first few weeks of life and persist. Initially the jaundice may be due to indirect hyperbilirubinemia, only later to be associated with an elevation of direct bilirubin as well. While on lactose, many infants with galactosemia present in the first 2 to 3 weeks with only poor feeding and growth, jaundice, and mild irritability or lethargy. With continual ingestion, multiorgan toxicity syndrome ensues, associated with liver disease that may progress to cirrhosis with portal hypertension, splenomegaly, ascites, renal tubular dysfunction, sometimes the full-blown renal Fanconi syndrome, anemia primarily due to decreased red blood cell (RBC) survival, lethargy, and brain edema associated with a bulging fontanel. Two clinical phenomena deserve further mention: cataracts and *Escherichia coli* sepsis. Cataracts may be evident in the first few weeks of life but often they are detected after 2 weeks of age. However, some infants are born with congenital cataracts that are associated with abnormalities of the embryonal lens: these are central in nature and require slit-lamp examination for documentation. *E. coli* sepsis is the most devastating complication in the newborn period; the mortality rate is higher than 50%. The reason that *E. coli* or gram-negative bacteria are so hazardous for newborns with GALT deficiency remains unknown.

After initiation of a lactose-free diet in the newborn period, usually the problems related to liver and kidney disease, anemia, and brain edema disappear unless there has been severe organ damage such as hepatic cirrhosis. Most infants begin to grow and develop at a normal rate. Even prospectively treated patients may manifest long-term complications. They relate to speech defects, delays in language acquisition, learning problems in school, and hypergonadotropic hypogonadism in most of the females. The cause of dietary-independent complications is unknown. Patients with galactosemia must stay on a lactose-restricted diet for their entire lives. When the infant is initially diagnosed, either through the newborn screening program or because of the recognition of clinical signs, blood galactose levels may be as high as 5 to 20 mM, RBC galactose-1-phosphate level is significantly elevated, as are urine galactitol levels. During this phase of severe hypergalactosemia, positive reducing substances are present in the urine. One of the first abnormalities to be detected—albuminuria—reflects a poorly understood renal glomerular component. This develops within 24 to 48 hours of ingestion of lactose and disappears as quickly following galactose elimination. In addition to hyperbilirubinemia there may be mild to severe elevations of serum alanine transferase (ALT) and aspartate transaminase (AST) levels and various abnormalities related to renal tubular dysfunction, such as hyperchloremic metabolic acidosis, hypophosphatemia, glucosuria, and generalized aminoaciduria. Vitreous hemorrhages are newly recognized complications in the newborn period. After the patient is placed on a lactose-free diet, the RBC galactose-1-phosphate levels in patients with classic galactosemia fall but never return to the normal range and remain mildly elevated for the lifetime of the patient. This is also true for the urinary metabolite galactitol and may be related to endogenous galactose production.

The deficiency of the enzyme GALT may be detected in RBCs in patients with most common forms of galactosemia. The newborn screening programs in various states use either an enzymatic and/or a metabolite screening method. When metabolites are assayed, the level of galactose-1-phosphate or total galactose and galactose-1-phosphate in RBCs are usually measured. Most of the gene defects that produce galactosemia are now known; therefore, some patients or siblings may be screened for the disease or for being a carrier by genotype analyses. Liver disease of any cause and congenital hepatic vascular shunts may lead to impaired galactose tolerance and a positive newborn screening test for galactosemia.

Glycogen Storage Diseases

The glycogen storage diseases (GSD) may be divided between those types that primarily affect the liver and those that affect striated muscle. With some forms, such as GSD Type 3, or debrancher disease, both striated muscle as well as the liver may be affected. According to European prevalence data, the overall frequency of GSD is 1 in 20,000 to 25,000. With the exception of GSD Type 2, or Pompe disease (a lysosomal defect), most of the patients with glycogenosis do not come to clinical attention in the newborn period. Patients with the three most common forms of GSD—Types I, III, and VI—have a phenotype that mimics a small-molecule disorder because glucose homeostasis is affected.

Glucose-6-Phosphatase Deficiency

Glucose-6-Phosphate + H_2O → Glucose + Phosphate

Enzyme: Heterodimer (Catalytic and Regulatory Subunit)
Catalytic Subunit Gene Location: Chromosome 17
Frequency: 1/100,000

GSD Type 1 is due to a decreased activity of glucose-6-phosphatase, the enzyme that is perched at the terminus of both glycogenolysis and gluconeogenesis. Several different biochemical abnormalities can result in this phenotype, now classified as GSD Types 1a, 1b, and 1c. The enzyme that resides on the anticytoplasmic side of internal membrane spaces of the hepatocyte catalyzes the hydrolysis of glucose-6-phosphate to glucose and phosphate. Impairments in the transport of either glucose-6-phosphate or phosphate may result in decreased function of this enzyme. The major clinical findings are poor growth and enlarged abdominal girth, hepatomegaly, and any of the signs that may be related to hypoglycemia. The major laboratory findings are fasting hypoglycemia, ketosis, lactic acidosis, hyperlipidemia (specifically, hypertriglyceridemia), and hyperuricemia. The most important aspect of therapy is to prevent brain damage from hypoglycemia and growth failure. The mainstay of therapy is frequent feedings and restriction of lactose and sucrose. The use of continuous nasogastric feedings or uncooked cornstarch, particularly during the night, has significantly improved the care of these children, and although it does not correct all the biochemical perturbations, it does improve growth and can prevent hypoglycemic spells.

Lysosomal α-Glucosidase Deficiency

$$Glycogen_{(n)} + H_2O \rightarrow Glycogen_{(n-1)} + Glucose$$

> Enzyme: α-1,4-Glucosidase Monomer
> Location: Chromosome 17q23
> Frequency: 1/100,000

GSD Type 2, or Pompe disease, is a deficiency of the lysosomal enzyme alpha-glucosidase. In the newborn period the main clinical finding relates to heart disease. There is usually marked cardiomegaly and a typical abnormal electrocardiogram, with biventricular hypertrophy and a short PR interval. Decreased cardiac output may lead to heart failure and passive congestion. Infants may also have generalized hypotonia not just because of heart failure but also because of skeletal myopathy. There is increased deposition of glycogen within striated muscle. Except because of passive congestion, the liver is not usually enlarged. Diagnosis is based on muscle enzyme analysis. Cardiac transplantation has been performed to prevent death in infancy.

Hereditary Fructose Intolerance

Fructose-1,6-Bisphosphate Aldolase B Deficiency

Fructose-1-Phosphate + H_2O →
   Dihydroxyacetone Phosphate + Glyceraldehyde

Enzyme: Homotetramer
Gene Location: Chromosome 9q13-q32
Frequency: Very Rare, Except Approximately 1/20,000 in Swiss

Hereditary fructose intolerance is secondary to a deficiency of the enzyme fructose-1,6-bisphosphate aldolase. There are different isoforms of aldolases in human tissues. The enzyme deficient in this disease results in an impairment in the conversion of fructose-1-phosphate to glyceraldehyde and dihydroxyacetone phosphate and, to a much lesser degree, fructose-1,6-bisphosphate to glyceraldehyde-3-phosphate and dihydroxyacetone phosphate. It is inherited as an autosomal recessive trait. Manifestations of clinical disease depend on sucrose or fructose ingestion. Thus, it usually does not come to clinical attention in the newborn period unless fruits are started early in the diet or the patients are placed on a formula that contains sucrose or fructose. The major clinical findings include poor feeding, vomiting, loose stools, poor growth, hepatomegaly, and any sign that could be related to hypoglycemia. Classically, the infants become ill soon after ingesting fructose. The acute signs may include pallor and lethargy, an altered state of central nervous system (CNS) function due to hypoglycemia. The major laboratory findings consist of hypoglycemia; hypophosphatemia; elevations of serum ALT and AST, including any of the findings that may be associated with hepatocellular disease per se; and reducing substances in the urine. The liver disease may be severe. Patients may be jaundiced with hyperbilirubinemia. There may be a bleeding diathesis. In addition to liver disease, renal tubular dysfunction may lead to full-blown renal Fanconi syndrome. Thus, one may detect metabolic acidosis due to a renal tubular acidosis, hypophosphatemia, impaired urate handling, spillage of glucose as well as fructose into the urine, and generalized aminoaciduria. It is believed that the severity of the clinical findings is related to the amount of fructose ingested. Infants, however, probably because of decreased intake, may manifest only the signs of poor growth and have few findings related to liver disease, except perhaps intermittent hypertransaminasemia. The suspicion of the physician is crucial in establishing the diagnosis. An intravenous fructose test may be performed under controlled circumstances, such as in the neonatal intensive care unit (NICU) or clinical research center, to determine whether after 15 to 30 minutes of fructose administration there is a decrease in serum phosphate and glucose levels and an elevation in the serum AST and ALT levels. In the past, diagnosis depended on enzyme analysis, but molecular diagnostic testing is more available now. The treatment consists of elimination of dietary fructose and sucrose.

Fructose-1,6-Bisphosphatase Deficiency

Fructose-1,6-Bisphosphatase Deficiency

Fructose-1,6-Bisphosphate + $H_2O \rightarrow$
   Fructose-6-Phosphate + Phosphate

Enzyme: Homotetramer
Gene Location: Unknown
Frequency: Very Rare

The deficiency of the enzyme fructose-1,6-bisphosphatase results in an inability to hydrolyze fructose-1,6-bisphosphate to fructose-6-phosphate. This is a key enzyme in gluconeogenesis. The main clinical features of this disease are hypoglycemia and the signs related to glucose deprivation in the CNS. The disease is primarily brought on by fasting, not by fructose ingestion, although fructose may exacerbate the abnormalities induced by fasting adaptation. Enlargement of the liver due to diffuse steatosis may be present only during periods of fasting and enhanced gluconeogenesis. The laboratory findings consist of hypoglycemia, ketosis, and lactic acidosis. The acidosis due to accumulation of lactic, 3-hydroxybutyric, and acetoacetic acids may be severe in this disease. Diagnosis depends on enzymatic analysis. The therapy primarily consists of avoidance of fasting.

INBORN ERRORS OF AMMONIA METABOLISM

Ornithine Transcarbamylase (OTC) Deficiency

Ornithine + Carbamylphosphate $\xrightarrow{OTC}$ Citrulline

> Enzyme: Homotrimer
> Gene Location: Chromosome X p21.1
> Frequency: 1/70,000–100,000

Argininosuccinate Lyase (ASAL) Deficiency

Argininosuccinate $\xrightarrow{ASAL}$ Arginine + Fumarate

> Enzyme: Homotetramer
> Gene Location: Chromosome 7 cen-p21
> Frequency: 1/70,000–100,000

Argininosuccinate Synthetase (ASAS) Deficiency

Citrulline + Aspartate $\xrightarrow{ASAS}$ Argininosuccinate

> Enzyme: Homotetramer
> Gene Location: Chromosome 9q34
> Frequency: 1/70,000–100,000

Carbamylphosphate Synthetase I (CPSI) Deficiency

NH_3 + Adenosine triphosphate (ATP) + HCO_3 $\xrightarrow{CPSI}$ Carbamylphosphate

Enzyme: Homodimer
Gene Location: Chromosome 2p
Frequency: 1/70,000–100,000

Genetic diseases involving each of the five enzymes of the hepatic mitochondrial urea cycle have been described. In the urea cycle, carbamylphosphate, which carries the nitrogen atom from ammonia, condenses with ornithine to form citrulline in a reaction catalyzed by the enzyme ornithine transcarbamylase (OTC), which is the most common defect among the inborn errors of the urea cycle. Citrulline subsequently interacts with aspartate to form argininosuccinate (ASA) and, in the process, another waste nitrogen atom is shuttled into the urea cycle substrate. Arginine is formed from ASA and the terminal enzyme in this cycle, arginase, converts arginine to urea for urinary excretion while regenerating ornithine to complete the cycle. The first step in this cycle involves the synthesis of carbamylphosphate, and this reaction, catalyzed by carbamylphosphate synthetase Type I (CPS-I), requires an activator, N-acetylglutamate, which is synthesized from acetyl coenzyme A (CoA) and glutamate via the enzyme N-acetylglutamate synthetase (NAGS). Rare patients may have reduced activity of NAGS. With the exception of arginase deficiency, each of these enzymes has been associated with disease in the newborn period. Clinical presentation in the newborn period is similar for all these defects. Almost all the infants are well in the first 12 to 24 hours of life and then begin to manifest poor feeding, vomiting, hyperventilation, lethargy, and coma, usually with seizures. When these diseases are untreated, they are almost always fatal. The treatment requires specific therapy to lower the waste nitrogen burden, including the toxic substance ammonia. Additional clinical findings include increased intracranial pressure. As with maple syrup urine disease the severe encephalopathic and life-threatening features may be related to brain edema. Chronic hepatomegaly has been reported in patients with argininosuccinicaciduria, whereas in the other urea cycle disorders, hepatomegaly is evident only during hyperammonemic episodes. Histologic examination of the liver shows modest fatty infiltration and fibrosis. Children with argininosuccinicaciduria may also manifest a specific abnormality of the hair, termed *trichorrhexis nodosa*.

The main laboratory finding in the urea cycle enzyme defects (UCEDs) is an elevated plasma ammonium level. Plasma ammonium levels may vary in different laboratories. In general, however, with automated chemistry testing for ammonia, the normal plasma values in older infants, children, and adults range between 10 and 35 μmol/L. However, in the Clinical Chemistry Laboratory at Children's Hospital of Philadelphia, the normal plasma ammonium value in newborns may be as high as 110 μmol/L. In patients with newborn-onset UCEDs, the plasma ammonium levels are often higher than 1000 or 2000 μmol/L when they are acutely ill. Patients with UCED usually do not have metabolic acidosis unless they are in a terminal state with vascular collapse or respiratory failure. Instead, the characteristic acid-base abnormality associated with hyperammonemia is respiratory alkalosis due to the effect of ammonia on the respiratory control centers in the brain stem. The various UCEDs can usually be distinguished by the pattern and levels of plasma amino acids. Because citrulline is the product of the CPS-I and OTC reactions and the substrate for argininosuccinate synthetase (ASAS), its value is critical. In newborn-onset CPS-I and OTC deficiencies, plasma citrulline concentrations are zero to trace. With *OTC deficiency* there is increased urinary orotate excretion secondary to carbamylphosphate accumulation and pyrimidine synthesis. With *CPS-I deficiency*, carbamylphosphate production is decreased or absent and orotate excretion is decreased. Theoretically, a defect in the production of the activator of CPS-I, namely N-acetylglutamate (NAG), resembles a partial CPS-I deficiency. In citrullinemia, the plasma citrulline concentrations are markedly elevated. With argininosuccinicaciduria, plasma citrulline concentration is moderately elevated in the 100 to 300 μmol/L range and can be readily detected during an analysis of plasma by amino acid column chromatography.

Excessive protein leads to hyperammonemia.

However, too great a restriction of protein during long-term therapy leads to poor growth. Actually, this approach fails when the patient is in negative nitrogen balance, as occurs in the catastrophically ill infant presenting in the first week of life with massive hyperammonemia. For such an infant with hyperammonemia and coma, the mainstay of therapy is dialysis treatment. Hemodialysis is the most effective way of reducing plasma ammonium levels because the clearance of ammonia is greatest. Next in efficacy is continuous arteriovenous hemofiltration (CAVH). Ammonia clearance with peritoneal dialysis is only approximately one tenth that of CAVH and is not recommended for specific UCED therapy in the newborn period.

While waiting for dialysis therapy, alternate waste nitrogen therapy using intravenous sodium benzoate, sodium phenylacetate, and for patients with ASAS and ASAL deficiencies, arginine hydrochloride should be initiated. In addition, patients with OTC and CPS-I deficiency should also receive intravenous arginine hydrochloride, since body arginine pools can begin to deplete as arginine becomes an essential amino acid with a complete block in cycle function. The plasma arginine levels are usually low in all sick newborns with UCED. Unless corrected, arginine deficiency accentuates the hyperammonemia by promoting negative nitrogen balance and, theoretically, by failing to provide its usual stimulation of NAGS. A second role of arginine is to stimulate alternate pathways of waste nitrogen excretion.

The outcome for patients with severe newborn-onset CPS-I and OTC deficiency is poor. Sometimes, even dialysis therapy cannot rescue severely affected male infants with X-linked OTC deficiency in the first few days of life. Prospectively administered alternate pathway therapy in conjunction with high calorie administration usually prevents death and severe hyperammonemia in these patients. Even after institution of successful therapy, the morbidity and mortality are high in such patients. At the present time, liver transplantation is recommended for patients with CPS and OTC deficiencies who present in the newborn period and have almost no residual enzyme activity. Alternate pathway therapy has led to a 92% 1-year survival rate in newborns who recover from hyperammonemic coma, but most of the survivors are mentally retarded.

Transient Hyperammonemia of the Newborn

Transient hyperammonemia of the newborn (THAN) is a distinct clinical syndrome that was first identified by Ballard and colleagues in 1978. The disease usually develops in premature infants during the course of treatment for respiratory distress syndrome. The plasma ammonium level may be enormously elevated, as high as that found in any of the patients with the most severe type of UCED. Its onset is usually in the first 24 hours after birth when the infant is undergoing mechanical ventilatory support. The babies can manifest all the signs associated with hyperammonemic coma. The diagnosis may be difficult to determine, however, because many of these same infants are receiving sedatives and muscle relaxants to optimize therapy of their life-threatening pulmonary disease. Important clues are the absence of deep tendon reflexes, absence of the normal newborn reflexes, and decreased or absent response to painful stimuli. As with hyperammonemic coma in the UCED, this medical emergency requires dialysis therapy.

The cause of this disease is unknown. The plasma amino acid levels are similar to those found in CPS-I or OTC deficiency. Investigators have hypothesized that the disorder may be caused by impaired hepatic mitochondrial energy production or shunting of portal blood away from the liver, such as in patent ductus venosus. However, patients with congenital portal shunting defects have been described with disturbances in liver function such as impaired galactose metabolism but who are not premature and who do not have life-threatening hyperammonemia. The mortality rate in THAN is high. If the patients can be treated early and aggressively, they may survive the episode. There is no evidence that any of the survivors have suffered any further episodes of hyperammonemia; nor has there been any further evidence of impaired ammonia metabolism.

INBORN ERRORS OF AMINO ACID METABOLISM
Maple Syrup Urine Disease
Branched-Chain 2-Keto Dehydrogenase (BCKAD) Complex Deficiency

Leucine $\leftrightarrow$ 2-Ketoisocaproate $\xrightarrow{BCKAD}$ Isovalerlyl-CoA
Isoleucine $\leftrightarrow$ 2-Keto-3-Methylvalerate $\xrightarrow{BCKAD}$
2-Methylbutyryl-CoA
Valine $\leftrightarrow$ 2-Ketoisovalerate $\xrightarrow{BCKAD}$ Isobutyryl-CoA

Enzyme: 6 Subunits
    BCKA Decarboxylase Subunits (E_1)
        2 α Subunits
        2 β Subunits
    1 Dihydrolipoyl Transacylase (E_2) Subunit
    1 Dihydrolipoyl Dehydrogenase (E_3) Subunit
    1 BCKAD Kinase Subunit
    1 BCKAD Phosphatase Subunit

Gene Locations: $E_1\alpha$ on Chromosome 1q13.1-q13.2
                  $E_1\beta$ on Chromosome 6p21-p22
                  E_2 on Chromosome 2p31
                  E_3 on Chromosome 7q31-q32

Frequency: For MSUD, 1/185,000, Except for $E_1\alpha$ Deficiency, Approximately 1/176 in Pennsylvania Mennonites

Maple syrup urine disease (MSUD) is a rare inborn error of amino acid metabolism. It is inherited as an autosomal recessive trait and secondary to a deficiency of the enzyme BCKAD complex. This enzyme catalyzes the conversion of each of the 3-ketoacid derivatives of the branched-chain amino acids into their decarboxylated coenzyme metabolites within the mitochondria. The disease occurs in fewer than 1 in 200,000 newborn infants around the world, but in the Mennonite communities of the United States it has a frequency somewhat higher than 1 in 200 due to a founder effect for a point mutation in the $E_1\alpha$ gene. In most of the patients around the world, as well as in the Mennonite community, the classic form of the disease occurs. This is associated with severe and catastrophic illness in the newborn period and usually results in death without specific medical intervention. Typically, the infants are well at birth and only after 2 or 3 days of ingestion of breast milk or formula do the babies begin to manifest poor feeding and spitting up. Lethargy becomes evident; the cry may be shrill and high pitched. There may be hypotonia alternating with hypertonia and opisthotonic posturing. The odor of maple syrup may be detected in the saliva, on the breath, in the urine and feces, and in cerumen obtained from the ear. The babies become more and more obtunded and eventually lapse into a deep coma. The anterior fontanel may be bulging. Seizures may develop. The life-threatening encephalopathic features may simply be related to brain edema. Laboratory findings consist of metabolic acidosis. The anion gap may be raised but not necessarily so. There is almost always ketonuria. The plasma ammonium levels are not usually elevated. The levels of the plasma branched-chain amino acids, leucine, isoleucine, and valine, are elevated, with striking elevation in leucine.

A nutritional approach works just as well as peritoneal dialysis in newborns. This includes the use of a branched-chain amino acid–free modified parenteral nutrition therapy for infants as well as older children with acute metabolic decompensation. Usually, insulin therapy is also necessary to curtail the effects of catabolic stress. Based on the rate of plasma leucine decline, we have found that this nutritional therapy is comparable to peritoneal dialysis when the plasma leucine levels are as high as 25 to 40 mg/dL. Patients whose diagnosis and therapy, however, are delayed, or perhaps even in those diagnosed in the first week of life but who have suffered such severe damage because of increased intracranial pressure, often have substantial decreases in their developmental quotient or I.Q., as well as signs compatible with spastic diplegia or quadriplegia.

The mainstay of long-term therapy for patients who survive the newborn period is a special formula devoid of the branched-chain amino acids.

Hereditary Tyrosinemia Type 1

Fumarylacetoacetate Hydrolase (FAH) Deficiency

Fumarylacetoacetate $\xrightarrow{FAH}$ Fumarate + Acetoacetate

Enzyme: Homodimer
Gene Location: Chromosome 15q23-q25
Frequency: Very Rare, Except in French-Canadians in Quebec

This is a rare disease inherited in an autosomal recessive manner. The highest incidence is found in those of French-Canadian ancestry due to a founder effect. Two clinical phenotypes may be detected. The first occurs in early infancy and is a severe, usually fatal disease in which liver disease dominates the clinical picture. The second is a more chronic phenotype, with patients presenting with hypophosphatemic rickets related to renal Fanconi syndrome. These patients usually also have evidence of liver disease, albeit milder. Most of the patients with the severe liver disease phenotype do not come to clinical attention in the newborn period. Careful search, however, may reveal the laboratory findings compatible with this disease even in newborn infants. When the disease does present in the newborn period, the abnormalities are related to liver disease. Like hereditary fructose intolerance and hereditary galactosemia, this is one of the inborn errors of metabolism in which hepatocellular disease is also associated with renal Fanconi syndrome. In the phenotype seen in early infancy, the clinical findings include hepatomegaly, bleeding from coagulation defects, and jaundice. Ascites is not uncommon. The laboratory findings consist of abnormal liver function tests with increased serum AST, ALT, and direct and indirect bilirubin; prolonged prothrombin time (PT) and partial thromboplastin time (PTT); and the findings related to renal Fanconi syndrome, such as glycosuria, hypophosphatemia, hypouricemia, proteinuria due to $beta_2$-microglobulin hyperexcretion, and generalized aminoaciduria and organic aciduria.

Nonketotic Hyperglycinemia

Glycine Cleavage Complex (GCC) Deficiency

Glycine + Tetrahydrofolate $\xrightarrow{GCC}$ CO_2 + NH_3 + Methylenetetrahydrofolate

Enzyme Complex: 4 Subunits
   1 Pyridoxal-Phosphate–Dependent Glycine Decarboxylase P Protein
   1 Lipoate-Containing Hydrogen Carrier H Protein
   1 Tetrahydrofolate-Dependent T Protein
   1 Lipoamide Dehydrogenase L Protein
P Protein Gene Location: Chromosome 9p13
Frequency: 1/250,000, Except 1/12,000 for P Protein Gene Mutation in Finns

Nonketotic hyperglycinemia is inherited as an autosomal recessive trait; it is due to deficient activity of the glycine cleavage enzyme complex (GCC). Its frequency is fewer than 1 in 200,000 newborn infants. Although several variant forms exist, most infants who come to clinical attention in the newborn period, presumably most patients with this disease, have a severe catastrophic type of disease that mimics the most acute forms of ammonia, amino acids, or organic acid metabolism. The infants, usually well at birth, begin to manifest hypotonia and seizures after 12 to 36 hours. Quickly, they become comatose and there is a loss of all the newborn reflexes, as well as the deep tendon reflexes. The clinical findings predominantly relate to those associated with CNS intoxication. The electroencephalogram (EEG) usually shows a characteristic pattern of spike and slow waves. The babies may manifest hiccups owing to diaphragmatic spasms.

The main laboratory finding is a massively elevated level of serum glycine. The urine glycine is usually also elevated. The cerebrospinal fluid (CSF) glycine is also elevated and out of proportion to the degree of elevation in blood. The amino acid serine, which is also a product of the defective enzyme reaction, is depressed in plasma and there is a corresponding increase in the glycine-to-serine ratio in body fluids.

Methionine Synthetase Deficiency

In humans, the essential amino acid methionine is converted to homocysteine and in the process a methyl group is transferred to an acceptor molecule from S-adenosylmethionine that serves as a donor for methyl groups in many different reactions. Subsequently, the homocysteine may either be completely metabolized through the cysteine pathway to sulfate or it may be remethylated back to methionine. Defective methionine remethylation or a deficiency in methionine synthetase leads to an uncommon remethylation form of homocystinuria.

The clinical findings associated with methionine synthetase deficiency are poor growth and development. There may be severe cortical atrophy and possible brain lesions owing to thromboses of the arteries or veins, as in classic homocystinuria. The laboratory findings consist of an elevation in plasma homocysteine levels and a normal or decreased level of methionine. Often the levels of homocysteine are not as elevated as in classic cystathionine beta-synthetase deficiency.

Phenylketonuria

Phenylalanine Hydroxylase (PAH) Deficiency

$$\text{Phenylalanine} + O_2 + \text{Tetrahydrobiopterin} \xrightarrow{\text{PAH}} \text{Tyrosine} + \text{Biopterin} + H_2O$$

> Enzyme: Multimer, Identical Subunits
> Gene Location: Chromosome 12q22-q24.1
> Frequency: 1/10,000

Phenylketonuria (PKU) is the most common inborn error of amino acid metabolism that can result in mental retardation. It is due to a defect in the activity of the enzyme phenylalanine hydroxylase (PAH), which converts phenylalanine to tyrosine, a reaction that resides primarily in the liver. This disease, inherited as an autosomal recessive trait, has an overall frequency of about 1 in 12,000 newborns.

The cutoff for newborn screening in most states is 4 mg/dL of plasma phenylalanine with the upper range of normal being approximately 2 mg/dL. In the first 6 months of life, the affected babies may have difficulties with feeding and vomiting. In some instances, the persistent vomiting has been associated with the diagnosis of pyloric stenosis for which corrective surgery has been performed, perhaps inappropriately. Developmental delay is usually evident in the second 6 months of life. Patients may have seizures, sometimes infantile spasms in early infancy associated with a hypsarrhythmic EEG pattern. Persistent elevation of plasma phenylalanine levels above 10 mg/dL is sufficient to result in mental retardation. The mechanism of brain disease in PKU is still unknown.

The mainstay of therapy is a low-protein diet and the use of a special formula in which phenylalanine is absent. The diet should be for life. The phenylalanine hydroxylase gene has been cloned and sequenced, and the mutations that are responsible for most abnormalities in humans are known. DNA sequencing and mutational analysis may be used to determine carriers in families and to provide a scientific rationale during family counseling.

INBORN ERRORS OF ORGANIC ACID METABOLISM

Methylmalonic Acidemia

L-Methylmalonyl-CoA Mutase (MCM) Deficiency

$$\text{L-Methylmalonyl CoA} \xrightarrow[\substack{\text{adenosylcobalamin} \\ \text{(or vitamin B}_{12}\text{)}}]{\text{MCM}} \text{Succinyl-CoA}$$

Enzyme: Homodimer
Gene Location: 6p12-p21.2
Frequency: 1/20,000

Methylmalonic acidemia, along with propionic acidemia, is the most common of the disorders of organic acid metabolism. Although more than one enzyme defect may result in methylmalonic acidemia, all are inherited as autosomal recessive traits. The enzyme that is most often deficient is L-methylmalonyl-CoA mutase. Some patients, but not usually newborn infants with methylmalonic acidemia, are responsive to pharmacologic therapy with vitamin B_{12}. Methylmalonic acidemia, therefore, is one of the important disorders that can be considered to be a vitamin-responsive inborn error of metabolism.

The most striking presentation is in the second or third day of life. The baby is usually well at birth, as in the UCEDs, but then gradually begins to manifest problems with feeding, vomiting, lethargy, and perhaps seizures. There may be respiratory distress as a manifestation of metabolic acidosis. The liver may be enlarged as a consequence of diffuse steatosis. The important laboratory findings include a metabolic acidosis usually associated with an increased anion gap, ketosis, and hyperammonemia. The elevation of plasma ammonium levels may be as high as in the severe newborn-onset hyperammonemic syndromes. Since ketonuria is relatively uncommon in newborn infants, even in stressed infants with hypoglycemia because of poor feeding, and because diabetes mellitus is so uncommon in the newborn period, the physician caring for newborn infants must always consider an inborn error of organic acid metabolism when confronted with the acutely ill baby with ketosis. Other laboratory findings include thrombocytopenia, leukopenia, and anemia due to effects of the metabolite on the hematopoietic elements in bone marrow. Methylmalonic acid may be detected in urine. The diagnosis can be confirmed by assaying the activity of L-methylmalonyl-CoA mutase enzyme in cultured skin fibroblasts.

The treatment of acute disease consists of protein restriction, empiric therapy with vitamin B_{12}

(1 mg IM per day); intravenous fluids with 10% glucose and sodium bicarbonate to correct dehydration; electrolyte imbalance and acidosis; high-calorie feeds via a nasogastric tube; and, often, dialysis. The use of carnitine, 25 to 200 mg/kg/day, intravenously or orally, is controversial. The treatment of the chronic state centers around the judicious use of a low-protein diet and alkali to eliminate any acid-base imbalance.

Propionic Acidemia
Propionyl CoA Carboxylase (PCC) Deficiency

Propionyl CoA + ATP + $HCO_3 \xrightarrow[\text{biotin}]{\text{PCC}}$
D-Methylmalonyl CoA + AMP + Pyrophosphate

> Enzyme: 6 α Subunits
> 6 β Subunits
> α Subunit Gene Location: 13q32
> β Subunit Gene Location: 3q13.3-q22
> Frequency: Rare

Propionic acidemia is due to a selective deficiency of propionyl-CoA carboxylase and is inherited as an autosomal recessive trait. This disorder was originally called *ketotic hyperglycinemia* because of the elevation of plasma glycine levels in conjunction with ketosis. The precursors of propionyl CoA include the amino acids, isoleucine, and valine, plus methionine, threonine, the pyrimidine compound, thymine, and odd-chain fatty acids. Of the several hundred patients described with this disease, most present in the newborn period with poor feeding, vomiting, lethargy, and hypotonia. Not uncommonly, the patients manifest seizures and hepatomegaly due to steatosis. The metabolic acidosis may be severe with or without an increase in the anion gap. Ketosis is almost always present. Patients who survive may often manifest choreoathetosis because of persistent damage to the basal ganglia.

Therapy consists of a low-protein diet and adequate calories. As in L-methylmalonyl-CoA mutase deficiency, there is secondary carnitine deficiency with elevated levels of propionylcarnitine. The use of L-carnitine to relieve a deficiency of free carnitine and promote increased urinary excretion of propionylcarnitine to lower mitochondrial propionyl CoA levels is controversial.

Isovaleric Acidemia

Isovaleryl-CoA Dehydrogenase (IVCD) Deficiency

Isovaleryl CoA $\xrightarrow{\text{IVCD}}$ 3-Methylcrotonyl CoA

Enzyme: Homotetramer
Gene Location: Chromosome 15q14-q15
Frequency: Very Rare

Isovaleric acidemia is caused by a selective deficiency of the enzyme isovaleryl-CoA dehydrogenase. It is inherited as an autosomal recessive trait. There are two major phenotypes: an acute form that presents with catastrophic disease in the newborn period and a late-onset type characterized by chronic, intermittent episodes of metabolic decompensation. In the acute form the infants become extremely sick in the first week of life. There is usually a history of poor feeding, vomiting, lethargy, and often seizures. The characteristic odor of sweaty feet or rancid cheese due to isovaleric acid is noted. Metabolic acidosis usually with an elevated anion gap and ketosis is present. There may be secondary hyperammonemia, thrombocytopenia, neutropenia, and sometimes anemia, resulting in pancytopenia. The babies usually lapse into a coma. Dialysis therapy may be necessary. As with other organic acid disorders for which an amino acid determines organic acid production, treatment also consists of protein or total parenteral nutrition restriction, intravenous fluids with glucose and perhaps sodium bicarbonate, protein-free formula with calories via nasogastric tube administration, and glycine 250 mg/kg/day. Intravenous L-carnitine may be beneficial. In the chronic, intermittent form, the patients have repeated episodes of metabolic decompensation precipitated by infections or protein intake.

Multiple Carboxylase Deficiency

There are two specific forms of multiple carboxylase deficiency. The first is holocarboxylase synthetase deficiency and the second is biotinidase deficiency. The biotinidase deficiency does not usually present in the newborn period. Patients with the holocarboxylase synthetase deficiency have a severe disease and are characteristically catastrophically ill in the newborn period. Fewer than 20 cases have been reported. They have severe metabolic acidosis with lactic acidosis and are in coma. As with the biotinidase deficiency, biotin administration is lifesaving. This is one of the few disorders of organic acid metabolism for which the administration of a vitamin in megadoses produces a dramatic turnabout in the clinical and laboratory findings.

Glutaric Acidemia Type 1

Glutaryl-CoA Dehydrogenase (GCDH) Deficiency

$$\text{Glutaryl-CoA} + \text{Flavin adenine dinucleotide (FAD)} \xrightarrow{\text{GDCH}} \text{Crotonyl CoA} + CO_2 + FADH_2$$

Enzyme: Homotetramer
Gene Location: Chromosome 19p13.2
Frequency: Very Rare, Except in Saulteaux-Ojibway Canadian Indians and Pennsylvania Old-Order Amish

An isolated deficiency of GCDH causes glutaric acidemia Type 1 (GA-1). Multiple phenotypes are known. In the most dramatic presentation, which accounts for less than half of the known patients with GA-1, the illness develops acutely in the first year of life, usually following an infection. Acute encephalopathy is followed by the development of what appears to be a severe form of extrapyramidal cerebral palsy. These infants had developed bilateral damage to the caudate and putamen in the basal ganglia, resulting in an incapacitating dystonic syndrome. Some patients have a slowly progressive course with developmental delay, hypotonia, dystonia, and dyskinesia in the first couple years of life.

Other patients are relatively asymptomatic. In general, this is not a disorder that is associated with acute disease in the newborn period. However, macrocephaly at birth is common. The etiology of any of the CNS lesions is unknown. The magnetic resonance image (MRI) scan of the head typically shows bilateral widening of the sylvian fissures associated with hypo-opercularization, resulting in the "bat wing" appearance.

Glutaric Acidemia Type 2

The mitochondrial acyl-CoA dehydrogenases include the very-long-chain acyl-CoA dehydrogenase, the medium-chain acyl-CoA dehydrogenase, the short-chain acyl-CoA dehydrogenase (all of which are involved in fatty acid oxidation), the isovaleryl-CoA dehydrogenase and 2-methylbutaryl-CoA dehydrogenase (important in branched-chain amino acid catabolism), glutaryl-CoA dehydrogenase (important in lysine, hydroxylysine, and tryptophan metabolism), and the dimethylglycine and sarcosine dehydrogenases (important in choline degradation). All these dehydrogenase proteins have in common the binding of a protein called *electron transfer flavoprotein* (ETF). This protein is responsible for accepting the electrons in any of these oxidative dehydrogenation reactions, and it is a deficiency of either ETF or the ETF dehydrogenase enzyme, responsible for further transferring the electrons from ETF to coenzyme Q_{10} within the mitochondria, that causes glutaric acidemia Type 2 (GA-2). There are essentially three phenotypes of GA-2: (1) a newborn-onset type with congenital anomalies; (2) a newborn-onset type without anomalies; and (3) a milder or later-onset type, sometimes called *mild acyl-CoA dehydrogenase deficiency* or *ethylmalonic adipic aciduria*.

Patients with GA-2 who have multiple malformations are often premature; severe disease is usually evident in the first week of life. The patients develop hypotonia, encephalopathy, hepatomegaly, hypoglycemia, and metabolic acidosis; often the odor of isovaleric acid (IVA) is present since these patients also have a defect in metabolism of isovaleryl CoA as in isolated IVA. There may be facial dysmorphism consisting of a high forehead, low-set ears, hypertelorism, and a hypoplastic mid-face. The kidneys may be palpably enlarged associated with large renal cysts, rocker-bottom feet, muscular defects of the inferior abdominal wall, and anomalies of the external genitalia, including hypospadias and cordee. Most of the patients with this disease do not survive the first weeks of life. In some, the malformations are not so noticeable and only renal cysts are identified at autopsy. Infants without the congenital abnormalities usually present in the first 24 to 48 hours of life with hypotonia, tachypnea due to a metabolic acidosis, liver enlargement, hypoglycemia, and the sweaty feet odor. Some of these patients develop cardiomyopathy. In contrast, some of these infants can survive the newborn period. The phenotype in the third form is quite variable. Some patients are relatively disease free and have intermittent episodes of vomiting, dehydration, hypoglycemia, and acidosis during childhood or adult life.

Medium-Chain Acyl-CoA Dehydrogenase (MCAD) Deficiency

Medium-Chain Acyl-CoA Dehydrogenase Deficiency

$$R\text{-}CH=CH\text{-}\overset{O}{\overset{\|}{C}}\text{-}S\,CoA + FAD \xrightarrow{MCAD}$$

$$R\text{-}CH=CH\text{-}\overset{O}{\overset{\|}{C}}\text{-}S\,CoA + FADH_2$$

Enzyme: Homotetramer
Gene Location: Chromosome 1p31
Frequency: Approximately 1/20,000

The most common of the CoA dehydrogenase deficiencies is the MCAD deficiency. More than 200 patients with this disorder have been described. Most patients do not present until late infancy. The typical patient is an older infant who, following an infection, develops anorexia, vomiting, dehydration, lethargy, and hypoglycemia that may be associated with seizures. Similarly, older patients have features that mimic Reye syndrome and can die because of brain edema. Onset of symptoms in the newborn period is rare. However, some patients in the extended newborn period or in the first 6 months of life were originally believed to have sudden infant death syndrome but in retrospect turned out to have nonketotic hypoglycemia with coma following the development of fasting associated with an infection. In MCAD deficiency, there is a high mortality rate associated with the initial episode. The laboratory studies usually reveal hypoglycemia and an absence of moderate to large ketones in urine that would be expected to accompany hypoglycemia. The plasma ammonium level may be mildly elevated, the liver may be enlarged, and the serum ALT and AST levels may be slightly increased. During an acute episode, urine gas chromatography–mass spectrometry (GC-MS) analysis of organic acids characteristically shows increased levels of adipic, suberic, and sebacic acids, as well as the unsaturated analogues of these medium-chain dicarboxylic acids. Increased urinary excretion of dicarboxylic acids is common in many of the defects of carnitine or fatty acid metabolism. However, this is not pathognomonic of a disorder of fat metabolism because infants fed medium-chain triglyceride–enriched formulas also manifest dicarboxylic aciduria. Fatty acid analysis of plasma from patients with MCAD deficiency reveals increased levels of octanoic and 4-decenedioic acids. Urine also contains glycine conjugates such as suberylglycine and hexanoylglycine. A secondary carnitine deficiency can be present.

Very-Long-Chain Acyl-CoA Dehydrogenase (LCAD) Deficiency

Patients with LCAD deficiency may be ill in the newborn period because of liver disease with hypoglycemia, cardiomyopathy, and skeletal myopathy.

The membrane-bound very-long-chain acyl-Co dehydrogenase, as opposed to the soluble LCAD, whose specific metabolic role is unknown, is the main enzyme for initiating the oxidation of free fatty acids that are derived from adipose stores. This includes palmitic, stearic, and oleic acids. The fasting state may include coma. Even in its absence, however, the patients may exhibit hypotonia, hepatomegaly, and cardiomegaly. With an acute metabolic decompensation, urine organic acid analysis may reveal dicarboxylic aciduria. However, acylglycine excretion is not usually present. There may be a secondary carnitine deficiency with increased concentrations of the long-chain fatty acids bound to carnitine. This disorder may be fatal; sudden death in early infancy has been reported. Therapy is directed toward replenishment of glucose, calorie administration, and treatment of any potential brain edema. The myopathy and cardiomyopathy, however, may proceed even in the absence of fasting.

Short-Chain Acyl-CoA Dehydrogenase (SCAD) Deficiency

SCAD deficiency is a rare disorder. Laboratory findings reveal metabolic acidosis, hypoglycemia, and moderate hyperammonemia. The organic analysis shows increased levels of lactate, ketone bodies, butyrate, ethylmalonate, and adipic acid. Diagnosis can be made by assaying the SCAD enzyme in cultured skin fibroblasts. The human gene has been cloned and sequenced and mutations have been described. This should enable a more rapid genetic diagnosis as well as make prenatal diagnosis feasible.

Long-Chain 3-Hydroxy Acyl-CoA Dehydrogenase (LCHAD) Deficiency

LCHAD deficiency is associated with acute illness, fasting-induced hypoketosis, hypoglycemia, cardiomegaly, and muscle weakness. As with long-chain fatty acid oxidative abnormalities, some older patients may have episodes of illness associated with elevated serum creatine phosphokinase levels and myoglobinuria. A few patients have had sensory motor neuropathy and pigmentary retinopathy. Half of the patients have not survived. Some patients may develop severe liver disease with fibrosis in addition to necrosis and steatosis. Women who are carriers for this disease may also develop acute fatty liver of pregnancy syndrome. The diagnosis may be suggested by the demonstration of 3-hydroxydicarboxylic acids on urine organic analysis. However, some patients with liver disease per se may also manifest 3-hydroxydicarboxylic aciduria. Treatment of this disorder has involved frequent high-carbohydrate feedings, dietary fat restriction, and supplementation with uncooked cornstarch. Medium-chain triglyceride may be helpful. Carnitine and riboflavin have also been tried without benefit. The treatment of the acute episode is, as in the other defects of fatty acid oxidation, associated with hypoglycemia and potential brain swelling. Liver and neurologic disease may progress despite any intervention.

Carnitine Transporter Defect, Carnitine Palmitoyltransferase I and II, and Acylcarnitine Translocase Deficiencies

Since the first report of the carnitine transporter defect in 1988, more than 25 cases have been reported. However, many other cases previously reported as having cardiomyopathy or Reye syndrome may have had the transporter defect. Patients with the transporter defect may present in infancy or in childhood. Earliest reports concern the extended newborn period or early infancy. The disease is characterized by hypoketotic hypoglycemia, hyperammonemia, elevated transaminases, cardiomyopathy, and skeletal muscle weakness. In some of the older patients, cardiomyopathy may be the presenting sign. The characteristic laboratory finding in this disease is extremely low plasma carnitine levels. The total carnitine levels are usually less than 10 μM in plasma. A dicarboxylic aciduria is not usually evident on urine organic acid analysis. This is probably the only disorder in which pharmacologic administration of carnitine has dramatic effects on the clinical and laboratory abnormalities. The treatment is 100 to 200 mg of L-carnitine/kg/day.

Pyruvate Dehydrogenase Deficiency

Pyruvate Dehydrogenase Complex Deficiency

$$\text{Pyruvate} + \text{CoA} \xrightarrow{\text{PDH}} \text{Acetyl CoA} + CO_2$$

Enzyme: 12 Subunits per Functional Component
    4 Pyruvate Decarboxylase (E_1) Subunits
        2 $E_1\alpha$ Subunits
        2 $E_1\beta$ Subunits
    1 Dihydrolipoyl Transacylase (E_2) Subunit
    1 X-lipoate component
    2 Dihydrolipoyl Dehydrogenase (E_3) Subunits
    2 PDH Kinase Subunits
    2 PDH Phosphatase Subunits
Gene Location: $E_1\alpha$ on Chromosome X p22.1-22.2
        $E_1\beta$ on Chromosome 3p13-q23
        E_3 on Chromosome 7q31-32
Frequency: <1/250,000

There are several different phenotypes of PDH complex deficiency, based on the severity of the enzyme deficiency. Most of the patients with less than 20% residual enzyme activity in cultured skin fibroblasts present in the newborn period with overwhelming lactic acidosis. Some patients, but perhaps those without life-threatening acidosis, even have congenital lesions associated with cystic lesions in the cerebral hemisphere; cerebral atrophy; cystic lesions in the basal ganglia; and facial dysmorphism, including features that resemble fetal alcohol syndrome, such as a narrowed head, frontal bossing, wide nasal bridge and upturned nose, a long poorly developed philtrum, and flared nostrils. In addition, there may be partial or complete agenesis of the corpus callosum and impaired migration of neurons within the cerebral hemispheres, identified as heterotopic dysplasia on neuropathologic examination of brain tissue. Patients with less severe defects manifest progressive psychomotor retardation.

Pyruvate Carboxylase (PC) Deficiency

Pyruvate Carboxylase (PC) Deficiency

$$\text{Pyruvate} + \text{ATP} + \text{HCO}_3 \underset{}{\overset{PC}{\rightleftarrows}} \text{Oxaloacetate} + \text{AMP} + \text{PP}_1$$

Enzyme: Homotetramer
Gene Location: Chromosome 11q13
Frequency: 1/250,000

PC is a biotin-containing enzyme. Most of the patients presenting with a Type B form of PC deficiency were of French or English origin. Unlike patients with a Type A defect, in whom the blood lactate/pyruvate (L/P) ratio is normal because both lactate and pyruvate are comparably elevated, patients with the B defect form often have an elevated L/P ratio. Although PC is also an important enzyme in gluconeogenesis, hypoglycemia has not been a frequently reported finding. The liver may be enlarged. There is no effective treatment for PC deficiency when it is associated with progressive neurodegeneration. The gene that encodes the PC subunits, of which four combine to make an active enzyme, has been cloned and sequenced.

Phosphoenolpyruvate Carboxykinase Deficiency

Phosphoenolpyruvate carboxykinase (PEPCK) enzyme also functions in gluconeogenesis, and there are two forms in liver: one in the cytosol and the other in the mitochondrial compartment. Only three cases of PEPCK deficiency have been documented. Patients do not usually come to attention until childhood with hypotonia, failure to thrive, hepatomegaly, lactic acidosis, and hypoglycemia.

Benign Infantile Mitochondrial Myopathy and/or Cardiomyopathy

Benign infantile mitochondrial myopathy is associated with congenital hypotonia and weakness at birth, feeding difficulties, respiratory difficulties, and lactic acidosis. In this poorly understood, developmental-like disorder, only skeletal muscle appears to be affected, and histochemical analyses reveal a cytochrome c oxidase deficiency that returns to normal levels after 1 to 3 years of age. A nuclear DNA mutation in a gene important in a fetal isoform of an ETC polypeptide specific for muscle oxidative phosphorylation may be the cause of this problem. A developmental switch from the defective fetal gene to the adult form may be responsible for the gradual improvement. This disorder may be an inherited autosomal recessive or autosomal dominant fashion and is the only example of a developmental defect in oxidative phosphorylation that is probably nuclear encoded and in which the treatment is only support during the early newborn period to prevent death from respiratory disease.

Lethal Infantile Mitochondrial Disease

Infants with lethal infantile mitochondrial disease are severely ill in the first few weeks of life or in the extended newborn period. They present with hypotonia, muscle weakness, failure to thrive, and severe lactic acidosis. Death occurs by 6 months of age and almost always is associated with overwhelming lactic acidosis. Skeletal muscle shows lipid and glycogen accumulation and abnormally shaped mitochondria on electron microscopic examination.

Barth Syndrome

Barth syndrome is an X-linked disorder associated with cardiomyopathy, skeletal muscle disease, and neutropenia. Skeletal muscle shows abnormal mitochondrial morphology. Important laboratory findings include decreased plasma free carnitine, increased urinary excretion of 3-methylglutaconate on GC-MS analysis of urine organic acids, and decreased levels of serum cholesterol in early infancy.

Subacute Necrotizing Encephalomyelopathy (Leigh Disease)

Probably because of a failure to recognize the clinical signs, infants with subacute necrotizing encephalomyelopathy (SNE) or Leigh disease usually come to clinical attention after the newborn period. This disease is best characterized as a progressive neurodegenerative disorder with severe hypotonia, seizures, extrapyramidal movement disorders, optic atrophy, and defects in automatic ventilation or respiratory control. It is clear that there are many causes of SNE. As discussed earlier, PDH complex deficiency may lead to Leigh disease. Patients with defects in the ETC have also been reported with findings compatible with SNE. Many neuropathologists believe that the diagnosis of SNE depends on an analysis of CNS tissue at autopsy. However, MRI scanning characteristically reveals bilateral symmetric lesions of the basal ganglia. There is no effective treatment for this disease. It is possible that most of the patients with Leigh disease have disturbances in nuclear-encoded genes.

Early Lethal Lactic Acidosis

In an unknown fraction of patients with primary disturbances in mitochondrial oxidative phosphorylation or ETC defects, massive lactic acidosis develops within 24 to 72 hours after birth. Not uncommonly, it is untreatable, because it is relentless and unresponsive to alkali therapy. Dialysis is a remedy but not a cure. Often, these infants have no obvious organ damage early in the course or evidence of malformations. This is also true for the PDH complex deficiency, which is probably a more common cause of overwhelming acidosis in the first week of life. In addition, acidemia per se can easily explain the coma or impaired cardiac contractility that may be encountered. Some infants have survived with aggressive therapy. Anecdotal reports also suggest the existence of a transient disease process. The care of babies with these different forms of severe lactic acidosis almost always brings an ethical and moral dilemma to the forefront for the physicians and nurses of the NICU, as well as for the babies' families. To further complicate the issues, enzymatic and molecular analyses are usually not immediately available. The disease in most patients probably remains idiopathic and no DNA mutation, nuclear or mitochondrial, can be identified. Decisions regarding management need to be individualized because the mitochondrial dysfunction and resultant pathophysiology may vary among infants.

NEWBORN SCREENING

SCREENING PROGRAMS

Table 2–9 lists the frequencies of the disorders for which newborn screening is currently performed or considered. The specimen should be obtained from every newborn infant before nursery discharge or by the 4th day of life (whichever is first). With the practice of early nursery discharge, often during the 1st or 2nd day of life, there is concern that some infants with metabolic disorders will not have ingested sufficient protein for an amino acid elevation

TABLE 2–9

Approximate Frequencies in the United States of Disorders Included in or Considered for Newborn Screening

Disorder	Frequency
Congenital hypothyroidism	1 : 4000
Phenylketonuria	1 : 12,000
Galactosemia	1 : 60,000
Maple syrup urine disease	1 : 200,000
Homocystinuria	1 : 200,000
Biotinidase deficiency	1 : 70,000
Congenital adrenal hyperplasia	1 : 19,000
Sickle cell disease	1 : 4000
Cystic fibrosis	1 : 4000
Duchenne muscular dystrophy	1 : 8000*
Congenital toxoplasmosis	1 : 10,000
Hyperlipidemia	1 : 500
Alpha$_1$-antitrypsin deficiency	1 : 8000
Neuroblastoma	1 : 4000

*For males, 1 : 4000.

to occur and, therefore, may not be identified. Lack of amino acid elevation is unlikely for severe forms of phenylketonuria (PKU) but could occur in mild PKU and in disorders such as homocystinuria. In addition, an early specimen could result in missing an infant with congenital hypothyroidism in programs that use a low thyroxine (T_4) level as the indicator of this disorder. Consequently, to be certain that an infant with a disorder is not missed, a repeat blood specimen should be obtained no later than 2 weeks of age from infants whose initial specimen was obtained within the first 24 hours of life.

Special circumstances require specific attention to newborn blood specimen collection. In a newborn who is to receive a blood transfusion, a screening specimen should be collected before transfusion and a repeat specimen 2 days after the transfusion. This latter specimen is for metabolite testing because the pretransfusion specimen might have been obtained within the first 24 hours of life. In addition, a third screening specimen should be obtained 2 months after the transfusion, when most of the donor red cells have been replaced. This practice ensures reliable testing for analytes present in red cells, should a pretransfusion specimen not have been obtained. Infants transferred to a neonatal intensive care unit should have a blood specimen collected before transfer, regardless of age, and a second specimen collected in the neonatal intensive care unit by 4 days of age. This dual collection avoids the possibility that a newborn specimen will not have been obtained in the turmoil that frequently accompanies hospital transfer.

PHENYLKETONURIA

This metabolic disorder should always be identified by newborn screening. Most newborns with an elevated blood phenylalanine level have PKU, a variant such as non-PKU hyperphenylalaninemia, a pterin defect with secondary hyperphenylalaninemia, or a transient elevation of phenylalanine. Infants with severe liver disease or who are acutely ill from galactosemia may also have an increased concentration of phenylalanine.

Urine screening, either by ferric chloride testing for phenylketone identification or by Guthrie bacterial assay, should never be used to identify PKU in the newborn. Phenylketones usually do not appear in sufficient quantity in the urine to be identifiable by the ferric chloride test until the infant is 2 months or older. Increased phenylalanine may also not be detectable in urine because phenylalanine is readily reabsorbed by the kidney. Moreover, the urine of the newborn infant is usually dilute, further reducing the phenylalanine concentration.

Treatment for PKU should never be given on the basis of a positive screening test alone. The dietary therapy is complicated and can be hazardous to an infant who does not have PKU. Only after repeat testing and confirmation of PKU should treatment be given and then only in collaboration with or directly by a metabolic center.

CONGENITAL HYPOTHYROIDISM

Congenital hypothyroidism is the most frequent disorder identified by routine newborn screening. It occurs in 1:3000 to 1:5000 screened infants. This may be compared with the PKU frequency of 1:12,000.

Two different approaches are used to screen for congenital hypothyroidism. One is primary screening for low thyroxine (T_4) with secondary screening for high thyroid-stimulating hormone (TSH). The other is primary screening for high TSH, often with secondary screening for low T_4. Either procedure reliably identifies congenital hypothyroidism. Nevertheless, affected infants can be missed. This may be due to lack of the marker (either low T_4 or high TSH). Specifically the T_4 level during the first 24 hours of life in an infant with congenital hypothyroidism might not yet be sufficiently decreased for identification, owing to an ectopic thyroid gland or to persistence of maternally transmitted T_4. In addition, the premature infant with congenital hypothyroidism can have a lag of 2 weeks or more in developing an elevated TSH level.

False-positive results occur with a frequency of

approximately 0.1% to 0.2%. These infants transiently have low T_4 or elevated TSH. Many of those with low T_4 are premature infants with a normal TSH concentration or infants with perinatal stress and elevated TSH. To avoid missing congenital hypothyroidism, screening programs require a repeat blood specimen from each of these infants.

Infants with a positive screening test should not be labeled *congenital hypothyroidism* or treated for this disorder until confirmatory testing is in progress. This is especially true if the TSH concentration reported by the screening program is normal. In addition to prematurity, a low T_4 with normal TSH can result from thyroxine-binding globulin deficiency or hypothyroidism secondary to pituitary deficiency.

GALACTOSEMIA

Newborn screening for this disorder is advisable. Without routine newborn screening, 20% of affected infants may die without being diagnosed or remain undiagnosed until they become terminally ill with sepsis. In addition, another disorder of galactose metabolism, galactokinase deficiency, may not be identified until the development of irreversible cataracts.

Some screening programs use a metabolite assay for *total* galactose (galactose and galactose-1-phosphate) to detect galactosemia. Other programs screen the newborn specimen by a specific enzyme assay for activity of galactose-1-phosphate uridyltransferase, which is deficient in galactosemia. The enzyme assay identifies only galactosemia, whereas the metabolite assay identifies galactokinase and epimerase deficiencies as well as galactosemia. Several conditions other than the galactose metabolic disorders can produce increased galactose. These include severe neonatal liver disease, portosystemic shunting as a result of anomalies, and partial galactose-1-phosphate uridyltransferase deficiency.

The most rapid confirmatory test for a positive result in galactosemia screening is urine testing for reducing substance. In almost all cases of galactosemia, this test produces a strongly positive reaction. This is also true in galactokinase deficiency. If the urine contains reducing substance and the infant has clinical signs of galactosemia, a blood specimen for confirmatory testing should be immediately collected and milk feeding (breast or formula) discontinued. The confirmatory tests should include the measurement of blood galactose and galactose-1-phosphate and of galactose-1-phosphate uridyltransferase activity. If the urine is negative for reducing substance, the newborn screening result is likely to be false-positive or to indicate a galactose-1-phosphate uridyltransferase enzyme variant, probably one that is benign. Nevertheless, repeat blood testing should be performed.

HOMOCYSTINURIA

The newborn blood screening marker for detection of homocystinuria is an increased level of methionine. This screening test is included in some programs, and affected newborns have been detected. Infants with homocystinuria have also been missed, however, usually because their blood methionine concentration was not increased at the time the newborn specimen was collected. In addition, methionine is not increased in some forms of homocystinuria.

A high methionine level by itself is not diagnostic of homocystinuria. Liver disease can produce a strikingly increased methionine as can a metabolic disorder known as isolated hypermethioninemia, which may be benign. Tyrosinemia Type I (hereditary tyrosinemia) is also associated with high methionine. Furthermore, transient hypermethioninemia may occur in newborn infants. The initial action required for a newborn screening report of increased methionine is collection and submission of a repeat blood specimen. If the methionine level is again increased, quantitative amino acid analysis of plasma and urine should be performed. In the homocystinuric infant, homocystine is usually detectable in plasma and urine, methionine is usually increased in plasma, and cystine is reduced. In isolated hypermethioninemia, methionine is markedly increased in plasma, but there is no detectable homocystine in plasma or urine, and the plasma cystine concentration is normal.

Treatment of homocystinuria is complicated and should be administered and monitored by a metabolic center. The treatment is dietary and consists of a special formula and low-protein foods as well as other nutrient considerations.

MAPLE SYRUP URINE DISEASE

The marker for maple syrup urine disease (MSUD) is increased leucine in the newborn blood specimen. Newborns with classic MSUD almost always have at least a fourfold elevation of leucine. Transient increases in the blood leucine concentration are infrequent and usually no more than twice the normal concentration.

MSUD can be a fulminant disease associated with severe ketoacidosis and profound neurologic effects. Consequently the finding of a substantially increased leucine level in the newborn blood specimen should prompt an immediate call from the screening program to the attending physician. If the infant is ill, confirmatory plasma and urine specimens should be obtained and emergency therapy initiated. If the infant has MSUD, the plasma contains markedly increased concentrations of leucine, isoleucine, and valine (the branched-chain amino acids). In addition, the urine is strongly positive for ketones and contains large quantities of the branched-chain ketoacids and amino acids. The characteristic odor reminiscent of maple syrup may not yet be present.

Milder variants of MSUD can be missed in newborn screening. The newborn with the intermediate variant may not have an elevated blood leucine level, or the increase may be mild and overlooked. In the intermittent variant, the blood leucine concentration is normal in the newborn period and elevated only in later infancy or childhood during acute metabolic episodes precipitated by febrile illness or surgery.

CONGENITAL ADRENAL HYPERPLASIA

A decidedly increased level of 17-alpha-hydroxyprogesterone (17-OHP) suggests CAH owing to 21-hydroxylase deficiency. Infants with the salt-losing form of this disorder can die precipitously, often without a specific diagnosis. The clinical diagnosis may be suspected in the female newborn because of ambiguous genitalia but is rarely suspected on clinical grounds in male newborns or in females with atypical forms of CAH in which ambiguous genitalia may not occur. Even females with ambiguous genitalia may be clinically unrecognized in infancy, if the ambiguity is not obvious, or may be gender misassigned as males, if the ambiguity is advanced. Because accurate gender assignment and initiation of hormone therapy as soon as possible are critical to a favorable prognosis in CAH, newborn screening in leading to early diagnosis and prompt therapy is important. Consequently, screening for CAH has been added to routine newborn screening in a number of programs in North America, Europe, and Asia.

False-positive results in newborn screening for CAH are relatively frequent, often at a rate as high as 0.6%. Prematurity and low birth weight are the most common causes. The elevated level may be truly 17-OHP or may be due to cross-reacting steroids. These steroids are produced by residual fetal adrenal cortex or result from decreased metabolic clearance by an immature liver. Perinatal stress and early specimen collection (within the first 24 hours of life) are frequent causes of high 17-OHP.

Repeat blood specimens are required from all infants with increased 17-OHP. If CAH seems likely on clinical grounds, serum electrolytes should be measured, and if this reveals hyponatremia and hyperkalemia, the electrolyte imbalance should be immediately corrected with intravenous fluids. In addition, pediatric endocrinology consultation should be sought.

BIOTINIDASE DEFICIENCY

Biotin recycling is necessary for maintaining sufficient intracellular biotin to activate carboxylase enzymes. Biotinidase is a key enzyme in biotin recycling. Lack of biotinidase activity results in carboxylase inactivities and an organic acid disorder known as *multiple carboxylase deficiency*. The clinical features of the disorder include developmental delay, seizures, hearing loss, alopecia, and dermatitis. The developmental delay and seizures usually present at 3 to 4 months of age. Death during infancy has also been reported.

The initiation of biotin therapy in early infancy, when the disorder is presymptomatic, prevents all of the features of biotinidase deficiency. For this reason, a screening test has been developed and added to the newborn blood specimen in a number of newborn screening programs throughout the world. The frequency of identified newborns in these programs has a wide range, from 1:30,000 to 1:235,000. The average frequency is about 1:70,000. Almost all infants have been asymptomatic when identified and have remained normal on biotin treatment.

SICKLE CELL DISEASE

In a number of state newborn screening programs, the blood specimen is tested for hemoglobin abnormalities. The major goal of this testing is to identify infants with sickle cell disease so that they can be given penicillin prophylaxis to prevent pneumococcal septicemia. Additional benefits of early detection include early referral to a comprehensive sickle cell program and early education and genetic counseling for parents.

Sickle cell screening is usually performed by hemoglobin electrophoresis of blood eluted from a disc of the newborn specimen. This procedure identifies not only sickle cell disease, but also sickle cell trait and the presence of several other abnormal hemoglobins. Other than sickle cell disease, most of these abnormalities are benign. Consequently, whenever a hemoglobin abnormality is found by screening, it is important to perform confirmatory testing. This testing is especially critical in differentiating the frequent and benign sickle cell trait from the much rarer sickle cell disease. For instance, sickle cell disease (homozygosity for S hemoglobin) affects approximately 1:600 of the black population, whereas sickle cell trait (carrier status for S hemoglobin) is present in 1:12 blacks. Infants with sickle cell trait do not develop complications and should not be stigmatized as having sickle cell disease.

When sickle cell disease is confirmed, the infant should be started on penicillin prophylaxis as soon as possible and referred to a sickle cell disease center or hematologist. This combination of screening and careful follow-up has been effective. In Massachusetts, for instance, no infant with sickle cell disease is known to have developed pneumococcal sepsis since newborn screening for hemoglobinopathies began.

OTHER DISORDERS SCREENED
Cystic Fibrosis

The frequency and severity of cystic fibrosis explain its consideration for routine newborn detection. Similar to sickle cell disease, therapy that can prevent the ultimate complications is not yet available. Again similar to sickle cell disease, however, there is benefit from early and usually presymptomatic diagnosis. This benefit includes early nutritional therapy, pancreatic enzyme replacement, and antibiotic prophylaxis for pulmonary infection. Other benefits of newborn screening include identifying the genetic *set-up* for producing additional children with cystic fibrosis before subsequent pregnancies occur and, through presymptomatic identification, allowing the family to avoid months or years of delay in the correct diagnosis of a child with chronic respiratory problems or poor growth.

The analyte marker in newborn screening for cystic fibrosis is increased immunoreactive trypsinogen (IRT) in the newborn blood specimen. Increased IRT can also occur in normal newborns as a transient finding as a result of perinatal stress or for unknown reasons. Consequently the false-positive rate in cystic fibrosis screening is relatively high. To reduce this rate, screening programs have adopted a *second-tier* DNA analysis for one or more of the mutations associated with cystic fibrosis in specimens with increased IRT. Despite this expanded approach to screening detection, a substantial number of infants who do not have cystic fibrosis must have a sweat test before the diagnosis of cystic fibrosis can be eliminated. Because of this relatively high false-positive rate and the need for a somewhat interventive test for follow-up, screening for cystic fibrosis has not yet been adopted by most programs. It is offered in some states that also give parents the option to decline.

Congenital Toxoplasmosis

Screening for congenital toxoplasmosis has been added to the newborn blood specimen in two states, Massachusetts and New Hampshire. The test is an enzyme-linked immunosorbent assay (ELISA) that captures *Toxoplasma*-specific gamma M immunoglobulin (IgM) antibodies. The objective is to identify the majority of newborns with prenatally acquired toxoplasmosis who are asymptomatic at birth. It is believed that many, or perhaps most, of these infants develop neurologic sequelae or hearing loss or suffer recurrent chorioretinitis with progressive visual impairment and blindness unless treated in early infancy. Treatment with sulfadiazine, pyrimethamine, and leucovorin (folinic acid) is effective against actively multiplying parasites and may prevent the development of these clinical sequelae. Among 1 million newborns screened for congenital toxoplasmosis, the frequency has been about 1:10,000. Most of these infants were asymptomatic and, on treatment, have remained asymptomatic.

Medium-Chain Acyl-Coenzyme A Dehydrogenase Deficiency

Medium-chain acyl-coenzyme A (CoA) dehydrogenase deficiency is the most frequent disorder of fatty acid oxidation, occurring in 1:10,000 to 1:20,000 individuals. Under conditions of fasting or stress, these infants can develop hypoketotic hypoglycemia and metabolic acidosis, hepatomegaly, and hyperammonemia. The presentation can be identical to Reye syndrome. Sudden infant death can occur. The mainstay of treatment is prevention of metabolic episodes by avoidance of fasting and restricting fat intake. This treatment is effective in allowing these children to maintain a normal life. Consequently, screening for medium-chain acyl-CoA dehydrogenase deficiency would be a valuable addition to newborn screening. Two methods are available. One is a direct analysis for the specific genetic mutation that is present in greater than 90% of affected individuals. The other is an analysis for the major metabolites that accumulate. Either method can be performed on the newborn blood specimen. Presently a newborn screening program in Pennsylvania includes this disorder using tandem mass spectrometry to identify increased metabolites. Among the first 80,000 infants screened, 9 (1:9000) were found to have medium-chain acyl-CoA dehydrogenase deficiency.

Duchenne Muscular Dystrophy

Duchenne muscular dystrophy is an X-linked recessive muscle disorder that affects approximately 1:4000 male infants. It is progressive and produces profound muscle weakness leading to early death. It can be detected by newborn screening. The screening test is an assay that identifies increased creatinine phosphokinase activity. Several areas in France and Germany and a large screening program in Manitoba include this test. Increased creatinine phosphokinase, however, is not specific for Duchenne muscular dystrophy but also occurs in other muscular dystrophies and transiently in infants with perinatal stress or muscle trauma. Both the gene and the protein (dystrophin) defects in this disorder have been identified, but there is as yet no therapy that prevents the clinical manifestations. Nevertheless, presymptomatic diagnosis can lead to early information for these families and allow them to obtain support in preparing for the disabilities in the affected child. In addition, these families can receive genetic counseling before subsequent pregnancies.

Neuroblastoma

Neuroblastoma is the most frequent solid tumor of childhood, accounting for a significant number of deaths in preschool children. It is characterized by the excretion of increased vanillylmandelic acid (VMA) and homovanillic acid (HVA). In Japan and in several European programs, screening for neuroblastoma is conducted with filter paper urine specimens collected when the infant is 6 months old. VMA and HVA are measured by high-performance liquid chromatography in the urine eluted from the paper. In Quebec, Canada, filter paper urine specimens collected at 3 weeks and again at 6 months of age are initially screened for VMA and HVA by thin-layer chromatography with confirmatory follow-up by gas chromatography–mass spectrometry. Both types of screening have resulted in the early detection of neuroblastoma in many clinically normal infants. In most, the tumor was localized and could be completely removed at surgery. These infants have remained well. Only a few infants already had advanced and inoperable cancer.

A study of the program in Quebec, however, has shown that the screening has not reduced the mortality rate from neuroblastoma. Notably, most children clinically diagnosed with poor prognosis disease have had false-negative screening results, whereas most of the infants identified by screening have had good prognosis neuroblastoma, which either spontaneously regresses or can be effectively treated after clinical detection and probably does not require detection by screening. Consequently, screening for neuroblastoma not only may be unnecessary but also may cause inappropriate intervention. In Japan, however, screening continues in the belief that it has significantly reduced the mortality from neuroblastoma. Debate on this subject continues.

Alpha₁-Antitrypsin Deficiency

In the 1970s, there was much interest in newborn screening for alpha₁-antitrypsin deficiency. The association of this deficiency with infantile cirrhosis in infants and obstructive lung disease in young adults had been discovered in the 1960s, and it seemed that presymptomatic identification such as in newborns could lead to measures that might at least reduce the risk of lung disease. The prophylactic measures that were suggested included the avoidance of areas in which the air is polluted or smoke filled. In Sweden, 200,000 infants were screened by electroimmunoassay applied to the newborn blood specimen, and approximately 1:2000 were found to have PiZZ, the type of alpha₁-antitrypsin deficiency associated with disease. Only three of these infants, however, developed cirrhosis; it is still too early to determine the frequency of lung disease in this identified population. Uncertainty over the risk of disease, even in PiZZ alpha₁-antitrypsin–deficient individuals, and the absence of clearly preventive therapy for either the hepatic or pulmonary sequelae caused the interest in newborn screening for alpha₁-antitrypsin deficiency to wane. Presently, no newborn screening programs include this disorder.

Human Immunodeficiency Virus

A high percentage of newborns infected by human immunodeficiency virus (HIV) from the mother develop acquired immunodeficiency syndrome (AIDS). To determine the frequency and distribution of HIV seropositivity in pregnant women as reflective of the general population, newborn blood specimens were tested for HIV-specific IgG in most newborn screening programs in the United States. This screening was anonymous, and consequently the affected infants and their mothers were not identified. There is a movement in the United States to require routine newborn screening of HIV for the identification and treatment of affected infants. This movement is controversial. Only in New York State is there such linked newborn screening, but a parent must provide informed consent for the result to be provided.

Hyperlipidemia

Recognition that hyperlipidemia, particularly increased low-density lipoprotein, is a major cause of premature cardiovascular disease has led to an interest in general population screening so as to identify those at risk. Although most of this interest has focused on children and adolescents, screening of the newborn has been considered. Evidence that hyperlipidemia can be controlled with medication as well as diet has increased this interest. Until recently, however, there was no reliable marker for newborn screening. For instance, the cholesterol level varies widely in early infancy and was found not to correlate with later serum cholesterol levels. Investigators are now studying increased apolipoprotein B in the newborn as a marker for genetically determined hyperlipoproteinemia. Apolipoprotein B, the major carrier of low-density lipoproteins, can be measured in the newborn blood specimen by an ELISA method. This could become an important addition to routine newborn screening.

Cord Blood

Umbilical cord blood can be screened for maternal metabolic disorders that secondarily affect the fetus and produce neonatal abnormalities. Paramount among these abnormalities is maternal PKU. Cord blood contains the increased phenylalanine transferred from the mother. Disorders intrinsic to the infant can also be screened in cord blood when the abnormality is present in erythrocytes. Among these disorders is galactosemia, in which cord blood has increased galactose-1-phosphate and no activity of galactose-1-phosphate uridyltransferase.

Routine cord blood screening was conducted in Massachusetts for more than 10 years. A filter paper card was soaked with umbilical cord blood at delivery of the infant and sent to the state screening laboratory. Initially, this specimen was screened for galactosemia and maternal PKU. Subsequently, galactosemia screening was discontinued because this disease could be effectively screened in the newborn blood specimen. Screening for maternal PKU continued, and screening for other maternal metabolic disorders, such as maternal histidinemia, was added. This screening led to valuable genetic and biochemical information about these disorders and their relation to the fetus. The information was of limited value to the families, however, and cord blood screening has been discontinued.

Cord blood is currently used for congenital hypothyroidism screening in several newborn screening programs. This specimen may be collected in filter paper or submitted as a tube of cord serum. If TSH elevation is the indicator, this may constitute effective screening for congenital hypothyroidism. A newborn blood specimen must then be collected for PKU screening, however, because in PKU (as distinguished from maternal PKU) the phenylalanine level in cord blood is normal and does not become elevated until at least several hours after birth.

CHAPTER 3

Newborn Stabilization and Initial Evaluation

RESUSCITATION IN THE DELIVERY ROOM

MANAGEMENT AT DELIVERY

Assessment of Degree of Asphyxia

Asphyxia is defined as a combination of *hypoxemia*, *hypercapnia*, and *metabolic acidemia*. If lung expansion does not occur in the minutes following birth and the infant is unable to establish ventilation and pulmonary perfusion, a progressive cycle of worsening hypoxemia, hypercapnia, and metabolic acidemia evolves.

The Apgar score was originally introduced to help quantitate the initial evaluation of newborn infants. Apgar scores should be assigned at 1, 5, and 10 minutes, and, if the infant still requires resuscitation, at 15 and 20 minutes as well. The scoring process requires the discipline to evaluate several aspects of the infant at once within the 1st minute of life. It serves as a framework around which to gear resuscitative efforts, because the score is an indicator of responsiveness to therapy as well as a way of defining infants who are at high risk for further difficulty. The score at 5 minutes and later is more predictive of survival and neurologic status than the 1-minute score, because the ability to interrupt and reverse the process indicates not only successful intervention but also that the process was not established for a long period in utero.

TABLE 3–1
Apgar Scoring System

Features Evaluated	0 Points	1 Point	2 Points
Heart rate	0	<100	>100
Respiratory effort	Apnea	Irregular, shallow, or gasping respirations	Vigorous and crying
Color	Pale, blue	Pale or blue extremities	Pink
Muscle tone	Absent	Weak, passive tone	Active movement
Reflex irritability	Absent	Grimace	Active avoidance

Overview of Resuscitation

Initial resuscitation of the depressed newborn always includes maintenance of body temperature and rapidly drying and placing the infant under a radiant heater. Clearing the airway is essential; this may be done using a bulb syringe, or, in the case of the infant born through thick particulate material, by endotracheal suction. The infant is placed on an open bed near a table with all of the resuscitative equipment available and then assessed for further intervention. A double-clamped segment of umbilical cord should be obtained for cord blood gas analysis.

American Heart Association–American Academy of Pediatrics Approach to Resuscitation

The AHA-AAP approach to resuscitation of the newborn takes the same type of clinical information that is gathered from the Apgar score and uses it to develop a schema for approaching resuscitation of the term infant. Even though these are guidelines developed by experienced physicians, they have not undergone any clinical trials. Recently, concerns have been raised about the value of resuscitation with 100% oxygen versus room air as well as the need for chest compressions and medications.

Infants with an Apgar Score of 7 or More

Vigorous infants generally do not require resuscitation other than perhaps a brief period of oxygen blown over the face. In approaching these infants who are not at risk for retrolental fibroplasia, it is important to remember (1) that administration of oxygen is accompanied by decreased pulmonary vascular resistance and increased pulmonary blood flow, and (2) that at birth, the newborn infant's lungs are normally full of fluid, which is cleared by resorption into the pulmonary arterial system. Excessive suctioning of clear fluid from the nasopharynx is not helpful and may contribute to atelectasis.

Infants with an Apgar Score of 4 to 6

Infants with an Apgar score of 4 to 6 require stimulation and often administration of oxygen by face mask; in addition, they may require some use of bag and mask ventilation to expand the lungs. Most infants respond to these measures and begin spontaneous respiration. It is important to empty the stomach of any infant who is receiving bag and mask ventilation.

Infants with an Apgar Score of 1 to 3

Infants with an Apgar score of 1 to 3 usually require intubation and expansion of the lung. However, if staff skilled in intubation and the appropriate equipment are not immediately available, initial bag and mask ventilation usually is adequate to sustain the infant. Further resuscitative steps depend on the heart rate response to ventilation.

Infants with an Apgar Score of 0

Virtually no liveborn infant should be assigned a score of 0, and resuscitation of an infant who truly has an Apgar score of 0, indicative of cardiac arrest before delivery, is probably a subject for ethical discussion. However, it is frequently impossible in the excitement that surrounds the delivery of an asphyxiated infant to make absolutely certain that there is no heartbeat, and, in such circumstances, resuscitation should proceed immediately as for an infant with an Apgar score of 1 to 3, with the addition of cardiac compression.

The primer for resuscitation techniques is the manual prepared by the American Heart Association in conjunction with the American Academy of Pediatrics. It provides complete, well-illustrated instructions on how to proceed with mask ventilation, intubation, and cardiac compressions if necessary. If an infant does not respond to adequate ventilation and cardiac compression with an increase in heart rate to greater than 80 after 30 seconds of positive-pressure insufflation, then the administration of medications should be considered. However, the most likely explanation for failure to respond is inadequate ventilatory support. Table 3–2 provides the recommended drug dosages for neonatal resuscitation.

Expansion of the Lungs

Usually, the only requirement for initiation of resuscitation of the newborn is adequate expansion of the lung. The airway must be cleared before attempts to expand the lung are made. Initial inflation of the gasless, fluid-filled lung is best accomplished by application of a relatively high inflation pressure (sufficient to move the chest, usually 25 to 40 cm H_2O) over a relatively long time (0.5 to 1 second) The object is to inflate the lung as well as to trap some gas during exhalation, thereby creating a functional residual capacity. This process occurs over a series of breaths. The term infant with a strong chest wall and larger terminal airways is better able to generate the necessary forces to achieve lung inflation than is the premature infant who may need to be assisted. Lung inflation also stimulates surfactant secretion in mature lungs, and this response is enhanced by large-volume inflation. No attempt at intubation should last longer than 30 to 45 seconds before returning to bag and mask ventilation to support the child.

Administration of Epinephrine

If the infant does not respond to intubation and ventilation with an increase in heart rate, and it is certain that the endotracheal tube is in good position, epinephrine should be administered either endotracheally or preferably intravenously.

Umbilical Vessel Catheterization

In the high-risk or significantly asphyxiated infant, it is important to place an umbilical catheter, preferably in the umbilical artery (although frequently a

TABLE 3-2
Medications for Neonatal Resuscitation

Medication	Concentration to Administer	Preparation	Dosage/Route	Total Dose/Infant			Rate/Precautions
Epinephrine	1:10,000	1 mL	0.1–0.3 mL/kg IV or ET	*Weight*		*Total mL*	Give rapidly
				1 kg		0.1–0.3 mL	May dilute with normal saline to 1–2 mL if giving ET
				2 kg		0.2–0.6 mL	
				3 kg		0.3–0.9 mL	
				4 kg		0.4–1.2 mL	
Volume expanders	5% Albumin-saline Normal saline Ringer's lactate		10 mL/kg IV	*Weight*		*Total mL*	Give over 5–10 minutes
				1 kg		10 mL	
				2 kg		20 mL	
				3 kg		30 mL	
				4 kg		40 mL	
Sodium bicarbonate	0.5 mEq/mL (4.2% solution)	20 mL or two 10-mL prefilled syringes	2 mEq/kg IV	*Weight*	*Total Dose*	*Total mL*	Give *slowly*, over at least 2 minutes
				1 kg	2 mEq	4 mL	Give only if infant is being effectively ventilated
				2 kg	4 mEq	8 mL	
				3 kg	6 mEq	12 mL	
				4 kg	8 mEq	16 mL	

			Weight	Total Dose	Total mL	
Naloxone hydrochloride	0.4 mg/mL	1 mL	1 kg	0.1 mg	0.25 mL	Give rapidly
		0.1 mg/kg (0.25 mL/kg) IV, ET IM, SQ	2 kg	0.2 mg	0.50 mL	IV, ET preferred
			3 kg	0.3 mg	0.75 mL	IM, SQ acceptable
			4 kg	0.4 mg	1.00 mL	
	1.0 mg/mL	1 mL	1 kg	0.1 mg	0.1 mL	
		0.1 mL/kg (0.1 mL/kg) IV, ET IM, SQ	2 kg	0.2 mg	0.2 mL	
			3 kg	0.3 mg	0.3 mL	
			4 kg	0.4 mg	0.4 mL	
			Weight	Total µg/min		
Dopamine			1 kg	5–20 µg/min		Give as a continuous infusion using an infusion pump
		Begin at 5 µg/kg/min (may increase to 20 µg/kg/min if necessary)* IV	2 kg	10–40 µg/min		Monitor heart rate and blood pressure closely
			3 kg	15–60 µg/min		Seek consultation
			4 kg	20–80 µg/min		

$$\frac{\text{Weight (kg)} \times \text{Desired dose } (\mu g/kg/min)}{\text{Desired fluid (mL/h)}} \times 6 = \text{mg of dopamine per 100 mL of solution}$$

*There is evidence that 2–3 µg/kg/min may be adequate in many infants.
IM, intramuscular; ET, endotracheal; IV, intravenous, SQ, subcutaneous.
From Bloom RS, Cropley CS: American Heart Association–American Academy of Pediatrics Textbook of Neonatal Resuscitation. Dallas, American Heart Association National Center, 1994. Reproduced with permission. Copyright American Heart Association.

venous catheter can be placed more rapidly), to obtain arterial blood gases and other samples as well as to monitor arterial pressure. Changes in arterial pulse pressure and mean pressure can thus be followed up during the resuscitation, providing important indicators of cardiovascular responsiveness. In addition, appropriate medications can be administered easily through the catheter.

Correcting Metabolic Acidosis

Whenever possible, samples for cord blood gas determination should be obtained. In addition, the infant's blood gases should be measured immediately and the results known before the infusion of sodium bicarbonate. No bicarbonate should be given unless ventilation has been established and $PaCO_2$ is normal or low. The most severely asphyxiated infants are those with an arterial pH of 7.0 or less and a calculated base deficit of 25 mEq/L or greater in the presence of a marked elevation of $PaCO_2$. By means of artificial ventilation alone, this calculated deficit can be reduced by approximately 10 mEq/L if the infant's circulation is normal and oxygenation is achieved. This effect results from a significant bicarbonate shift that occurs when $PaCO_2$ exceeds 70 mm Hg and therefore must be taken into consideration in calculations for correcting base deficit. Some additional correction occurs with ventilation at pH levels above 7.0, and therefore, the dose of bicarbonate administered should always be no more than one fourth of the initially calculated value. Blood gas studies should be repeated before giving additional increments of bicarbonate. The equation for calculation of base replacement is:

$$\text{mEq Base} = \frac{0.3 \times \text{weight in kg} \times \text{base deficit in mEq/L}}{4}$$

Bicarbonate should always be diluted 1:1 with sterile water and administered very slowly. Arterial blood pressure should be measured both before and after bicarbonate is given, because the administration of sodium bicarbonate may unmask hypovolemia that has not been apparent because of peripheral vasoconstriction.

Support of the Cardiovascular System

Many conditions that produce asphyxia or preterm birth may be associated with loss of a large volume of blood, and the asphyxiated infant is even less able to compensate for large losses of blood volume than the normal infant. However, most asphyxiated infants are *not* hypovolemic, and it is often a challenge to assess the infant's circulatory status to determine whether hypovolemia is the cause of hypotension or whether the infant is suffering cardiovascular depression because of some other problem. Physiologic variables to be remembered are as follows:

1. There is an association of falsely high arterial blood pressure readings with acidosis (which may respond to sodium bicarbonate administration).
2. There is an association of hypocapnia with hypotension, so that infants who are being overventilated may have falsely low arterial blood pressure readings.
3. An infant with normal blood pressure who has poor perfusion may be maximally vasoconstricted; therefore, significant hypotension may be masked.
4. An infant who is distressed and in pain may have a falsely elevated blood pressure level.
5. The normal range of blood pressure for very small premature infants may be low. The physician should assume that the blood pressure is normal in infants with good oxygenation and good peripheral perfusion and no signs of circulatory collapse, particularly if the infant passes urine. In the infant who is not voiding, use of low-dose dopamine (2–5 μg/kg per minute) may help establish normotension.
6. Monitoring an infant's hematocrit levels over time can be enormously helpful. A decrease in hematocrit during the first 2 hours after birth may be an indication of hypovolemia, because infants have the ability to mobilize fluid rapidly.

7. Preterm newborn infants ordinarily do not exhibit tachycardia as a sign of shock; therefore, a rapid heart rate generally is not useful as an indicator of volume status.

Support of the circulatory system and treatment of hypovolemic shock may be accomplished by the administration of small (10 mL/kg) transfusions of packed red blood cells. However, it is usually appropriate to give an initial infusion of 10 mL/kg of normal saline and to note the infant's response in blood pressure, peripheral perfusion, and oxygenation. Five percent albumin in saline may also be used while awaiting the availability of packed red cells. In administering volume replacement, it is of the utmost importance that it be given slowly, because some vascular beds (particularly those of the brain) may already be maximally dilated in response to systemic hypotension, and excessive pressure may be transmitted to the fragile capillaries, leading to intracranial hemorrhage.

In infants who have had prolonged or severe asphyxia, myocardial failure resulting from poor contractility may occur, evidenced by hypotension that persists after initial resuscitation. Such infants may respond to dopamine at a starting dose of 2.5 to 5 μg/kg per minute and increased as needed up to 15 to 20 μg/kg per minute to produce an adequate response. Rarely, dobutamine may be added at 5 μg/kg per minute (up to 15 μg/kg per minute). It may be useful in these infants to pass a second umbilical catheter through the umbilical vein, via the ductus venosus, into the right atrium to monitor central venous pressure in addition to arterial pressure.

Continuation of Support after Resuscitation

One of the factors essential to successful resuscitation is the ability to identify the infant who has continuing difficulties after resuscitation and, thus, to facilitate prevention of a relapse. This applies particularly to the premature infant with respiratory distress syndrome who initially responds favorably to treatment with ventilation and sodium bicarbonate but then requires continued cardiorespiratory support to prevent respiratory distress from becoming severe and causing another cycle of hypoxia and acidosis. Another example is in the infant born after undergoing an episode of fetal distress, who may have reactive pulmonary vasculature. If such an infant is allowed to become hypoxic, pulmonary vasoconstriction may occur (or worsen) and progress to persistent pulmonary hypertension of the newborn.

THINGS TO AVOID IN RESUSCITATION

Successful resuscitation of a newborn infant involves not only interrupting the cycle of hypoxia and acidemia and bringing the infant back toward the physiologic norm but also avoiding iatrogenic damage. There are, therefore, some important "rules" of resuscitation:

1. *Don't panic if an endotracheal tube cannot be placed immediately.* Concentrate on bag and mask ventilation and call for help. Do not assume that medication is a substitute for ventilation.
2. *Don't do excessive suctioning of clear fluid from the infant's nasopharynx.* Fluid is normally absorbed into the lungs.
3. *Don't use excessive oxygen concentrations to resuscitate the premature infant unless the infant clearly requires it.*
4. *Don't use too much ventilatory pressure to expand the infant's lungs.* Initially this may briefly be significantly higher than it is within just 15 to 30 minutes after birth. Use good clinical judgment. Watch the infant's chest and listen to breath sounds. Try reducing ventilation with hand ventilation to ensure that the lowest pressure necessary is being used. Excessive pressure on lungs that are normalizing may decrease venous return to the heart and decrease cardiac output and cause injury to lung tissue.
5. *Avoid hypocapnia.* There is evidence that

even brief overdistention of the lung may increase risk of bronchopulmonary dysplasia.
6. *Don't give volume or sodium bicarbonate automatically.* Each of these agents has been associated with production of intracranial hemorrhage in animal models.
7. *Don't focus or rely too heavily on cardiac resuscitation*, because, by far, the most likely problem in neonatal resuscitation is the need for ventilatory support.
8. *Don't withhold oxygen from the term or postterm infant with meconium aspiration or asphyxia*, who needs it because these infants may have reactive pulmonary blood vessels and pulmonary vasoconstriction may develop if oxygen administration is not generous.

SPECIAL CONDITIONS REQUIRING ATTENTION DURING RESUSCITATION
Extremely Premature Infant (<1000 g)

Resuscitation of the very premature infant begins in utero; therefore, whenever possible, such infants should be born in a perinatal center with skilled staff from the obstetric, anesthetic, and neonatal teams in attendance. The fragility of these infants requires gentleness in handling and a high level of skill in the staff performing the resuscitation. Because of their relatively large surface area, attention to immediate drying and temperature control is of even greater importance for these infants than for the normal newborn. When possible, they should be moved to a small warm room adjacent to the delivery room and carefully dried and placed under a radiant warmer for resuscitation. It is essential that the gas used for very small infants, even for resuscitation, be warmed and humidified. Many of these infants require immediate intubation as part of their resuscitation, and, in many centers, such infants are intubated routinely to enhance the clearance of lung water and the release of surfactant. If infants are intubated routinely, it is of great importance to avoid overventilation, which may cause interstitial emphysema or pneumothoraces as well as interfere with cardiac output. Other centers observe tiny infants briefly and provide respiratory support, particularly in the form of oxygen and continuous distending pressure via nasal prongs, if there is any evidence of respiratory deterioration. Particularly if the infants are known to be surfactant deficient, it would appear appropriate to initially intubate these tiny infants, give them surfactant, and then carefully evaluate their status to determine whether further respiratory support is needed. In resuscitating very small infants, it is also important to avoid hyperoxia; therefore, it is recommended that the oxygen blender be set at 40% when resuscitation is begun, then turned down as rapidly as possible, and thereafter increased only if the infant has clinical signs of cyanosis.

Most of these tiny infants also benefit from having an umbilical artery catheter placed so that the initial monitoring of their blood gases does not require painful procedures for obtaining blood or for the administration of fluid, drugs, or volume. At many centers, umbilical venous lines are also placed. Arterial blood pressure monitoring is important in this group of infants as an adjunct to assessing adequacy of circulating blood volume. The range of mean blood pressure for the tiny infant is wide and initially may be as low as 28 to 30 mm Hg. In an infant who is well oxygenated at low inspired oxygen concentrations and who has good peripheral perfusion, low blood pressure alone should never be used as the basis for volume administration. These infants should, however, have initial blood pressure support with low-dose dopamine (2 to 5 μg/kg per minute). Careful administration and monitoring of blood glucose concentrations are also critical.

Finally, it is important to move these infants from the resuscitation area to the nursery with as little disruption of their support systems as possible. Therefore, a resuscitation bed that is fully equipped to be moved from the delivery area to the nursery is essential to maintain stabilization. It also enables continuous observation of these fragile infants whose course may change rapidly during the first few hours after birth.

Meconium Aspiration

It is estimated that approximately 11% of all pregnancies are complicated by passage of meconium and that 2% of infants have some degree of aspiration syndrome, ranging from some minor initial tachypnea to very severe meconium aspiration pneumonia with pulmonary hypertension. There are two reasons why it is essential that skilled personnel are present at the delivery of an infant born through meconium:

1. It is critical that any *particulate* matter be removed from the infant's airway as rapidly as possible. A combined approach of suctioning of the nasopharynx on the perineum, followed by intubation and gentle tracheal suction, appears to be the most effective procedure for preventing obstruction of the airway and pneumonitis. It is *not* necessary to intubate an infant who is simply born through fluid that is stained with meconium but does not contain particulate material. Unnecessary intubation can cause iatrogenic damage. The most severe meconium aspiration pneumonias occur when an infant has passed a large amount of meconium in utero and is asphyxiated and gasping, thus moving large amounts of meconium into the thoracic airways before birth.

2. The passage of meconium indicates that an infant has been in trouble at some period in time. This group of infants is more susceptible to having reactive pulmonary vessels, which may reconstrict with hypoxia. They require careful initial evaluation and close observation to ensure that oxygenation is adequate and to prevent the gradual development of hypoxia and consequent pulmonary vasoconstriction, setting off the cycle that ultimately may result in persistent pulmonary hypertension of the newborn.

Hydrops

The evaluation and resuscitation of the infant with hydrops, as for very small premature infants, begins with interdisciplinary management by the perinatal team to assess the fetus and to arrive at decisions as to optimal time of delivery. It is always appropriate to administer antenatal corticosteroids before delivery of these infants. Ultrasound evaluation is recommended to determine whether the infant would benefit from removal of excessive fluid from either the abdominal or thoracic cavity before delivery. In preparing for resuscitation of a hydropic infant, it is critical that equipment be set up and a member of the team assigned to perform either paracentesis or thoracentesis, or both, immediately after the birth, if the amount of fluid should interfere with the ability to ventilate the infant. In addition, it is essential to have packed red cells available at the resuscitation site if the cause of the hydrops is related to anemia. Hydropic infants have extremely stiff lungs and may require high ventilatory pressures, including high end expiratory pressure, for initial stabilization. It is usually necessary to continue administering oxygen at high pressures until the infant begins to mobilize and clear fluid. It is always appropriate to administer surfactant as soon as possible after delivery. In severe cases, it may also be appropriate to have a dose of diuretic already drawn up and ready to administer in the delivery room. It is always appropriate to catheterize both the umbilical vein and umbilical artery so that central venous pressure, as well as systemic pressures, can be measured for evaluation of volume status. In addition, for severely anemic infants, the hematocrit can be augmented by immediate, isovolemic exchange transfusion through the two catheters. Staff should be aware that skin electrodes and saturation monitors frequently do not function accurately when used for infants with hydrops.

Infants with Severe Malformations

Sometimes the resuscitation team is faced with an infant who has severe malformations. Resuscitation should proceed in a normal fashion unless (1) the staff present at the delivery have enough experience and skill to recognize that the malformations are associated with conditions incompatible with life, and (2) there has been some foreknowledge of the possibility of malformations and the family has requested that there be no resuscitation of a severely malformed infant. Otherwise, it is appropriate to proceed with the resuscitation and stabilize the infant so that an accurate diagnosis can be made and the family can see the baby and participate in further decision making about their child.

CONTROVERSIES IN RESUSCITATION
Administration of Sodium Bicarbonate

The routine use of sodium bicarbonate to treat asphyxiation in infants is clearly fraught with danger ranging from problems associated with hypernatremia and high osmotic load to those related to rapid shifts in volume and circulatory status of the infant. Complete avoidance of sodium bicarbonate, however, may delay an infant's recovery from severe asphyxia. Therefore, it is probably most reasonable to give bicarbonate with extreme caution.

Intubation of the Extremely Low-Birth-Weight Infant

Although many centers have adopted a policy to intubate and ventilate at birth all infants weighing less than 1000 g, there remains some controversy. Other centers prefer to stabilize and watch vigorous, extremely low-birth-weight infants and only give respiratory support if signs of respiratory distress syndrome develop. Such centers recommend that an infant who is having retractions and other signs of distress have nasal prongs inserted for continuous positive airway pressure and oxygen administration to facilitate stabilization of the chest wall. As discussed previously, however, it has become standard procedure to give extremely low-birth-weight infants surfactant if they have any early evidence of distress, in which case intubation is necessary.

Resuscitation with Room Air Versus 100% Oxygen

Saugstad and other researchers have recently raised concerns about the possibility that oxygen radicals produced in excess in the posthypoxic reoxygenation period may cause tissue damage, particularly to the brain. Animal data and some preliminary human clinical studies suggest that resuscitation with room air may be both effective and possibly even safer than with 100% oxygen.

Duration of Resuscitation

Resuscitation should rarely be continued beyond 15 to 20 minutes in an infant whose initial Apgar score is truly 0 and who does not respond rapidly to adequate ventilation, appropriate cardiac compression, and drugs. In infants who respond after this period of time, the incidence of death or very severe, irreversible, neurologic damage is unacceptably high.

CHAPTER 4

Newborn: General Principles of Care

TEMPERATURE REGULATION OF THE PREMATURE INFANT

THERMAL NEUTRAL ZONE

The thermal neutral zone is a narrow range of environmental temperatures within which newborn babies do not alter their metabolic rate in response to either peripheral cold stimulation or core hyperthermia. Rather, infants regulate temperature through vasomotor tone alone. A range of "critical" environmental temperatures relevant to modern incubators was identified in 1970 by Hey and Katz. Below this range, an increase in the infant's minimal metabolic rate was observed. This range, therefore, was defined as the optimal incubator temperature. Several important considerations in regulating incubator temperature were included in these studies: (1) incubator wall temperature was maintained identical to air temperature, (2) relative humidity was controlled near 50%, and (3) the environment was maintained in a steady state, uninterrupted by turbulence.

Many modern incubators, however, incorporate a single-walled design that results in higher radiant heat loss because the incubator's outside wall is exposed to cooler room air. Moreover, many nurseries do not humidify incubators artificially, fearing the occurrence of bacterial colonization. Finally, the incubator's steady state is frequently interrupted for nursing and medical procedures that require that doors be open to care for the infant. Although a useful concept, the thermal neutral zone must be rigorously defined in practical terms. Silverman and colleagues used a modified concept of the thermal neutral zone to simplify clinical application. Reasoning that infants sense environmental temperature first on the skin, electronic negative-feedback (servocontrolled) regulation of the incubator heater in response to skin temperature was used. These authors demonstrated minimal metabolic expenditure near 36.5° C (97.7° F) abdominal skin temperature measured by a shielded thermistor in a less rigidly defined incubator environment. The importance of frequently checking core temperatures (axillary or rectal) must be emphasized, however, before delegating the infant's environment to such thermostatic control. In addition, Chessex and associates have demonstrated that incubator temperature may vary by more than 2° C when skin temperature servocontrol rather than air temperature control is used.

Finally, with the modern use of open radiant warmer beds (improving the means of access to the critically ill premature infant without interrupting heat delivery), skin temperature servocontrol has become the only practical method for approximating the thermal neutral zone. These variations in incubator design and technique, and the extension of infant warming to include very-low-birth-weight, critically ill premature babies have generated new problems for determining a universally accepted optimal environment.

ACID-BASE, FLUID, AND ELECTROLYTE MANAGEMENT

DEVELOPMENTAL CHANGES IN BODY COMPOSITION AND FLUID COMPARTMENTS

In early gestation, body composition is characterized by a high proportion of total body water and a large extracellular compartment. There also appears to be a prolactin-mediated increase in the water-binding capacity of fetal cells and perhaps the interstitium, which contributes to the maintenance of increased total fetal body water content. As gestation advances, the rapid cellular growth, accretion of body solids, and fat deposition result in gradual decreases in total body water content and extracellular water volume while the intracellular fluid compartment increases. In the 16-week fetus, total body water represents approximately 94% of total body weight with roughly two thirds of the total body water being distributed in the extracellular compartment and one third in the intracellular compartment. In the full-term newborn, total body water is only about 75% of total body weight with almost half of it located in the intracellular space. Thus, infants born prematurely are in a state of total body water excess and extracellular volume expansion compared with their full-term counterparts, and the majority of the expanded extracellular volume is distributed in the interstitium.

During intrauterine development, the placenta provides ample supply of nutrients and electrolytes for the fetus. To maintain normal fetal weight gain, especially during the third trimester when an acceleration of fetal mass accumulation occurs, the fetus must be in a positive electrolyte balance.

Additional, more acute changes in total body water and its distribution take place during labor and delivery. Arterial blood pressure increases a few days before delivery in response to increases in catecholamine, vasopressin, and cortisol plasma concentrations and translocation of blood from the placenta into the fetus. The rise in arterial blood pressure and the changes in the fetal hormonal milieu along with the borderline intrapartum hypoxia-induced increase in capillary permeability result in a shift of fluid from the intravascular to the interstitial compartment. This fluid shift results in an approximately 25% reduction in circulating plasma volume in the human fetus during labor and delivery. Because the expanded interstitial fluid is not immediately accessible for filtration and excretion by the kidneys after birth, it may serve as a source of volume supply until maternal milk production becomes adequate. Thus, the translocation of fluid from the intravascular to the interstitial compartment during labor and delivery is part of the physiologic adaptation for the transition to extrauterine life. The postnatal increase in oxygenation and the concurrent changes in vasoactive hormone production then restore capillary membrane integrity and favor absorption of interstitial fluid into the intravascular compartment. The ensuing gradual movement of fluid from the expanded interstitial space into the vessels aids in maintaining intravascular volume during the first 24 to 48 hours when oral fluid intake may be limited. Prematurity or pathologic conditions may disrupt this delicate process, however, and interfere with the physiologic contraction of the extracellular fluid compartment in the immediate postnatal period.

In the fetus, body composition and fluid balance depend on the electrolyte and water exchange between the mother, fetus, and amniotic space. Therefore, several antenatal events influencing this exchange may exert significant effects on the postnatal fluid balance. Maternal indomethacin treatment or excessive intravenous fluid administration during labor may result in neonatal hyponatremia with an expanded extracellular water content.

The timing of cord clamping after delivery is another important factor significantly affecting total circulating blood volume and extracellular volume in the newborn. Immediate clamping of the cord results in an average hematocrit of 48% to 51%, and there is little change in the newborn's hematocrit over the next days. If the cord is clamped only 3 to 4 minutes after delivery with the newborn being positioned at or below the level of the placenta, however, 25 to 50 mL/kg of blood is transfused into the newborn representing an approximately 25% to 50% increase in the total blood volume.

Although the exact mechanisms of the extracellular fluid contraction are unknown, several studies have suggested that atrial natriuretic peptide may play a role in this process. The postnatal increase in capillary membrane integrity favors absorption of the interstitial fluid into the intravascular compartment. The ensuing increase in circulating blood volume stimulates atrial natriuretic peptide release from the heart, which, in turn, may contribute to the postnatal enhancement of renal sodium and water excretion. In addition, the concomitant decrease in the release of vasoconstrictive and antidiuretic hormones also may play a role in the postnatal extracellular volume contraction.

The total body water excess and extracellular volume expansion of preterm infants imply that their negative water and sodium balance during the first 5 to 10 days of life represents an appropriate adaptation to extrauterine life and should not be compensated for by increased fluid administration and sodium supplementation. If this principle is not followed and a positive fluid balance (i.e., weight gain) is achieved during the transitional period, preterm infants are at higher risk to present with a more severe course of hyaline membrane disease as well as with an increased incidence of patent ductus arteriosus, congestive heart failure, pulmonary edema, necrotizing enterocolitis, and bronchopulmonary dysplasia.

Healthy full-term newborns lose an average of 5% to 10% of their body weight during the first 4 to 7 days of life. Thereafter they establish a steady weight gain pattern. Because preterm infants have an increased total body water content and extracellular volume, they lose on average 15% of their body weight during transition, and depending on the degree of prematurity and associated pathologic conditions, these newborns regain their birth weight only by 10 to 20 days after birth. Because total body water content at birth is also influenced by factors other than maturity, however, physiologic weight loss may significantly differ among patients of the same gestational age, and there is no established optimal rate or extent of weight loss in infants born prematurely.

PHYSIOLOGY OF REGULATION OF BODY COMPOSITION

Although human cells have the ability to adjust their intracellular composition, ultimate regulation of the intracellular volume and osmolality relies on the control of the extracellular compartment. Therefore, the human body must be able to monitor the volume and osmolality of the extracellular compartment and to correct the changes resulting from its interaction with the environment.

The major intracellular solutes are the cellular proteins necessary for cell function, the organic phosphates associated with cellular energy production and storage, and the equivalent cations balancing the phosphate and protein anions. As a result of the activity of the cell membrane–bound sodium-potassium (Na^+-K^+) pump, potassium is the major intracellular cation, and sodium is the major extracellular cation. The energy derived from the concentration differences for sodium and potassium between the intracellular and extracellular compartments is used for cellular work.

Because changes in osmolality of the extracellular compartment are reflected as net movements of water in or out of the cell, regulation of extracellular fluid concentration ultimately controls the osmolality and size of the intracellular compartment. This physiologic principle must be kept in mind by the neonatologist when managing sick term and preterm newborns with disturbances of sodium homeostasis. Rapid changes in serum sodium concentration and thus in extracellular osmolality directly affect the osmolality and size of the intracellular compartment and may lead to irreversible cell damage, especially in the central nervous system (see later).

There are small but important differences in the composition of the interstitial and intravascular fluid compartments that allow the movement of water, solute, and nutrients from the blood into the interstitium and the transport of cellular waste products into the circulation for final elimination. The tightly regulated differences in the composition of the interstitium and the intravascular fluid space result from the interaction of the intravascular and interstitial hydrostatic and oncotic pressures. According to this principle, water movement across the capillary wall can be described by the following equation:

$$J_V = K_F [(P_C - P_T) - \delta (\pi_P - \pi_T)]$$

where J_V = the net flow across the capillary, K_F = filtration coefficient, P_C = capillary hydrostatic pressure, P_T = interstitial hydrostatic pressure, δ = protein reflection coefficient, π_P = plasma oncotic pressure, and π_T = interstitial oncotic pressure. Thus, the movement of fluid out of the capillary is determined by the product of the water permeability characteristics of the capillary wall (K_F) and the net driving pressure $[(P_C - P_T) - \delta(\pi_P - \pi_T)]$ that forces fluid out from the capillary. The net driving pressure is the difference between the hydrostatic ($P_C - P_T$) and oncotic ($\pi_P - \pi_T$) pressures on either side of the capillary wall. Under physiologic conditions, the balance of these forces results in a small amount of fluid leaving the plasma at the arterial end of the capillary circulation. As capillary hydrostatic pressure falls and plasma oncotic pressure increases along the capillary bed, filtration ceases, and much of the filtered fluid re-enters at the venous end of the capillary circulation. The difference between the filtered and reabsorbed fluid is cleared from the interstitium by the lymphatic system.

In the healthy full-term newborn, hydrostatic and oncotic pressures are well balanced, being roughly half of those in the adult. Pathologic conditions readily disturb the delicate balance between the hydrostatic and oncotic forces and result in an expansion of the interstitial compartment at the expense of the intravascular volume. The increased interstitial fluid volume (edema) then further affects tissue perfusion by altering the normal function of the extracellular/intracellular interface.

The sick newborn has a limited capacity to maintain appropriate intravascular volume and to regulate the volume and composition of the interstitium. The ensuing intravascular hypovolemia and edema formation result in vasoconstriction and disturbances in tissue perfusion and cellular function with further impairments in the regulation of extracellular volume distribution.

The heart, the kidneys, the skin, and the endocrine system play the most important role in the regulation of extracellular (and thus intracellular) fluid and electrolyte balance in the newborn. Immaturity of these organ systems, especially in the very-low-birth-weight infant, results in a compromised regulatory capacity, which must be remembered when estimating daily fluid and electrolyte requirements in these patients. Other organs, including the gastrointestinal tract, are also involved in the physiologic regulation of fluid and electrolyte homeostasis. The impact of the maturational state of these organs, however, is less significant on fluid and electrolyte management in the critically ill preterm and term newborn.

Although term infants have a well-developed cornified layer of the epidermis, extremely immature newborns have only two to three cell layers in the epidermis. Because of the lack of an effective barrier to diffusion of water through the immature skin, transepidermal free water losses in the immature infant may be extremely high during the first few days of life. Gestational age, postnatal age, pattern of intrauterine growth, and environmental factors play a crucial role in the magnitude of transepidermal free water losses. Although skin cornification rapidly increases even in the extremely immature 23- to 26-week preterm infant during the first few days of life, full maturation of the epidermis occurs only after 28 days of postnatal age.

HORMONE REGULATORS

Renin-Angiotensin-Aldosterone System. Decreases in renal capillary blood flow and tubular sodium delivery to the juxtaglomerular apparatus stimulate renin secretion, which, in turn, initiates the production of angiotensin. Angiotensin induces vasoconstriction, increased tubular sodium and water reabsorption, and aldosterone release. Aldosterone increases potassium secretion and further enhances sodium reabsorption in the distal tubule. Thus, the primary function of this system is to protect the volume of the extracellular compartment and maintain adequate tissue perfusion. Its effectiveness in the newborn is somewhat limited, however, by the decreased responsiveness of the immature kidney to the sodium-retaining and water-retaining effects of these hormones. This insensitivity is also one of the reasons why this system remains activated for several weeks to months, especially in the more immature or the critically ill newborn.

Vasodilatory and natriuretic prostaglandins generated in the kidney are the main counter-regulatory hormones balancing the renal actions of renin-angiotensin-aldosterone. Therefore, when prostaglandin production is inhibited by indomethacin, unopposed vasoconstrictive and sodium-retentive actions of the activated renin-angiotensin-aldosterone system contribute to the development of the drug-induced renal failure in the preterm infant.

Vasopressin (Antidiuretic Hormone). The increase in serum osmolality is a much more potent stimulus for vasopressin secretion than the decrease in systemic blood pressure. This fact indicates that vasopressin is more important for maintaining the osmolality of the extracellular compartment than it is for regulating total extracellular volume and effective circulating blood volume. By midgestation, the fetus is able to respond to both osmotic and baroreceptor stimulation as well as to hypoxia with increased vasopressin release. The primary renal action of vasopressin is to increase free water reabsorption selectively via the insertion of water channels into the luminal membrane of the distal tubular and collecting duct epithelium. The hormone-induced free water retention is counterbalanced by locally generated prostaglandins. Indomethacin administration abolishes this regulatory effect, and the unopposed vasopressin-induced free water reabsorption contributes to the development of the drug-induced renal side effects.

Atrial Natriuretic Peptide. Via its direct vasodilatory and renal natriuretic actions, atrial natriuretic peptide regulates the volume of the extracellular compartment in the fetus and newborn in a fashion opposite to that of the renin-angiotensin-aldosterone system. This opposing action is further reflected by the direct inhibitory effect of atrial natriuretic peptide on renin production and aldosterone release. The stretch of the atrial wall caused by an increase in the circulating blood volume is the most potent stimulus for the release of this hormone. During early development, atrial natriuretic peptide is produced by all the chambers of the heart, and plasma levels are high in the fetus.

Dopamine, Noradrenaline, and Adrenaline. Dopamine, produced in the renal proximal tubule cells and the dopaminergic nerve endings of the kidneys, regulates total extracellular fluid volume by enhancing sodium excretion and selectively increasing blood flow to the kidney. In general, adrenaline and locally produced noradrenaline exert opposite renal vascular and tubular effects in the fetus and newborn. Both the dopaminergic and the alpha-adrenergic systems appear to be functionally mature even in the preterm newborn as evidenced by their cardiovascular and renal response to dopamine treatment.

Prostaglandins. Prostaglandins play a well documented counter-regulatory role for the renal vascular and tubular effects of renin-angiotensin-aldosterone and vasopressin. The inhibition of these actions of prostaglandins by indomethacin results in clinically important and sometimes detrimental renal vascular and tubular effects in the preterm infant. The actions of prostaglandins modulating the effects of the other regulatory hormones of the neonatal fluid and electrolyte homeostasis are less well studied.

Kallikrein-Kinin System. The renal cortical enzyme, kallikrein, catalyzes the formation of the vasodilator and natriuretic hormone bradykinin. The kallikrein-kinin system is activated at birth and stimulates renal prostaglandin production. Bradykinin also antagonizes the renal actions of vasopressin, renin, and angiotensin.

Prolactin. Prolactin plays a permissive role in the regulation of fetal and neonatal water homeostasis.

The high fetal plasma prolactin levels contribute to the increased tissue water content of the fetus. Interestingly, postnatal prolactin levels remain high in the preterm newborn until the 40th postconceptional week. Dopamine inhibits prolactin secretion in the preterm and term newborn resulting in a decreased water-binding capacity of the tissues. A clinical significance for this hypolactotropic effect in the dopamine-treated edematous preterm infant remains to be demonstrated.

FLUID AND ELECTROLYTE MANAGEMENT

Water and electrolyte requirements depend on the daily losses and the state of metabolic activity. Water requirement should be estimated based on the volume status and the sensible and insensible losses in the given infant. Because abrupt alterations in serum sodium concentration are associated with similar changes in serum osmolality, they may result in severe central nervous system sequelae.

Hyponatremia (<130 mEq/L) is most frequently caused by excessive free water administration or retention in the sick preterm and term newborn. In these cases, the diagnosis is based on the clinical signs of edema and weight gain and on the history of increased free water administration and medical conditions associated with enhanced vasopressin production. The appropriate restriction of free water intake is the treatment of choice in these cases. Less frequently, hyponatremia develops secondary to increased renal sodium losses. This may occur in the immature preterm infant with improving cardiovascular status and renal perfusion after the immediate postnatal period and in the recovering term infant following a cardiovascular and renal compromise. These infants usually lose weight, and supplementation of the calculated sodium deficit and that of the ongoing sodium losses leads to normalization of serum sodium concentration.

Hypernatremia (>150 mEq/L) most frequently occurs in the extremely immature newborn as a result of excessive transepidermal free water losses.

The diagnosis is based on the decrease in body weight and clinical signs of severe extracellular volume contraction. The treatment of choice is the replacement of free water losses. Hypernatremia may also develop in response to excessive sodium supplementation, mainly in the sick newborn receiving repeated volume boluses for cardiovascular support. In these cases, clinical signs of edema, increased body weight, and history of volume boluses help to establish the diagnosis. Management is more complex in these cases because the underlying severe illness and cardiovascular compromise limit the physician's ability to restrict fluid (and sodium) boluses. Appropriate fluid and sodium restriction and early support of cardiovascular and renal functions with dopamine may be of value in these patients by buying time to allow recovery from the underlying pathologic process.

The following calculations may be used to govern fluid and electrolyte replacement therapy in newborns with abnormal fluid and electrolyte status. Sodium deficit (or excess) may be calculated using the formula:

Na^+ deficit (or excess)
$$= (0.6 \times BW) \times ([Na^+]_{desired} - [Na^+]_{actual})$$

In this formula, sodium deficit (or excess) and body weight (BW) are expressed in mEq/L and kg, and $(0.6 \times BW)$ is the estimation of the extracellular volume. Similarly, free water deficit (or excess) may be calculated as:

H_2O deficit (or excess)
$$= (0.6 \times BW) \times ([Na^+]_{desired}/[Na^+]_{actual} - 1)$$

In this formula, H_2O deficit (or excess) and body weight (BW) are given in L and kg, and $(0.6 \times BW)$ is the estimation of the extracellular volume. Finally, serum osmolality may be calculated by the formula:

Serum osmolality
$$= 2[Na^+_{plasma}] + BUN/2.8 + blood\ glucose/18$$

Serum osmolality, $[Na^+_{plasma}]$, BUN, and blood glucose should be expressed in mOsm/L, mEq/L, mg/dL, and mg/dL. Although use of the above-listed calculations has limitations, these formulas may be helpful in the initiation of the appropriate therapeutic measure, while strict monitoring of the changes in the clinical condition, body weight, and laboratory findings provide the ultimate guidance in clinical management.

To estimate the daily free water requirements of the sick newborn appropriately, all sources of water losses must be taken into account, which include the insensible, sensible, and surgical water losses. Free water losses occurring through the skin and the respiratory tract are considered insensible losses, whereas sensible water losses are compromised of urinary and fecal free water losses.

As described earlier, gestational age, postnatal age, and environmental factors determine the amount of daily insensible water losses through the skin. During the first few days of life, transepidermal water losses may be 15 times higher in extremely premature infants born at 24 to 26 weeks of gestation than in full-term newborns. Although the skin rapidly matures in the early postnatal period even in extremely immature infants, insensible water losses in these infants is still somewhat higher at the end of the first months of life than those of their full-term counterparts. Among the environmental factors, ambient humidity has the greatest impact on transepidermal water loss. In extremely immature newborns, an increase in the ambient humidity of the isolette from 20% to 80% decreases the transepidermal water loss by approximately 75%. The difference in daily free water losses between the 20% and 80% ambient humidity is around 150 mL/kg. The use of an open radiant warmer more than doubles transepidermal water losses. If a plastic heat shield is applied while the infant is under the warmer, however, transepidermal water loss may be decreased by 30% to 50%. At low ambient humidity, phototherapy increases transepidermal water losses by approximately 30%. In infants older than 28 weeks, phototherapy does not increase the transepidermal water loss if the ambient humidity is 50% in the isolette. Other factors, including activity, air flow, and prenatal steroid treatment, also influence the magnitude of transepidermal free water losses. Recently, newer incubator design has allowed precise control of humidity. When very small premature babies are maintained in greater than 80% relative humidity ("swamp care"), insensible losses of water are *markedly* reduced. Fluid overload rapidly occurs unless the clinician is aware of this issue.

Insensible water losses from the respiratory tract depend mainly on the temperature and humidity of the inspired gas mixture and on the respiratory rate, tidal volume, and dead space ventilation. In a healthy full-term newborn, the water loss through the respiratory tract is approximately half of the total insensible water loss if the ambient air temperature is 32.5° C and humidity is 50%. The respiratory water loss in critically ill preterm and full-term infants on mechanical ventilation is zero if the gas mixture is saturated with water at body temperature.

Free water loss in the urine is the most important form of sensible water loss. Smaller preterm infants without systemic hypotension and prerenal renal failure usually lose 30 to 40 mL/kg per day water in the urine during the 1st day of life and around 120 mL/kg per day on the 3rd day after birth. In stable, more mature preterm infants born after the 28th week of gestation, the values are around 90 and 150 mL/kg per day. Because of their renal immaturity, preterm newborns have a tendency to produce dilute urine, which increases their obligatory free water losses.

Water losses in the stool are less significant and amount to approximately 10 and 7 mL/kg per day in term and preterm infants during the 1st week of life. Water losses in the stool increase thereafter and are influenced by the type of feeding and the frequency of stooling.

The most frequently encountered surgical water losses occur when a nasogastric tube is placed under continuous suction to provide relief for the gastrointestinal tract with conditions such as necrotizing enterocolitis and postoperative management after abdominal surgery. Because these losses may be significant, their replacement every 8 to 12 hours is necessary to maintain appropriate water and electrolyte balance. Because free water retention often develops after surgery, full replacement of the nasogastric free water loss is not recommended. The composition of the replacement solution depends on the electrolyte concentration of the fluid loss. Gastric fluid usually contains 50 to 60 mEq/L of sodium chloride, and it should also be replaced.

In the preterm infant, sodium chloride supplementation should be started only after the completion of the postnatal extracellular volume contraction. In general, as long as the infant's fluid balance is stable, daily sodium requirement does not exceed 3 to 4 mEq/kg per day, and provision of this amount usually ensures a positive sodium balance necessary for adequate growth. Extreme prematurity and pathologic conditions associated with delayed transition or disturbed fluid and electrolyte balance may significantly reduce or increase the infant's daily sodium requirement. Newborns recovering from an acute renal insult or preterm infants with immature proximal tubule functions who are in a state of extracellular volume expansion may require daily sodium bicarbonate supplementation to compensate for their increased renal bicarbonate losses.

In the early postnatal period, newborns, especially immature preterm infants, have higher serum potassium concentrations than older age groups. The cause of the relative hyperkalemia of the newborn is multifactorial and includes developmentally regulated differences in renal functions, Na^+/K^+-ATPase activity, and hormonal milieu. In general, potassium chloride supplementation should be started after urine output has been established, usually during the 2nd day of life. In the majority of cases, potassium requirement is 2 to 3 mEq/kg per day. After the completion of the postnatal volume contraction, however, preterm infants may require more potassium because of increased plasma aldosterone concentrations, prostaglandin excretion, disproportionately high urine flow rates, and use of diuretics.

Infants born between 23 and 27 weeks of gestation are at a particular risk to develop acute abnormalities of fluid and electrolyte status. These infants, when cared for in an open warmer without the use of a plastic heat shield, may lose 150 to 300 mL/kg per day free water through their skin during the first 3 to 5 days of life. Although the insensible water loss primarily affects extracellular volume, the intracellular compartment ultimately shares the loss of free water as osmotic pressure in the extracellular compartment rises. As water leaves the cells, intracellular osmolality increases, and cell volume decreases. In many organs, including the central nervous system, these changes stimulate the generation of osmoprotective amino acids (*idiogenic osmoles*). These molecules selectively increase intracellular osmolality and thus prevent further intracellular water and volume losses. This protective mechanism has significant clinical implications for the rate at which hypernatremia should be corrected. If large amounts of idiogenic osmoles have been generated, a rapid lowering of the extracellular sodium concentration places the infant at high risk for development of acute cerebral edema. This iatrogenic central nervous system compromise then further increases the high underlying risk for neurologic sequelae in the immature preterm newborn, including the development of periventricular leukomalacia. Because effective generation of idiogenic osmoles takes several days, however, a more rapid decrease in serum sodium concentration during the first 2 days of life may, at least in theory, be less harmful than that after a more prolonged period of hypernatremia. Nevertheless, the decrease in serum sodium concentration should not exceed 10 mEq/L per 24 hours during the correction of hypernatremia in the immature newborn.

Because serum sodium concentration is a reliable clinical indicator of extracellular osmolality, monitoring of serum sodium concentration every 6 to 8 hours during the first 2 to 3 days of life coupled with daily measurements of body weight provides valuable information and appropriate guidance for the fluid and electrolyte management of the extremely immature preterm newborn. The critically ill, extremely immature infant may tolerate daily measurements of body weight only if a built-in scale is available in the incubator or on the radiant warmer. Serum osmolality should be directly measured in cases in which calculated serum osmolality is greater than 300 to 320 mOsm/L.

Because immature newborns cared for in an incubator with an ambient air humidity of 50% to 80% require significantly less free water and less frequent serum electrolyte and osmolality measurements, open radiant warmers should be used only for critically ill, extremely labile preterm infants requiring frequent hands-on medical management. In these cases, the use of a protective plastic heat shield decreases excessive evaporative losses, and total daily fluid intake may be started at 80 to 100 mL/kg per day with 5% dextrose in water. Daily fluid intake is then increased by 10 to 30 mL/kg per day every 6 to 8 hours if serum sodium concentration rises from the baseline, with the goal being to maintain serum sodium concentration below 150 mEq/L. As skin integrity increases during the course of the 2nd to 3rd days, serum sodium concentration starts to decrease. At this time, a significant stepwise limitation of total fluid intake is obligatory to allow for a complete contraction of the extracellular volume to occur and to minimize the possibility of free water overload with its attendant risks for the development of ductal patency, pulmonary edema, and worsening underlying lung disease. Prenatal steroid administration may also decrease the rate of transepidermal water evaporation during the immediate postnatal period.

Potassium chloride supplementation may be started as soon as urine output has been established and serum potassium is below 5 mEq/L. Because extremely premature infants are at risk for the development of both oliguric and nonoliguric hyperkalemia, serum potassium should be monitored closely and potassium chloride supplementation discontinued if changes in serum potassium values or in renal function indicate. Critically ill, extremely immature newborns usually receive excess sodium with volume boluses, medications, and maintenance infusion of arterial lines. Therefore, extra sodium supplementation should not be started during the first few days of life to prevent an increase in total body sodium and thus extracellular volume. Many critically ill infants, however, retain their originally high extracellular volume during the course of the disease even when sodium and water intake are restricted. Such preterm newborns also tend to lose more bicarbonate in the urine. Interestingly, despite the immaturity of their renal functions, proximal tubular bicarbonate reabsorption may be appropriate even in the very-low-birth-weight infant as long as extracellular volume contraction takes place. Therefore, it appears that the presence of extracellular volume expansion is necessary for the manifestation of the renal bicarbonate wasting in these infants. Moreover, the diagnosis of functional proximal tubular acidosis in such cases should not rely solely on the finding of an alkaline urine pH because the distal tubular function is usually mature enough to acidify the urine once serum bicarbonate has decreased to its new threshold. Daily supplementation of bicarbonate in the form of sodium acetate or potassium acetate normalizes blood pH and serum bicarbonate in these infants and increases urine pH, aiding in the diagnosis. Once extracellular volume contraction occurs, these newborns generally achieve a positive bicarbonate balance, and supplementation therapy becomes unnecessary.

Other general guidelines in the fluid and electrolyte management of the immature preterm infant during the 1st week of life include calculation of fluid balance and estimation of sodium balance every day; testing of all urine samples for glucose, albumin, hemoglobin, and osmolality or specific gravity; and daily analyses of serum electrolytes, BUN, creatinine, and blood glucose. The frequency of testing and addition of other tests, including the measurement of serum albumin concentration and osmolality, depend on the clinical status, severity of underlying disease, and fluid and electrolyte disturbance of the given patient.

DISTURBANCES OF ACID-BASE BALANCE IN THE NEWBORN

Metabolic acidosis is a common problem, particularly in the critically ill newborn. Metabolic acidosis occurs when the fall in pH is caused by the accumulation of acid other than H_2CO_3 by the extracellular fluid resulting in loss of available HCO_3^- or by the direct loss of HCO_3^- from body fluids. Cases of metabolic acidosis are divided into those with an *elevated anion gap* and those with a *normal anion gap*.

The anion gap reflects the unaccounted for acidic anions and certain cations in the extracellular fluid. The unmeasured anions normally include the serum proteins, phosphates, sulfates, and organic acids, whereas the unaccounted for cations are the serum potassium, calcium, and magnesium. Thus, in clinical practice, the anion gap is estimated using the following formula:

Anion gap
$$= [Na^+]_{serum} - ([Cl^-]_{serum} + [HCO_3^-]_{serum})$$

The normal range of the serum anion gap in newborns is 8 to 16 mEq/L, with slightly higher values in very premature newborns. Accumulation of strong acids owing to increased intake or production or to decreased excretion results in an increased anion gap acidosis, whereas loss of HCO_3^- or accumulation of H^+ results in a normal anion gap acidosis. A decrease in serum potassium, calcium, and magnesium concentrations; an increase in serum protein concentration; or a falsely elevated serum sodium concentration may also result in an increased anion gap in the absence of metabolic acidosis.

An increased anion gap metabolic acidosis in the newborn is most frequently due to lactic acidosis secondary to tissue hypoxia as seen in asphyxia, hypothermia, severe respiratory distress, sepsis, and many other severe neonatal illnesses.

The syndrome of late metabolic acidosis of prematurity was first described in the 1960s, in which otherwise healthy premature infants at several weeks of age developed mild to moderate increased anion gap acidosis and decreased growth. All the infants were receiving high-protein cow's milk formula, and they demonstrated increased net acid excretion compared with controls. This type of late metabolic acidosis is now rarely seen, probably because of the use of special premature formulas and changes in regular formulas with decreased casein:whey ratios and lower fixed acid loads.

A normal anion gap metabolic acidosis most frequently occurs in the newborn as a result of HCO_3^- loss from the extracellular space through the kidneys or the gastrointestinal tract. Hyperchloremia develops with the HCO_3^- loss because a proportionate increase in serum chloride concentration must occur to maintain the ionic balance and/or to correct the volume depletion in the extracellular compartment. The most common cause of normal anion gap metabolic acidosis in the preterm newborn is a mild, developmentally regulated, proximal renal tubular acidosis with renal HCO_3^- wasting. In these infants, the serum HCO_3^- usually stabilizes at 14 to 18 mEq/L in the early postnatal period. The urinary pH is normal once the serum HCO_3^- falls to this level because the impairment in proximal tubular HCO_3^- reabsorption is not associated with an impaired distal tubular acidification of similar magnitude. The diagnosis of this temporary cause of acidosis can be established by the recurrence of a urinary alkaline pH when serum HCO_3^- is raised above the threshold after HCO_3^- or acetate supplementation. Even term newborns have a lower renal threshold for HCO_3^-, with normal plasma HCO_3^- levels in the range of 17 to 21 mEq/L. In most infants, plasma HCO_3^- increases to adult levels over the first year as the proximal tubule matures. Other common causes of normal anion gap metabolic acidosis seen in neonatal intensive care units include gastrointestinal HCO_3^- losses often owing to increased ileostomy drainage, diuretic treatment with carbonic anhydrase inhibitors, and dilutional acidosis with rapid expansion of the extracellular space using non-HCO_3^- solutions in the hypovolemic newborn.

The presence of metabolic acidosis in the newborn should be suspected from the clinical presentation and the history of predisposing conditions, including perinatal depression, respiratory distress, blood or volume loss, sepsis, and congenital heart disease associated with poor systemic perfusion or cyanosis. Metabolic acidosis is confirmed by blood gas measurements. The cause of metabolic acidosis is often readily discernible from the history and physical examination; specific laboratory evaluation of electrolytes, renal function, lactate, and serum and urine amino acids may be undertaken, depending on the diagnosis clinically suspected.

The morbidity and mortality of metabolic acidosis depend on the severity of the acidosis and the responsiveness of the underlying pathologic process to clinical management. Because experimental data suggest that even a very low pH is compatible with neurologically intact survival, and because a clear benefit of buffer therapy in the management of metabolic acidosis has not been demonstrated, indications for the use of buffers in newborns remain uncertain. At present, the judicious use of temporizing buffer therapy aimed at increasing the arterial pH to 7.25 to 7.30 in cases of severe acidosis is recommended and practiced by most neonatologists to avoid the complications of acidosis per se, which include arteriolar vasoconstriction followed by dilation, depression of cardiac contractility, systemic hypotension, pulmonary edema, and arrhythmias. This practice is supported by findings on the cardiovascular effects of sodium bicarbonate in preterm newborns with an arterial pH of less than 7.25 and term newborns with an arterial pH of less than 7.30. The use of sodium bicarbonate induced an increase in myocardial contractility and a reduction in afterload.

Sodium bicarbonate should be administered slowly and in its diluted form only to newborns with documented metabolic acidosis and adequate alveolar ventilation. Once a blood gas measurement has been obtained, the dose of sodium bicarbonate required to correct the pH can be estimated using the following formula:

$$\text{Dose of NaHCO}_3 \text{ (mEq)} = \text{base deficit (mEq/L)} \times \text{body weight (kg)} \times 0.3$$

Sodium bicarbonate is confined mostly to the extracellular fluid compartment, and the 0.3 value in the formula represents its volume of distribution.

Most clinicians would use half of the calculated total correction dose for initial therapy to avoid overcorrection of metabolic acidosis. Subsequent doses of sodium bicarbonate are then based on the results of repeated blood gas measurements.

In certain clinical situations, tromethamine (Tham) may be used as an alternative buffer to sodium bicarbonate. The theoretical advantages of tromethamine over sodium bicarbonate in the treatment of metabolic acidosis of the newborn include its more rapid intracellular buffering capability, its ability to lower $PaCO_2$ levels directly, and the lack of an increase in the sodium load. Tromethamine lowers $PaCO_2$ by directly reacting with plasma CO_2, resulting in formation of cations and one HCO_3^- ion per one molecule of tromethamine. Because the cations are excreted by the kidneys, oliguria is a contraindication to the repeated use of this buffer. Tromethamine administration also has been associated with the development of acute respiratory depression, most likely secondary to an abrupt decrease in $PaCO_2$ levels as well as from rapid intracellular correction of acidosis in the cells of the respiratory center. Furthermore, especially when large doses of tromethamine are administered, dilutional hyponatremia, hypoglycemia, hyperkalemia, an increase in hemoglobin oxygen affinity, and diuresis followed by oliguria may occur. Because the solution is hyperosmolal, and because rapid infusion of tromethamine may also lower blood pressure and intracranial pressure, slow infusion rates are recommended.

Despite these disadvantages, tromethamine has a major advantage over sodium bicarbonate in that it acts to increase pH by lowering $PaCO_2$. The suggested initial dose is 1 to 2 mEq/kg or 3.5 to 6 mL/kg intravenously using the 0.3 M solution, with the rate of administration not exceeding 1 mL/kg per minute. Once a blood gas measurement has been obtained, the dose of tromethamine required to increase the pH can be estimated using the following formula:

Dose of tromethamine in mL
    = base deficit (mEq/L) × body weight (kg)

Management of respiratory acidosis is directed toward improving alveolar ventilation and treating the underlying disorder. In the sick newborn, adequate ventilation often must be provided by mechanical ventilation. In severe respiratory acidosis, tromethamine, because it lowers CO_2, may be used to raise pH. Tromethamine, however, produces only a transient decrease in $Paco_2$, and toxic doses would quickly be reached if it were used to buffer all the CO_2 produced by metabolism over any sustained period of time. Therefore, tromethamine should be used only as a temporizing measure in severe respiratory acidosis until alveolar ventilation can be improved.

Metabolic alkalosis is characterized by a primary increase in the extracellular HCO_3^- concentration sufficient to raise the arterial pH above 7.45. In the newborn, metabolic alkalosis occurs when there is a loss of H^+, a gain of HCO_3^-, or a depletion of the extracellular volume with the loss of more chloride than HCO_3^-. It is important to understand that metabolic alkalosis generated by any of these mechanisms can be maintained only when factors limiting the renal excretion of HCO_3^- are also present.

Metabolic alkalosis can result from a *loss of H^+* from the body, either from the gastrointestinal tract or the kidneys, which induces an equivalent rise in the extracellular HCO_3^- concentration. The most common causes of this type of metabolic alkalosis in the newborn period are continuous nasogastric aspiration, persistent vomiting, and diuretic treatment. Less frequent causes of H^+ losses include congenital chloride-wasting diarrhea, certain forms of congenital adrenal hyperplasia, hyperaldosteronism, posthypercapnia, and Bartter syndrome.

Metabolic alkalosis can also result from a *gain of HCO_3^-*, such as occurs during the administration of buffer solutions to the newborn. In certain situations, the creation of a metabolic alkalosis is intentional, for example, in the use of sodium bicarbonate or tromethamine to raise pH and thus to decrease pulmonary vasoreactivity in infants with persistent pulmonary hypertension. At other times, however, iatrogenically produced metabolic alkalosis is unintentional and due to chronic excessive administration of HCO_3^-, lactate, citrate, or acetate in intravenous fluids. Because excretion of HCO_3^- is normally not limited in the newborn, metabolic alkalosis resulting from HCO_3^- gain alone should rapidly resolve following the discontinuation of HCO_3^- administration.

Metabolic alkalosis can also result from a *loss of extracellular fluid* containing disproportionally more chloride than HCO_3^-, so-called contraction alkalosis. During the diuretic phase of normal postnatal adaptation, preterm and term newborns retain relatively more HCO_3^- than chloride. The obvious clinical benefits of allowing this physiologic extracellular volume contraction to occur, especially in the critically ill newborn, clearly outweigh the clinical importance of a mild contraction alkalosis developing after recovery. No specific treatment is needed in such cases because with the stabilization of the extracellular volume and renal function after recovery, acid-base balance rapidly returns to normal. Contraction alkalosis due to other causes, however, may require treatment as discussed subsequently.

For metabolic alkalosis to persist, *factors limiting the renal excretion of HCO_3^-* must be present. The kidneys are usually effective in excreting excess HCO_3^-, but this ability can be limited under certain conditions, including a decreased glomerular filtration rate, an increased aldosterone production, and the more common clinical situation of volume contraction–triggered metabolic alkalosis with potassium deficiency. In the last-mentioned condition, there is a direct stimulation of Na^+ reabsorption coupled to H^+ loss in the proximal tubule, and an indirect stimulation of H^+ loss in the distal nephron by the increased activity of the renin-angiotensin-aldosterone system. Contraction alkalosis responds to saline administration to replete the intravascular volume and potassium supplementation. In the other disorders, however, the primary problem of reduced glomerular filtration rate or elevated aldosterone must be treated for the alkalosis to resolve.

One of the most frequently encountered clinical scenarios of chronic metabolic alkalosis actually occurs most often in the form of a mixed acid-base disorder in preterm newborns with bronchopulmonary dysplasia on long-term diuretic treatment. These newborns initially have a chronic respiratory acidosis that is partially compensated by renal HCO_3^- retention. Prolonged or aggressive diuretic use can lead to total-body potassium depletion and contraction of the extracellular volume, thus exacerbating the metabolic alkalosis. By stimulating proximal tubular Na^+ reabsorption and thus H^+ loss, distal tubular H^+ secretion, and renal ammonium production, the diuretic-induced hypokalemia contributes to the severity and maintenance of the metabolic alkalosis in these newborns. Furthermore, metabolic alkalosis per se worsens hypokalemia because potassium replaces intracellular hydrogen as the latter shifts into the extracellular space. Although serum potassium may be decreased, the serum levels in these newborns do not accurately reflect the degree of total-body potassium deficit because potassium is primarily an intracellular ion. In addition, the condition is often accompanied by marked hypochloremia and hyponatremia. Hyponatremia occurs in part because sodium shifts into the intracellular space to compensate for the depleted intracellular potassium. If the alkalosis is severe, alkalemia (pH >7.45) can supervene and result in hypoventilation. In this situation, potassium chloride and not sodium chloride supplementation reverses hyponatremia and hypochloremia, corrects hypokalemia and metabolic alkalosis, and increases the effectiveness of diuretic therapy. Because chloride deficiency is the predominant cause for the increased pH, ammonium chloride or arginine chloride also corrects the alkalosis. Because these agents do not affect the other electrolyte imbalances, they should not be used as the only therapy.

It is important to keep ahead of the potassium losses in infants on long-term diuretics, rather than attempt to replace potassium after intracellular depletion has occurred. Because the rate of potassium repletion is limited by the rate at which potassium moves intracellularly, correction of total body potassium deficits can take days to weeks. In addition, there is also a risk of acute hyperkalemia if serum potassium levels are driven too high during repletion, particularly in newborns in whom an acute respiratory deterioration may occur, with worsened respiratory acidosis and the subsequent movement of potassium from the intracellular to the extracellular space. The routine use of potassium chloride supplementation and close monitoring of serum sodium, chloride, and potassium are therefore recommended during long-term diuretic therapy to prevent these common iatrogenic problems.

When a primary decrease in $PaCO_2$ results in an increase in the arterial pH beyond 7.45, respiratory alkalosis develops. The initial hypocapnia is acutely titrated by the intracellular buffers, and metabolic compensation by the kidneys returns pH toward normal within 1 to 2 days. Interestingly, this is the only simple acid-base disorder in which, at least in the adult, the pH may completely be normalized by the compensatory mechanisms. The cause of respiratory alkalosis is hyperventilation, which in the spontaneously breathing newborn is most often caused by fever, sepsis, retained fetal lung fluid, mild aspiration pneumonia, or central nervous system disorders. In the neonatal intensive care unit, the most frequent cause of respiratory alkalosis is increased alveolar ventilation secondary to hyperventilation of the intubated newborn. Because findings suggest an association between hypocapnia and the development of periventricular leukomalacia and bronchopulmonary dysplasia in ventilated preterm infants, avoidance of hyperventilation during resuscitation and mechanical ventilation appears to be of utmost importance in the management of the sick preterm newborn. The treatment of neonatal respiratory alkalosis consists of the specific management of the underlying process causing hyperventilation.

CHAPTER 5

Infections and Immunologic Defense Mechanisms

HUMAN IMMUNODEFICIENCY VIRUS INFECTION

Since the first reported cases of HIV infection in children in 1982, more than 5700 cases of pediatric AIDS (children 13 years of age or younger) have been reported to the Centers for Disease Control and Prevention (CDC). These cases represent only a fraction of the total seropositive pediatric population with the most severe clinical manifestations.

Because the net seroprevalence rate among child-bearing women has been increasing, ongoing new infection of women in their child-bearing years has been occurring and will provide the most important contribution to increasing numbers of HIV-seropositive children who acquired the virus as a result of vertical transmission from chronically infected mothers. Women at high risk for acquiring HIV infection include those who received a blood transfusion before 1985, those who share needles for intravenous drug use, and those who have unprotected sexual intercourse with an infected partner. In 1992, the number of newly diagnosed AIDS cases among women infected through heterosexual contact exceeded those infected through intravenous drug use for the first time. Antenatal history-taking should include a careful transfusion history, history of intravenous drug use, and history of sexual contacts including bisexual or homosexual men, hemophiliacs, intravenous drug abusers, or males born in countries where heterosexual transmission of HIV is thought to play a major role.

In 1995 and 1996 more than 50 HIV-positive women delivered newborn infants after receiving zidovudine prenatally. None of the infants were found to be HIV positive after 8 months of follow-up. Because of the potential inaccuracy of risk histories, aggressive prenatal screening should be considered among all pregnant women. Because a substantial proportion of drug abuse is in inner city areas, racial minority groups or the socioeconomically disadvantaged are most affected.

Clinical categorization of HIV infection in children has been revised into four mutually exclusive clinical categories. The goal of this classification is to link prognosis and staging. All acquired immunodeficiency syndrome (AIDS)–defining conditions except lymphoid interstitial pneumonitis (LIP) are included in Category C.

From a management perspective, infants seropositive for or infected with HIV are members of a family whose other members are immunocompromised and may soon die. Therefore, HIV has been called a killer of families, not just of the infected children or adults. Thus, good therapy for this disease must begin with multidisciplinary, supportive care. Even though the physician plays an important role in this care, the needs of these children and families exceed the treatment capacity of a single discipline or individual. Nurses, social workers, physical therapists, educators, internists, infectious disease and neurology specialists, obstetricians, and many other professionals must be involved with the care of these children and families.

Medical care of the infant should also be prevention oriented. Voluntary antenatal screening for HIV infection in pregnant women permits identification of pregnancies in which vertical HIV transmission is a potential complication. Zidovudine, a thymidine analogue that inhibits replication of HIV in vitro by inhibiting the action of reverse transcriptase and possibly by other mechanisms, has been the best studied drug for interrupting vertical transmission. In a placebo-controlled trial performed on 477 pregnant women, zidovudine treatment was shown to lower the risk of vertical transmission from 25.5% to 8.3% ($P = .00006$). The treatment regimen used in this study consisted of zidovudine 100 mg orally five times a day beginning as early as 14 weeks of gestation plus intrapartum zidovudine (2 mg/kg of body weight given intravenously for 1 hour, followed by 1 mg/kg per hour until delivery) plus zidovudine for the infant (2 mg/kg orally every 6 hours for 6 weeks, beginning 8 to 12 hours after birth). The primary toxic effect on infants observed in this study was a statistically significant but clinically insignificant lower hemoglobin at birth in the zidovudine treated group. The applicability of these results to premature infants has not been rigorously evaluated. Because of the beneficial effects of this regimen on vertical HIV transmission, it was interrupted by the Data and Safety Monitoring Board of the National Institute of Allergy and Infectious Diseases. The study lacked sufficient statistical power to evaluate possible teratogenic effects of antenatally administered zidovudine.

Immunizations should also be administered. Killed poliomyelitis vaccine should be used. Exposure to varicella or measles should be treated with varicella zoster immune globulin or immune serum globulin, respectively. Family members should be screened for hepatitis B surface antigen, and HIV-positive children at risk should be vaccinated. Suspected infections should be aggressively diagnosed and treated. For example, treatment of severe thrush unresponsive to nystatin should be treated with ketoconazole (5 mg/kg per day) or severe, mucocutaneous herpes infections with oral (400 mg five times per day) or intravenous (5 to 10 mg/kg every 8 hours) acyclovir.

HIV infection among health care workers results primarily from exposures that occur outside the health care setting. Several prospective studies of health care workers who have had needle-stick exposure to known HIV-positive patients suggest that the risk of seroconversion is approximately 0.4%. The risk of mucous membrane or skin exposure to HIV-infected blood is less than 0.4%. Through June

1994, surveillance by the CDC has identified 42 health care workers who have documented occupational acquisition of AIDS/HIV infection. Of these individuals, 36 had percutaneous exposure to fluid thought to contain HIV, 4 had mucocutaneous exposure, 1 had both percutaneous and mucutaneous exposures, and 1 had an unknown route of exposure. AIDS developed in 15 of these individuals.

VIRAL INFECTIONS

The infant who is born with an infection acquired transplacentally during the first, second, or early third trimester may have what is termed "congenital infection." The most common causes are rubella virus, cytomegalovirus (CMV), *Toxoplasma gondii, Treponema pallidum*, human immunodeficiency virus (HIV), human parvovirus B19, and Epstein-Barr virus (EBV). The first four organisms are the so-called and somewhat misnamed TORCH group (*t*oxoplasmosis, *o*ther infections, *r*ubella, *c*ytomegalovirus infection, and *h*erpes simplex). The confusion generated by this acronym arises because herpes simplex so rarely belongs to the group and because syphilis and other infections are omitted. Owing to the increasing frequency and interest in HIV, parvovirus, and EBV, Kinney and Kumar have recommended their inclusion in the "other" category of TORCH infections. Certain other organisms may cause intrauterine infection but are usually transmitted just before delivery. This pattern is characteristic of herpes simplex virus, enteroviruses, group B streptococci, *Listeria*, and others, but these intrauterine infections differ little from those caused by the same organisms when acquired either just after delivery or during the 1st week or so of extrauterine life. For this reason, they are usually classified as "perinatal" rather than "congenital" infections.

Despite the extraordinary biologic heterogeneity

of the four TORCH organisms responsible for congenital infections, the syndromes they produce are remarkably similar.

Because the incidence of congenital infection in the fetus and newborn infant is high (0.5% to 2.5%), and a significant number of congenitally infected infants are asymptomatic, a high index of suspicion plus a sensitive, specific, and cost-effective approach to diagnosis is used. Evaluation begins with complete family and maternal history, including information on birth weights and medical problems of siblings, drug use, sexual orientation of sexual partners, maternal travel history, and blood transfusion history. Whether the children born with a birth weight less than the third percentile for gestational age (small for gestational age [SGA]) without other signs should be evaluated is unclear. Growth retardation has been described as the only manifestation of congenital infection with CMV, rubella, and toxoplasmosis. The clinician must rely on the history and the physical examination to identify infants for further evaluation.

If an infant is suspected of having a congenital infection, the infection may be confirmed through total cord IgM determination, although its efficacy is the subject of debate. Approximately 4% of newborn infants have elevated (>18 to 20 mg/dL) IgM in cord blood. Alford and associates showed that 42 of 123 infants with elevated IgM (>19.5 mg/dL) had identifiable infections.

CONGENITAL RUBELLA

Maternal rubella infection that occurs within 1 month before conception and through the second trimester may be associated with disease in the infant. The classic findings of congenital rubella predominate when the onset of maternal infection occurs during the first 8 weeks of gestation. Cataracts occur with maternal rubella before the 60th day after the 1st day of the last menstrual period; heart disease is found almost exclusively when maternal infection is before the 80th day (i.e., first trimester). Deafness, the most common manifestation, occurs, along with retinopathy as a consequence of both first and second trimester maternal infections. The incidence of congenital rubella defects following maternal rubella varies widely among series. A study of 1016 women with serologically confirmed rubella infection at different stages of pregnancy who were followed prospectively provides the most convincing estimate of the risks of congenital rubella infection. The frequency of congenital infection after maternal rubella with a rash was more than 80% during the first 12 weeks of pregnancy, 54% at 13 to 14 weeks, and 25% at the end of the second trimester. Rubella-associated defects (primarily congenital heart disease and deafness) were observed in all infants infected before the 11th week (n = 9) and in 35% of infants (9 of 26 infants) whose infections occurred at 13 to 16 weeks (deafness alone). The infected infant may excrete the virus for many months after birth despite the pressure of neutralizing antibody and, thus, pose a hazard to susceptible individuals in the environment. Only rarely can the virus be recovered by 1 year of age. An exception to this rule is the cataract, in which the virus may remain for as long as 3 years.

Infants infected with rubella are usually born at term but are of low birth weight. They may show only a few manifestations of the disease, such as glaucoma or cataracts, or they may have a systemic illness characterized by purpuric lesions, hepatosplenomegaly, cardiac defects, pneumonia, and meningoencephalitis. The skin lesions have been described as resembling a "blueberry muffin." These represent extramedullary hematopoietic tissue within the skin. Thrombocytopenia is commonly seen. Osseous lesions include a large anterior fontanel and striking lesions in the long bones. Linear areas of radiolucency and increased density are found in the metaphyses. The provisional zones of calcification are also irregular. These changes are not pathognomonic of rubella but resemble those of other congenital infections, such as cytomegalic inclusion disease.

Cardiac lesions include patent ductus arteriosus, septal defects, and stenosis of the peripheral pulmonary arteries. In one study of 18 patients with simple pulmonary artery stenosis, an association with rubella was found in 11.

Among the manifestations that may occur after the newborn period (late-onset disease) are a generalized rash with seborrheic features that may persist for weeks, interstitial pneumonia (either acute or chronic), defective hearing from involvement of the organ of Corti, central auditory imperception, or even complete autism. Infants with late-onset disease sometimes have immunologic abnormalities, with elevated total IgM and depressed total IgG. The principal immunologic perturbation in late-onset disease may be defective cytotoxic effector cell function that leads to defective virus elimination and immune complex disease. These patients may be susceptible to infection with unusual organisms such as *Pneumocystis carinii* or to development of histiocytosis.

Longitudinal studies of somatic growth reveal that most infants remain smaller than average throughout infancy but grow at a normal rate. Stunting of growth was more common after rubella in the first 8 weeks of pregnancy than after later infection. A higher than expected incidence of diabetes mellitus has been reported after congenital rubella.

Antirubella IgM can be determined with one of several immunofluorescence or enzyme immunoassays. Not all congenitally infected infants have detectable IgM antirubella antibody in the 1st month of life. If suspicion is high, repeat serologic examination and culture should be performed.

The virus is most often isolated from throat swabs but may also be found in the spinal fluid or urine. In late-onset disease, the virus is found in affected skin and lung.

There is no specific therapy for congenital rubella. The infant may need a blood transfusion for anemia or active bleeding and general supportive measures. The best therapy is to ensure that women who are considering pregnancy are immune to rubella. Vaccination of nonimmune women during the postpartum period has become an established medical practice, although prolonged polyarticular arthritis, acute neurologic sequelae including carpal tunnel syndrome and multiple paresthesias, and chronic rubella viremia have been reported in some of these women.

The problem of management of the pregnant woman who is exposed to or who contracts the disease should be resolved after weighing the known risks. If, at the time of exposure, serum antibody is detectable, then the fetus probably is protected completely. Routine postexposure rubella prophylaxis with immunoglobulin is not recommended, because efficacy has not been shown. Decisions about the interruption of pregnancy should be made only after maternal infection has been proved. An increase in antibody must be measured in two or more sera samples in the same laboratory on the same day; test variation may account for apparent antibody "rises" measured on different days.

The consequences of fetal rubella infection may not be evident at birth. Infection in the first or second trimester may lead to deafness or persistent growth retardation. Although infection in the third trimester may also lead to fetal growth retardation, this growth problem does not persist, suggesting that the mechanism of growth retardation among infants infected in the first or second trimester is different from that of infants infected in the third trimester. Hardy and coworkers followed up 123 infants with documented congenital rubella and found that 85% of them were not clinically suspect until after discharge from the nursery. Communication disorders, hearing defects, some mental or motor retardation, and microcephaly by 1 to 3 years of age were among the major problems that were discovered after the newborn period. A predisposition to inguinal hernias was also noted. Even in the absence of mental retardation, neuromuscular development is frequently abnormal.

CYTOMEGALOVIRUS

Cytomegalovirus (CMV) infection at any age is usually asymptomatic. After a period of active replication, the virus usually becomes latent but retains the capability of reactivation under special circumstances. Such reactivation appears to occur frequently during pregnancy. The fetus can be infected by either a newly acquired maternal infection or a reactivated maternal infection. The newly acquired maternal infection, although less common than the reactivated maternal infection, appears to carry a much higher risk of severe disease in the fetus. In reactivated infections, newborns are normal on examination and, if defects appear, they do not apparently do so until some time later in childhood.

A newborn infant without congenital infection can be infected by his or her mother at the time of delivery, through breast milk, by acquisition from the nursery or home environment, or by transfusion of blood from a donor who is antibody positive (i.e., latently infected). Perinatal or postnatal acquisition from the mother appears to be benign and common. Postnatal acquisition from the environment is probably less common and may be benign, although lower respiratory illness may occur under these circumstances. Acquisition from blood transfusion often results in severe, sometimes fatal, generalized disease in a setting in which maternal antibody is lacking. Although neonatal intensive care units in the United States are providing CMV-negative blood for transfusion, antibody-negative women who require transfusion during pregnancy should also be considered for transfusion with CMV-negative blood.

Approximately 40,000 infants are born with congenital CMV infection annually in the United States. This 1% infection rate compares with 0.3% in Europe and 1.4% in Africa. Twelve percent of congenitally infected infants die, and more than 90% have late complications, the most common of which is sensorineural hearing loss. Approximately 90% of congenitally infected infants are asymptomatic at birth. In the United States, approximately 60% of adult women have complement-fixing antibody. The incidence of excretion in the cervix or urine appears to increase during pregnancy from 3% in the first trimester to as much as 12% at term, although such findings are variable. Congenital infection occurs more frequently (3.4% versus 1%) among women who were antibody positive before pregnancy, a finding that implies either that most intrauterine infections result from reactivated maternal infections or that primary infections with different serotypes can occur in sequential pregnancies.

CMV is a member of the herpesvirus family and has the largest DNA genome of any known virus. Although all strains are serologically related, there appear to be some variations in antigenicity, and it is not clear whether this heterogeneity affects the incidence of exogenous reinfections. The virus differs from herpes simplex and varicella viruses in that it lacks the enzyme thymidine kinase, which renders it resistant to those antiviral agents that depend on this enzyme for their action, such as acyclovir.

Infants infected with the virus are often prematurely delivered. In the classic form of the infection, cytomegalic inclusion disease, newborn infants have acute progressive disseminated disease. They show petechiae and ecchymoses and are jaundiced at birth, or jaundice appears within a few hours and becomes intense. The liver and spleen are enlarged and firm from the start and may increase in size for a number of days. Skull radiographs usually demonstrate periventricular calcifications. Temperature as high as 39° C (102° to 103° F) may be found. Tachypnea and moderate dyspnea suggesting pulmonary involvement may appear. Pallor may or may not be striking. Puncture wounds bleed for many minutes, and hemorrhage from internal organs may cause death.

It is clear from prospective studies that most infants with congenital CMV infections are asymptomatic at birth and that milder manifestations of infections are more common than the aforementioned classic syndrome. Petechiae, hepatosplenomegaly, and jaundice are the most common signs. Although microcephaly is seen in only half the infants with other signs at birth, a number of additional children become microcephalic as they grow older. In others, hearing or visual impairment develops.

The laboratory diagnosis of congenital CMV infection can be made with absolute certainty only through detection of the virus in organs or culture specimens at birth or within the first 3 weeks of life. The most sensitive detection system is growth of the virus from urine in tissue culture. Serologic tests are often difficult to interpret, because, at the time of delivery, 50% to 75% of women have anti-CMV IgG, which is transplacentally transmitted to the infant, and even serial antibody titers cannot differentiate between congenital infection and perinatally acquired infection. No reliable CMV IgM assay is available. Molecular probes may permit rapid and specific diagnosis in the future. Careful consideration should be given to obtaining urine CMV cultures immediately after birth from those infants likely to receive blood transfusions or those who are at risk for enhanced immunosusceptibility. Such cultures permit identification of infants who are congenitally infected and those who are postnatally infected.

The urine usually contains bile but no urobilin. Albumin is commonly present, as are some red and white blood cells. Sediment that has been dried, fixed, and stained with hematoxylin and eosin often demonstrates the characteristic inclusion bodies within desquamated renal epithelial cells, so-called "owl's eye cells." Virus may be cultivated from the urine for an extended length of time.

Attempts to treat CMV infection with idoxuridine, cytosine arabinoside, adenine arabinoside, and interferon inducers have failed. Transient reduction in the titer of virus excretion in the urine may be seen, but no clinical benefit has been detected. Corticosteroids and cytotoxic agents have been used without success. Transfusion is indicated for anemia. Multicenter trials are underway to examine the potential efficacy of ganciclovir (9-[2-hydroxy-1-(hydroxymethyl)ethoxymethyl]guanine), an acyclic nucleoside structurally related to acyclovir but with increased potency against CMV in vitro. In addition, alpha interferon and CMV immune globulin are being studied.

Of infants who are symptomatic at birth, older studies suggested that approximately 25% die within the first 3 months. Of the remainder, 60% to 75% have intellectual or developmental impairment, about one third have hearing loss, one third have neuromuscular disorders (spasticity or seizures), and a smaller proportion have visual impairment owing to chorioretinitis. Only 10% to 25% are normal late in childhood, and those who demonstrate minimal abnormalities at birth have the greatest chance of being normal at long-term follow-up.

The fate of the congenitally infected infant who is normal at birth is still not clear. Two series indicate variable risks of deafness and reduction of I.Q. scores. In both instances, however, the case finding method was measurement of cord IgM level; an increase in this value might be found only in more severely affected infants (possibly reflecting primary infection in the mother). In one other follow-up study, the children were found to be normal at 4 years, but audiometric screening was not performed.

ENTEROVIRUSES

All enterovirus infections are seasonal, occurring most frequently during the late summer and early autumn in temperate climates. The incidence varies from year to year, with outbreaks sometimes caused by a single coxsackie or echo serotype and sometimes by several serotypes. Disease in newborn infants is uncommon but reflects the frequency of infections in the population at large. Severe disease in infants is seen with a frequency equal to or greater than that of perinatal herpesvirus infection.

Any of the nonpolio enteroviruses can cause disease in the newborn infant. In a review of 24 newborn infants with enteroviral infections, 10 infants died, 12 had aseptic meningitis, and 5 had myocarditis. Of the 24 isolates, 7 were echovirus, 15 were coxsackie B virus, one was coxsackie A virus, and one was nontypable. A more recent review indicated more favorable outcomes. Coxsackie B virus is associated primarily with myocarditis and aseptic meningitis, or combinations of the two. Echoviruses, however, are seen more often with severe, nonspecific febrile illnesses with disseminated intravascular coagulation or hepatitis. With both coxsackie B and echoviruses, nonspecific febrile illnesses, with or without the presence of a rash, are commonly seen. Infection takes place either just before or just after birth. Because infected infants have been delivered by cesarean section with intact membranes, it seems likely that transplacental infection has occurred. Severe disease may result when the baby lacks antibody to the infecting strain. It is not clear why the newborn infant is so highly susceptible to overwhelming illness. Nursery outbreaks of both coxsackie B virus and echovirus infections have been reported in which severe, and sometimes fatal, illnesses have occurred.

The symptoms of myocarditis and heart failure must be treated by slow digitalization, diuretics, and other supportive measures. Both plasma infusions and exchange transfusions have been attempted in overwhelming enterovirus infections with little evidence of beneficial effect. The use of steroids should be discouraged unless there is a clear rationale.

HERPES SIMPLEX INFECTIONS

Herpes simplex viruses are classified into two types: type 1 causes approximately 98% of oral infections (gingivostomatitis and pharyngitis), 7% to 50% of primary genital herpes, and almost 100% of encephalitis outside of the newborn period; type 2 causes 90% of primary genital herpes, 99% of recurrent genital infections, and most cases of aseptic meningitis. Seventy percent to 85% of neonatal herpes simplex infections are due to herpes type 2. It is likely that most infections are acquired from the mother shortly before or at the time of delivery. Some, perhaps accounting for the slight excess of cases resulting from type 1 that are above the percentage found in the adult genital tract, must be acquired from other sources. Considering the frequency of labial herpes in the adult population, however, acquisition of herpes simplex from such lesions must be extremely rare.

Current estimates suggest an incidence of one case of neonatal herpes simplex infection in approximately 3500 deliveries. Primary maternal genital herpes infections result in an attack rate of 50%, whereas recurrent maternal infection results in less than a 5% attack rate.

Most infants acquire the herpes simplex virus from the maternal genital tract at the time of delivery. Lesions have been reported to develop at the site of intrapartum monitoring electrodes on the infant's scalp. A smaller number of infants are infected several days before delivery and are born with clinically evident disease. There are some cases described of infants with a syndrome more closely resembling congenital viral infection who were probably infected in utero during the first or second trimester.

Localized infections without central nervous system involvement represent approximately 20% of all cases of neonatal herpes. Despite undetectable central nervous system disease, in 25% of this group, neurologic abnormalities develop. Localized central nervous system disease with or without skin, eye, or oral cavity involvement is seen in approximately 33% of infants with neonatal herpes. The mortality rate in this group is from 17% to 50%, and 40% have long-term neurologic sequelae. Infants with disseminated disease represent approximately 50% of all neonatal herpes patients. Without antiviral therapy, 80% die and survivors have serious neurologic sequelae. With therapy, 15% to 20% die, but 40% to 55% suffer neurologic sequelae.

Disseminated disease usually begins toward the end of the 1st week of life. Skin vesicles may be the first or a later sign, but they do not appear at all in more than half of patients. Systemic symptoms, although insidious in onset, progress rapidly. Poor feeding, lethargy, and fever may be accompanied by irritability or convulsions if the central nervous system is involved. These symptoms are followed rapidly by jaundice, hypotension, disseminated intravascular coagulation, apnea, and shock. This form of disease is indistinguishable at its onset from both neonatal enterovirus infection and bacterial sepsis.

Localized disease may begin somewhat later,

with most cases appearing in the 2nd week of life. When the central nervous system is the primary site of infection, the skin or eyes may or may not be involved; if not, then brain biopsy may be the only mode of diagnosis, as with encephalitis in older subjects. The infants are lethargic, irritable, and tremulous, and seizures are frequent and difficult to control.

Eye infections usually take the form of keratoconjunctivitis or chorioretinitis. On the neonatal skill, herpes simplex virus produces the characteristic grouped vesicles seen in later life, although individual lesions may be large and even bullous and late lesions are typically eroded, flat, irregular ulcers with an erythematous base. Scrapings of skin vesicles show giant, multinucleated cells when stained with Wright or Giesma stain (the Tzanck smear), typical of either herpes or varicella virus infection. Demonstration of viral antigens in cytologic smears using monoclonal or polyclonal antibodies is a more sensitive tool than Tzanck smear. Definitive microbiologic diagnosis, however, requires growth of the virus in tissue culture. Fortunately, herpes simplex virus can be detected by its cytopathic effect in 24 to 48 hours in most instances. When herpes is suspected, viral cultures of the throat, conjunctival and cerebrospinal fluids, blood, and urine should all be obtained as should scrapings of any suspicious skin lesions. The mother's genital and respiratory tracts should also be sampled. Serologic assays are rarely helpful and are difficult to interpret in view of the cross-reactions between the two herpes serotypes.

If a mother has active genital herpes simplex infection at the time of delivery and if the membranes are either intact or have been ruptured for less than 4 hours, strong consideration should be given to delivery by cesarean section. The risk to the child is greatest if maternal infection is primary (i.e., if the mother has previously had no infection with either type 1 or type 2 virus). Recurrences, however, with infectious virus recoverable from the genital area at the time of delivery also pose a hazard.

As soon as this diagnosis is suspected, the infant

should receive adenine arabinoside (Vidarabine), 20 to 30 mg/kg per day administered intravenously over a 12-hour period for 10 days, or acyclovir, 10 to 30 mg/kg per day intravenously every 8 to 12 hours, depending on the degree of renal impairment, for 10 to 14 days. This treatment has been shown to be effective in all forms of the disease, reducing (but by no means eliminating) both mortality and sequelae.

Even with antiviral treatment, the prognosis for survivors is not good. Microcephaly, spasticity, paralysis, seizures, deafness, or blindness develop in more than half of infants with disseminated disease. Those with skill involvement often have recurrent crops of skin vesicles for several years.

VARICELLA

There is some confusion about the term "congenital varicella" that would probably be best resolved by reserving this term for the rare cases transmitted to the fetus in the first or second trimester of pregnancy. Also called "congenital varicella" but probably better termed "neonatal varicella" are those cases of perinatal varicella beginning before or on the 10th day of life and, therefore, because of the incubation period of the disease, acquired in utero.

Varicella zoster virus infections occur during pregnancy with a frequency of 7 per 10,000 pregnancies. Unlike mumps and rubella infection during the first trimester, first-trimester varicella does not result in a detectable increase in fetal wastage. For infants whose mothers contract varicella 5 days or less before delivery or up to 2 days after delivery, the infant attack rate is 17% to 31%.

Neonatal varicella is probably transplacentally acquired in most cases. Because the incubation period for varicella is between 10 and 21 days, those cases beginning in the first 10 days of life are considered to have been acquired in utero. The prognosis, however, differs markedly between those cases in which maternal illness began 5 or more days from delivery and those in which maternal illness occurred from 5 days before to 2 days after delivery.

In the first group, neonatal disease usually begins with the first 4 days of life, and the prognosis is good. Presumably, maternal immunity has appeared before delivery and has been transferred to the baby before birth. In the second group, neonatal disease begins between 5 and 10 days after delivery. Of 23 cases described by Brunell, 7 (30%) died of overwhelming varicella and two barely survived after severe disease. In those instances in which the infant's preillness antibody has been measured in severe disease, none has been found.

Presumably, the placenta acts as a partial barrier to infection at term as well as earlier during pregnancy. Only about one in six such maternal infections results in neonatal disease.

Neonatal varicella follows typical maternal varicella and thus can usually be anticipated. When the disease appears in the infant during the danger period (from 5 to 10 days of age), it resembles closely varicella in the immunodeficient or immunosuppressed host. Recurrent crops of skin vesicles develop over a prolonged period of time, reflecting the newborn infant's inability to control the infection. Visceral dissemination is common, with involvement of the liver, lung, and brain. Secondary bacterial infection may occur.

Disease that is evident at birth or that appears in the first 4 days of life is usually mild, presumably owing to modification of the illness by maternal immunity.

The laboratory may be helpful in confirming the diagnosis. Prenatal diagnosis has been performed on blood obtained by funicentesis by quantifying varicella-specific IgM with an immunofluorescent antibody assay. Similar serologic studies can be performed on infants. Scrapings of skin lesions, as with herpes simplex infections, show large multinucleated cells when stained with Wright or Giemsa stain (Tzanck smears). The virus can be grown in tissue culture from skin and visceral lesions.

Infants of mothers in whom varicella develops from 5 days before to 2 days after delivery should receive high-titered immune globulin as soon as possible (125 U). In approximately 50% of exposed and treated infants, varicella develops, but the disease often is less severe. Follow-up of exposed and treated infants should include consideration of serologic testing (enzyme immunoassay, latex agglutination, or indirect fluorescent antibody) to determine whether asymptomatic infection has elicited immune protection. Repeat exposure of exposed and treated infants in whom varicella did not develop more than 3 weeks after administration of varicella zoster immune globulin (VZIG) should prompt giving another dose of VZIG.

In the event of a significant exposure in a nursery situation, as defined by prolonged contact (greater than 20 minutes) with an infectious staff member, patient, or visitor, infants who have no maternal history of varicella and who have undetectable anti-varicella titers should be considered candidates for VZIG. All infants less than 28 weeks' gestational age regardless of maternal history should be considered. The recommended dosage is 125 units per 10 kg.

If severe disease develops, antiviral chemotherapy might be considered. Drugs that might be effective are adenine arabinoside (15 mg/kg per day) and acycloguanosine (acyclovir) (10 to 30 mg/kg per day).

VIRAL HEPATITIS

Owing to the alliance between molecular biology and virology and clinical medicine, dramatic advances were made during the 1980s in understanding the pathogenesis of viral hepatitis. Hepatitis B and hepatitis C are currently of greatest importance for the pediatrician.

Hepatitis B

Women with acute hepatitis B infection during the first or second trimester rarely transmit the virus to their infants. Besides the timing of the infection, the hepatitis B surface antigen (HBsAg) carriage rate varies from 0.1% in the United States and Europe to 15% in Taiwan and parts of Africa. Infants of hepatitis B e antigen (HBeAg)-positive mothers have an 80% to 90% chance of becoming

HBsAg carriers. Chronic neonatal infection occurs in less than 10% of infants of e antigen-negative mothers. Transplacental leakage of HBeAg-positive maternal blood is the most likely source of intrauterine infection. Although HBsAg has been found in breast milk, breast-feeding does not appear to have any influence, either positive or negative, on the rate of transmission.

Despite either acute or persistent viremia in the mother, the virus rarely crosses the placenta and infection in the neonatal period occurs at or shortly after birth, probably by means of virus carried in maternal blood. Most infants born to mothers infected with hepatitis B virus have negative test results at birth and become HBsAg-positive during the first 3 months of life.

Infants with hepatitis B infection do not show clinical or chemical signs of disease at birth. The usual pattern is the development of chronic antigenemia with mild and often persistent enzyme elevations, beginning at 2 to 6 months of age. Occasionally, the antigenemia is entirely missed, and the child is merely found to have antibody to HBsAg at 6 to 12 months of age. Sometimes, the infection becomes clinically manifest, with jaundice, fever, hepatomegaly, and anorexia, followed by either recovery or chronic active hepatitis. Rarely, fulminant hepatitis is seen.

Laboratory tests are essential in the diagnosis of hepatitis B infection. Evaluations of serum enzymes and of bilirubin reflect the extent of liver damage. HBsAg appears early, usually before liver disease is found, and may disappear or persist. Antibody to the hepatitis B core antigen (anti-HBc) usually appears during or shortly after the acute disease and lasts for years. The HBeAg appears concurrently with HBsAg and is indicative of an increased potential to transmit the infection. Antibody to HBeAg appears approximately 2 to 4 weeks after the disappearance of e antigen. The last factor to appear, usually several weeks or even months after the illness (and never if HBsAg persists), is antibody to the surface antigen, or anti-HBs. It is very unusual for all three of these tests to yield negative results in the presence of hepatitis B infection.

In 1991, the Advisory Committee on Immunization Practices of the United States Public Heath Service recommended universal childhood vaccination against hepatitis B virus to begin in the neonatal period. The three-dose vaccination schedule should be initiated in the neonatal period or by 2 months of age. The second dose is given 1 to 2 months after the first dose, and the third dose is given at 6 to 18 months of age. Vaccination may be delayed until just before hospital discharge in preterm (less than 2000 g birth weight) infants born to HBsAg-negative mothers. However, all infants born to HBsAg-positive women should receive both active and passive vaccination.

Hepatitis C

In 1989, hepatitis C virus (HCV) was found to be the main cause of non-A, non-B parenterally transmitted hepatitis and has been subsequently found to account for a significant portion of the cases of sporadic acute and chronic hepatitis. In contrast to hepatitis B virus, HCV is not easily transmitted by sexual contact. Risk factors for HCV infection include transfusion, especially with contaminated lots of intravenous immune globulin beginning in April 1993, intravenous drug use, frequent occupational exposure to blood products, and household or sexual contact with an infected person. The vertical transmission rate of HCV is low (10%) and correlates with the titer of HCV RNA in mothers. Transmission of HCV in breast milk appears to be rare, although large, prospective studies are not available. Treatment of potentially infected individuals with immune globulin has been equivocal at best. Because of exclusion of anti-HCV–positive persons by screening programs, immune globulin manufactured in the United States is unlikely to provide passive immunity against HCV. The risks and consequences of perinatal transmission have not been defined. Other viral hepatitides may rarely complicate pregnancy.

HUMAN PARVOVIRUS B19

Considerable interest in the role of human parvovirus B19 infection in neonatal hydrops fetalis (nonimmune) and fetal aplastic crisis has developed since two cases of fetal deaths in humans associated with maternal B19 infection were reported.

Approximately 30% to 60% of adults in the United States are seropositive for human parvovirus B19. A significant proportion of child-bearing women is thus presumably susceptible to human parvovirus B19 infection. Approximately 36 fetal deaths associated with maternal human parvovirus B19 infection have been reported, as have approximately 130 cases in which the fetus survived and was normal at birth. Although large studies are not available, the overall risk of maternal exposure or infection to the fetus appears low. Postexposure passive immunization is not currently recommended.

BACTERIAL INFECTIONS

SEPTICEMIA

Neonatal sepsis is a disease of infants who are younger than 1 month of age, are clinically ill, and have positive blood cultures. The presence of clinical manifestations distinguishes this condition from the transient bacteremia observed in some healthy newborns.

The incidence of neonatal sepsis is between 1 and 4 cases per 1000 live births for full-term and premature infants, respectively. Among very-low-birth-weight infants who are undergoing prolonged hospitalization, the incidence increases dramatically to 300 per 1000 very-low-birth-weight infants. These incidence rates vary from nursery to nursery and depend on the presence of conditions that predispose infants to infection.

Although multiple factors have been associated with increased risk of bacterial infection within the first 7 days of life, the most important factors are the degree of prematurity of the infant and maternal medical conditions that may predispose the infant to fetal or neonatal infection (e.g., preterm labor, maternal genitourinary tract infection, or chorioamnionitis). The more premature the infant, the higher the risk of infection. Maternal or fetal infection probably contributes to initiation of preterm labor and a significant proportion of preterm births. The considerable rates of morbidity and mortality associated with bacterial infection in the newborn infant have prompted multiple investigations to develop risk evaluation methods that use information on maternal infection, fetal problems, and the initial evaluation of the infant. Unfortunately, the spectrum of variables requires individualized decision making for each patient. For example, duration of rupture of membranes before onset of labor, the latent period, or time before delivery has been investigated by several authors. None was able to demonstrate a significant difference in culture-proven sepsis with prolongation of the interval from rupture to delivery. However, maternal medical risk factors should prompt suspicion of infection, more intense monitoring of vital signs, and active consideration of the need for cultures and antimicrobial therapy.

Antenatal treatment of fetuses at risk for infection has improved infant outcome by decreasing the frequency of bacteremia. Boyer and Gotoff reported that bacteremia developed in none of 85 infants whose high-risk mothers received ampicillin, whereas the disease did develop in 5 of 79 control subjects ($P = .024$). They suggested that selective intrapartum chemoprophylaxis can prevent early-onset neonatal group B streptococcal disease.

Among infants older than 7 days of age who require neonatal intensive care, maternal risk factors become less important in predicting the risk of sepsis than the degree of prematurity, the presence of central venous or arterial catheters, poor skin integrity, and malnutrition. Attempts at preventing infection in these high-risk infants through the use of systemic prophylactic antibiotics only increase the risk of selecting multiply resistant organisms and systemic opportunistic infection, especially with *Candida* species. As discussed later, the most common systemic isolate in this group is *Staphylococcus epidermidis*.

The early signs and symptoms of septicemia in term or preterm infants younger than and older than 7 days of age are usually nonspecific. Early temperature imbalance with transient hyperthermia or hypothermia occurs in approximately 66% of septic infants (Table 5–1). Respiratory distress or apnea occurs in 55% of septic infants. Other symptoms include tachycardia, lethargy, vomiting, or diarrhea, and unwillingness to breast-feed may be noted. Conjugated hyperbilirubinemia, petechiae, seizures, and hepatosplenomegaly are late signs that usually denote a poor prognosis. Severe unconjugated hyperbilirubinemia has recently been shown in a retrospective series of 306 infants to be rarely a single symptom of bacteremia or incipient sepsis.

TABLE 5–1

Clinical Signs of Bacterial Sepsis and Meningitis*

Clinical Sign	Percent of Infants with Sign — Sepsis	Percent of Infants with Sign — Meningitis
Hyperthermia	51	61
Hypothermia	15	—
Respiratory distress	33	47
Apnea	22	7
Cyanosis	24	—
Jaundice	35	28
Hepatomegaly	33	32
Anorexia	28	49
Vomiting	25	—
Abdominal distention	17	—
Diarrhea	11	17
Convulsions	—	40
Building or full fontanel	—	28
Nuchal rigidity	—	15

*Data from 455 infants studied at four medical centers.

From Klein JO: Current concepts of infectious diseases in the newborn infant. Curr Prob Pediatr 31:405–446, 1984.

Although it is tempting to recommend a workup for septicemia in all infants with nonspecific clinical manifestations, this approach is both impractical and unnecessary in many instances. A complete history and physical examination, longitudinal and regular (every 1 hour to every 4 hours) assessment of symptoms and vital signs, and clinical experience are the best guides in determining the timing and extent of evaluation. Infants who are deteriorating should be strongly considered for evaluation and treatment. For example, full-term infants who require increased ambient oxygen shortly after birth should be considered for evaluation and treatment if their respiratory distress does not improve or worsens by 6 hours of age.

The diagnosis of systemic bacterial infection must start with a careful evaluation of the infant's signs and symptoms, physical examination, information on longitudinal changes in vital signs and laboratory indicators, and history including maternal history and relevant recent nursery history. The diagnosis is predicated on recovery of the organism from the blood or other sites. Blood (usually a minimum of 0.5 mL) may be obtained from a peripheral vein or from the umbilical vessels immediately following sterile umbilical vessel catheterization. Femoral vein aspiration should be avoided because of both potential contamination with coliform organisms from the perineum and the danger of inadvertent penetration of the hip joint capsule. It is frequently helpful to obtain cultures from other sites (e.g., cerebrospinal fluid or urine) before initiating antimicrobial therapy. Microscopic examination and culture of material obtained from gastric aspiration for leukocytes and bacteria may identify infants who are at risk for development of systemic bacterial disease. The presence of amniotic fluid infection increases the risk of systemic infection in a full-term infant from 1 to 5 per 1000 live births to 5 per 100 live births.

Measuring the peripheral white blood cell count and differential is a useful and rapid test, but it is nonspecific. If the total count is less than 5000 or if the band-to-neutrophil ratio exceeds 0.2 or 0.3, bacterial sepsis should be strongly considered, especially if the blood is drawn when the newborn is older than 12 hours of age. Other tests, such as sedimentation rate, C-reactive protein, haptoglobin concentration, and nitroblue tetrazolium have been extensively evaluated but are rarely more useful than the history, the physical examination, and careful longitudinal evaluation of the infant's status.

Since the late 1950s, *Escherichia coli* has been an important cause of neonatal sepsis. The dramatic increase in incidence of group B streptococcal infections is notable and has been reflected in many neonatal centers. Both group D streptococci and *Klebsiella* are pathogens that have been found relatively recently, the latter accounting for a high proportion of antibiotic-resistant organisms that colonize and infect babies in neonatal intensive care units. During the 1980s and 1990s, *S. epidermidis* has been recovered from systemic cultures with increasing frequency. This organism is most commonly seen in infants who are premature and who have required prolonged maintenance with central vascular catheters, peritoneal dialysis, or thoracostomy tubes. In most intensive care nurseries, this organism is the most common nosocomial systemic isolate.

Streptococcal Disease

The group B streptococcus is the most common gram-positive organism that causes septicemia and meningitis during the 1st month of life in infants older than 37 weeks' gestational age. Vertical transmission of this organism from mother to infant is one route of infection. Nosocomial acquisition of infection has been implicated in some nurseries and may be more common than was thought previously. The incidence of group B streptococcal disease has varied widely. However, despite this variability, group B streptococcus has been noted as an important neonatal pathogen since 1938.

The most common clinical manifestations of group B streptococcal infections are septicemia, pneumonia, and meningitis, but other more localized syndromes also occur, including osteomyelitis and septic arthritis, otitis media, cellulitis, and conjunctivitis as well as asymptomatic bacteremia. Generalized disease takes two clinically and epidemiologically distinct forms, early- and late-onset infection. By definition the early form occurs in the first 7 days of life, usually within hours of delivery (mean age 20 hours) and up to 50% of affected infants are symptomatic at birth. Infants with the early form of the disease usually deteriorate within hours of delivery and may exhibit unexplained apnea or tachypnea, respiratory distress with hypoxia, and shock. Chest radiographs reveal a diffuse pulmonary infiltrate that may be indistinguishable from the pathologic findings characteristic of hyaline membrane disease. In some instances, disease that occurs in utero may precipitate premature delivery. In a recent population-based analysis of group B streptococcal mortality, a mortality rate of 5.7% was noted in early-onset disease and 6.0% in late-onset disease.

The late-onset meningitic form of disease (onset 1 to 12 weeks of age) is indistinguishable from the other forms of purulent meningitis. Group B streptococci are grown from cultures of blood and cerebrospinal fluid, and the mortality rate is 20% to 40%. The principal organism appears to be serotype III. The pathogenesis is uncertain. Recurrent group B streptococcal infections have been consistently noted in approximately 1% of infected infants.

As described by Semmelweiss and Holmes, the group A streptococcus was the cause of the most common, lethal perinatal infection of both mothers and infants in the late 19th century, puerperal fever. During the 1970s and 1980s, this organism was a relatively infrequent cause of perinatal infection. However, group A streptococcal disease has been noted to be increasing in both adults and children over the past decade. The severity of disease caused by this organism in the newborn period varies from a low-grade, chronic omphalitis to fulminant septicemia and meningitis. Vertical transmission has been documented by molecular techniques. Because of the explosive nature of outbreaks in nursery settings, surveillance for colonized infants is probably indicated at the time the organism is found or when infant infections are recognized.

Group D streptococci include the enterococci and several other species, particularly *Streptococcus bovis*, which have been found in neonatal infection. Enterococci tend to be resistant to penicillin; therefore ampicillin, with or without an aminoglycoside such as kanamycin or gentamicin, should be used. For nonenterococcal strains, penicillin may be adequate. The incidence of these infections appears to have increased in many centers, and they are recognized as often as, or more often than, those caused by *E. coli*. The clinical pattern of the disease is remarkably similar to that seen with group B streptococci and is frequently associated with complicated deliveries. With prompt and appropriate antibiotic therapy, however, prognosis appears to be somewhat better.

In contrast to infants with systemic group B streptococcal infection, infants with *Streptococcus viridans* disease present later (mean age 3.5 days), exhibit leukopenia less frequently, and are less likely to have respiratory distress.

Staphylococcal Disease

Clinical disease with *Staphylococcus* may take one of several forms, which include bullous impetigo, toxic epidermal necrolysis, Ritter disease, and non-streptococcal scarlatina. The initial findings in Ritter disease are intense, painful erythema that is similar to a severe sunburn. Over the next few hours, bullae may form that, when ruptured, leave a tender, weeping erythematous area. The characteristic desquamation of large epidermal sheets occurs approximately 3 to 5 days after the onset of the illness. A fine desquamation is commonly seen in the perioral region. Bullous impetigo has been the most common disease associated with nursery outbreaks of phage group II staphylococcal infections.

Two additional kinds of staphylococcal infections have been recognized as major contributors to nursery infections, namely methicillin-resistant *Staphylococcus aureus* (MRSA) and *S. epidermidis*. MRSA outbreaks have been reported with increasing frequency in neonatal intensive care units. Although standard infection control measures including contact isolation, hand-washing with chlorhexidine, and cohorting are frequently used to control outbreaks, eradication of MRSA may require hand-washing with hexachlorophene. The population at highest risk for colonization or infection include infants under 1500 g with long-standing central vascular catheters, thoracostomy tubes, or central nervous system shunts, or those infants undergoing prolonged hospitalization after surgical procedures. When colonization with MRSA is noted and clinical deterioration suggestive of systemic infection occurs, some authors have strongly suggested the inclusion of vancomycin in the initial antibiotic administration. Vancomycin has been shown to be effective therapy for systemic MRSA infection in both adults and children. However, regular use of vancomycin may cause the development of vancomycin-resistant organisms.

Commonly considered nuisance contaminants in blood cultures of older children, coagulase-negative staphylococci, collectively known as *S. epidermidis*, have also assumed considerable importance as troublesome nosocomial pathogens in the neonatal intensive care unit. Similar to MRSA, these organisms are most frequently isolated from the smallest and sickest infants, many of whom have indwelling central vascular catheters, thoracostomy tubes, or central nervous system shunts. In contrast to MRSA infection, infants infected with coagulase-negative staphylococci have indolent presentations and infrequently metastatic focal infection develops. Although central venous catheters and contaminated hyperalimentation solutions have both been associated with *S. epidermidis* bacteremia, the surface hydrophobicity of the organism as well as opsonic differences in neonatal sera are more likely pathogenic mechanisms. In addition, after adherence to a hydrophobic polymer used in biomaterials (e.g., Teflon), these organisms produce a thick layer of extracellular slime that may permit the organism to escape phagocytosis by polymorphonuclear leukocytes. Treatment of these infections is complicated by the high frequency of penicillin- and gentamicin-resistant strains. Most strains remain sensitive to vancomycin. In some cases, removal of all vascular catheters in conjunction with the administration of a penicillin and aminoglycoside is sufficient for sterilizing the bloodstream. Use of vancomycin should be reserved for those infections that involve a catheter or anatomic site that cannot be readily removed or surgically approached (e.g., a heart valve), or that does not respond to initial antibiotic therapy. Persistent staphylococcal bacteremia unresponsive to vancomycin may be treated with intravenous rifampin (2.5 to 10 mg/kg every 12 hours for 10 days).

Infection with *Listeria monocytogenes*

As with group B streptococcal infections, there are two forms of infection with *Listeria*, early- and late-onset infection. Early-onset infections are acquired transplacentally or during passage through the vaginal canal. In such instances, fetal death and abortion may result or the child may be born with hepatosplenomegaly, disseminated disease, and granulomatous papules on the trunk and oral mucous membranes. This form of the disease has been called "granulomatosis infantisepticum." Perinatal complications are common in this group, and the mortality rate may be as high as 14% among infected infants. In the United States, the annual incidence of listeriosis is estimated to be 7.4 cases per 1 million population. Between 30% and 50% of these cases occur among pregnant women or their newborn infants. For infants younger than 1 year of age, the annual incidence has been estimated to be approximately 5.2 per 100,000 population, considerably less frequent than group B streptococcal infection (180 per 100,000 population).

Late-onset disease takes the form of meningitis, which occurs usually in the 2nd week of life but also may occur as late as the 4th or 5th week. The cerebrospinal fluid is highly cellular, the glucose is almost always markedly depressed, and monocytes are often seen on the smear, although they are usually not the predominant cell type.

Diagnosis is predicated on isolation of the organism, because serologic tests do not provide adequate sensitivity. The early-onset type of listeriosis, as with group B streptococcal disease, reflects the genital colonization of the mother and can be one of several serotypes. Meningitis, on the other hand, is almost always caused by type IV B and is usually acquired from the environment. The prognosis of the meningitic form is relatively good with regard to both survival and sequelae. Ampicillin plus gentamicin or kanamycin should be given for the first 5 to 7 days, followed by ampicillin alone to complete a 2-week course. The combination of ampicillin and an aminoglycoside has been shown to kill *Listeria* more rapidly than either drug alone.

Infection with *Escherichia coli*

E. coli are the most common gram-negative bacteria that cause septicemia during the neonatal period. Approximately 40% of *E. coli* strains that cause septicemia possess K1 capsular antigen, and strains identical with that in blood can usually be identified in the patient's nasopharynx or rectal cultures. The clinical features of *E. coli* septicemia are generally similar to those observed in infants with disease caused by other pathogens.

Pseudomonas Septicemia

Pseudomonas septicemia may present with one or several characteristic violaceous papular lesions that, after several days, develop central necrosis. Although this condition is most commonly observed in *Pseudomonas* infection, it may also be associated with other pathogens. In the newborn who receives broad-spectrum antibiotics while in an environment that is potentially contaminated by bacteria from respirators or moist oxygen, disease is likely to be caused by *Pseudomonas* species or other fastidious organisms.

Nontypable *Haemophilus influenzae* Infection

Although fewer than 50 cases of neonatal sepsis resulting from nontypable *Haemophilus influenzae* were reported between 1909 and 1981, during the decade of the 1980s this organism became a well-recognized neonatal pathogen that accounts in some centers for up to 7.9% of all cases of neonatal sepsis. Infants infected with this organism generally present with fulminant infection, exhibit neutropenia, and are born prematurely. The most common biotypes recovered are biotypes II and III. Approximately 20% of *H. influenzae* isolates recovered from the newborns are encapsulated (biotype I).

Therapy

For initial therapy, ampicillin in combination with gentamicin is a reasonable choice. Ampicillin is active in vitro against *L. monocytogenes* and enterococci as well as against many strains of *E. coli*. When the historical experience of the nursery or the physical findings suggest *Pseudomonas* infection, carbenicillin in combination with gentamicin should be used. Once the pathogen is identified and its antimicrobial susceptibilities are known, the most effective and least toxic drug or combination of drugs should be used. The aminoglycosides tobramycin and amikacin should not be used except in therapy of disease caused by kanamycin- and gentamicin-resistant gram-negative organisms to minimize the risk of aminoglycoside-resistant bacteria.

BACTERIAL MENINGITIS

Group B streptococcal meningitis usually manifests after the first several days of life, and the principal organism encountered in these infants is serotype III. The mortality rate is 20% to 40%. Streptococcal disease that occurs in the first 48 hours after delivery usually becomes manifest as acute respiratory distress with or without shock. Although the organism is frequently isolated from postmortem cerebrospinal fluid cultures taken from these infants, histologic evidence of meningeal inflammation may be lacking.

Approximately 80% of all types of *E. coli* that cause meningitis possess K1 antigen. The 018 and 07 somatic types and H6 and H7 flagellar types are most commonly associated with K1 strains cultured from cerebrospinal fluid. The presence, concentration, and persistence of this capsular polysaccharide antigen in cerebrospinal fluid and blood of infants with meningitis correlate directly with the outcome of the disease. The concentration and persistence of interleukin 1 beta and tumor necrosis factor alpha, the principal mediators of meningeal inflammation, correlate with an adverse outcome. The mortality rates for neonatal *E. coli* meningitis vary from 20% to 30% in some centers to 50% to 60% in others. These figures have been relatively constant despite improvements in overall perinatal mortality. This lack of improvement in outcome among infants with meningitis probably reflects the decrease in size and gestational age of infants who are receiving medical interventions in neonatal intensive care units and the emergence of different organisms with increased antibiotic resistance.

The early signs and symptoms of neonatal meningitis are frequently indistinguishable from those of septicemia. Specific findings such as stiff neck and Kernig and Brudzinski signs are rarely found. Lethargy, feeding problems, and altered temperature are the most frequent presenting complaints, and respiratory distress, vomiting, diarrhea, and abdominal distention are common findings. A bulging fontanel may be a late sign of meningitis. Seizures are observed frequently and may be caused by direct central nervous system inflammation or may occur in association with hypoglycemia, hyponatremia, or hypocalcemia.

The interpretation of cerebrospinal fluid cell counts in newborn infants may be difficult. During the first several days of life, as many as 32 white blood cells/mm^3 (mean, 8 cells/mm^3) may be found in cerebrospinal fluid of healthy or high-risk, uninfected babies. Approximately 60% of these cells are polymorphonuclear leukocytes. During the 1st week, the cell count slowly diminishes in full-term infants but may remain high or even increase in premature babies. Cell counts in the range of 0 to 10 cells/mm^3 are observed at 1 month of age. The cerebrospinal fluid protein concentration may be as high as 170 mg/100 mL, and the cerebrospinal fluid glucose to blood glucose percentage ratio is 44% to greater than 100% in both preterm and term infants. Thus, it is apparent that total evaluation of the cerebrospinal fluid examination is necessary to make an early diagnosis of neonatal meningitis. Although the cerebrospinal fluid cell counts and protein and sugar concentrations from normal infants overlap with those from infants with meningitis, less than 1% of babies with proven meningitis have totally normal results from a cerebrospinal fluid study on the initial lumbar tap. Approximately 50% of all infants with positive cerebrospinal fluid cultures for bacteria have negative blood cultures.

Stained smears of cerebrospinal fluid must be examined carefully from every infant with suspected meningitis. Grossly clear fluid may contain few white blood cells and many bacteria. The stained smears from approximately 20% of newborns with proven meningitis are interpreted as showing no bacteria. As its name implies, *L. monocytogenes* commonly evokes a mononuclear cellular response in the cerebrospinal fluid.

Latex agglutination assays can also be helpful in the early identification of infants with meningitis and in infants with abnormal cerebrospinal fluid findings who have received systemic antibiotics before culture of cerebrospinal fluid. The disadvantage of these tests is the lack of the availability of antibiotic susceptibility testing to direct antimicrobial therapy. Blood and urine cultures should be obtained from every infant with suspected meningitis.

Infants with meningitis require multisystem, aggressive management in the setting of an intensive care unit. Besides requiring antibiotic administration, these infants frequently require mechanical ventilation, compulsive fluid management to minimize the effects of cerebral edema, seizure control, pressor support, and cardiopulmonary monitoring. The beneficial effects of early administration of dexamethasone in infants with bacterial meningitis have recently been described in a placebo-controlled, double-blind trial in 101 infants and children. Dexamethasone (0.15 mg/kg of body weight) was administered approximately 20 minutes before the first dose of antibiotics and continued every 6 hours for 4 days. The efficacy of this intervention may result from attenuation of induction of cytokines, which mediate meningeal inflammation.

In the United States, ampicillin and either gentamicin or kanamycin are recommended as the initial therapy for neonatal meningitis. The dosages of ampicillin are 100 mg/kg per day in two divided doses during the 1st week of life and 200 mg/kg per day in three divided doses thereafter. The dosages for gentamicin and kanamycin are the same as those used for septicemia. An alternative regimen of ampicillin and a cephalosporin (e.g., cefotaxime or ceftazidime) can be used, but frequent use of such a regimen may lead to emergence of cephalosporin-resistant gram-negative bacterial isolates. All infants should have a repeated spinal fluid examination and culture at 24 to 36 hours after initiation of therapy. If organisms are seen on methylene blue or Gram-stained smears of the fluid, modification of the therapeutic regimen should be considered. In general, approximately 3 days are required to sterilize the cerebrospinal fluid in infants with gram-negative meningitis. In infants with gram-positive meningitis, sterilization is usually seen within 36 to 48 hours. Neuroimaging to exclude parameningeal foci should be considered in infants with persistently positive cerebrospinal fluid cultures who are receiving appropriate antibiotic coverage.

Once the pathogen has been identified and the susceptibility studies are available, the single drug or combination of drugs that is most effective should be used. In general, penicillin or ampicillin is preferred for group B streptococcal infection, ampicillin with or without kanamycin or gentamicin for infection with *L. monocytogenes* and *Enterococcus*, ampicillin plus gentamicin or kanamycin for infection with coliform bacteria, and carbenicillin plus gentamicin for *Pseudomonas* infections. There is no precise method for determining the duration of antimicrobial therapy. A useful guide is to continue therapy for approximately 2 weeks after sterilization of cerebrospinal fluid cultures or for a minimum of 2 weeks for gram-positive meningitis and 3 weeks for gram-negative meningitis, whichever is longer.

The mortality in neonatal meningitis is high. The overall mortality rate is approximately 20% to 50%, depending on the etiologic agent, the high-risk factors predisposing the infant to illness, and the ability of nursery personnel and physicians to provide general supportive care. Short- and long-term sequelae of neonatal meningitis occur frequently. The complications include communicating or noncommunicating hydrocephalus, subdural effusions, ventriculitis, deafness, and blindness. Gross retardation may be obvious at discharge. However, many infants appear relatively normal at time of discharge, and only after prolonged and careful follow-up do perceptual difficulties, reading problems, or signs of minimal brain damage become apparent. Approximately 40% to 50% of survivors have some evidence of neurologic damage. Infants who survive neonatal meningitis should have regular audiology, language, and neurologic evaluations until matriculation into the school system.

OTITIS MEDIA

Neonatal otitis media occurs most often in premature infants and in bottle-fed babies. The exact incidence of this disease is unknown, but it has been estimated to occur in approximately 1% to 5% of infants from birth to 6 weeks of age. The onset of illness is insidious, and the most common complaints are rhinorrhea, irritability, and failure to thrive. The presence of a fever greater than 38° C (100.4° F) and tugging of the affected ear are unusual.

Of special importance is the examination of the infant who has required prolonged oral or nasotracheal intubation. These children are at high risk for the development of eustachian tube dysfunction. The bacteriology of their infections is more likely to reflect the hospital environment. Recent preliminary data from children not born prematurely suggest that *S. epidermidis* is as important as *H. influenzae, S. pneumoniae,* and *Branhamella catarrhalis* in otitis media of early infancy. Perinatal problems, especially prematurity, appear to increase the risk of otitis media in the first 6 months of life. *E. coli, S. aureus, Klebsiella pneumoniae,* and *S. epidermidis* cause approximately one half of the cases of otitis media outside of neonatal intensive care units. *Diplococcus pneumoniae* and *H. influenzae* are the most frequently encountered pathogens during the first 6 weeks of life, as they are during the entire period of infancy.

DIARRHEAL DISEASE

Infectious diarrhea in newborns may be caused by bacteria, yeast (*Candida*), and viruses, but the most frequent of these agents is rotavirus. Rotavirus infections in newborns differ from those observed in older infants in that most cases are asymptomatic. Although severe symptoms have been reported in rotavirus infected newborn infants (e.g., bowel perforation, necrotizing enterocolitis, and diarrhea), these manifestations are rare. Neonatal rotavirus infection provides significant immunologic protection against severe rotavirus disease later in childhood. Strains that infect newborn infants are characterized by a highly conserved outer capsid protein (VP4) that may play an important role in attenuated virulence of these strains. In nursery outbreaks of bacterial diarrhea, enteropathogenic *E. coli, Campylobacter jejuni,* and, much less commonly, *Shigella* and *Salmonella* have all been recognized.

Salmonellae produce diarrhea by mechanisms that are even less clearly understood. Many species invade the mucosa without destroying it and set up an inflammatory reaction in the lamina propria. From there, particularly in newborn infants, the bloodstream may be invaded. Finally, *Campylobacter fetus* subspecies *jejuni* (the form that most often causes diarrhea in older individuals) may sometimes be present in newborn infants and produce bloody diarrhea. The outcome is usually favorable. Both *Clostridium difficile* and *S. epidermidis* have been associated with a syndrome that resembles necrotizing enterocolitis. As a general rule, diarrhea caused by enteropathogenic strains of *E. coli* is insidious in onset and is associated with 7 to 10 green, watery stools a day, but does not contain blood or mucus. The infants do not appear acutely ill. Complications are rare and are related primarily to dehydration and electrolyte disturbances. *Salmonella* gastroenteritis is usually associated with 5 to 10 foul-smelling loose green stools a day that rarely contain mucus or blood. Complications, which are unusual, include extra-intestinal foci of infection such as septicemia, osteomyelitis, and septic arthritis. Shigellosis is rare in neonates, but when encountered, it is an acute illness associated with a profuse, watery, nonodorous diarrhea frequently containing blood and mucus. The infants may be very toxic, and illness in a small number of patients initially mimics meningitis or gram-negative shock. Suppurative complications are rare, but dehydration and electrolyte disturbances are common and need immediate and constant attention.

A useful procedure for differentiating enteropathogenic from enterotoxigenic diarrhea is examination of fecal material for polymorphonuclear cells. Feces from patients with dysentery have significant numbers of polymorphonuclear cells, whereas those from patients with enterotoxigenic disease have very few neutrophils. This test may be helpful in the selection of appropriate antimicrobial therapy.

The most important aspect of therapy for infantile diarrhea is maintenance of hydration and electrolyte balance. As a rule, oral electrolyte solutions with a carbohydrate-to-sodium ratio less than 2:1 should be administered during the time of active diarrhea, and the infant should be examined and weighed frequently to ensure proper rehydration and to prevent complications. If sepsis or shock is suspected, intravenous fluids are needed. Estimation of fluid loss from diarrhea and vomiting should be carefully recorded and used as a basis for replacement therapy.

The selection of an antimicrobial agent depends

in part on the mechanism of diarrhea. An absorbable antibiotic such as ampicillin or chloramphenicol is indicated for disease caused by invasive bacteria, whereas orally administered nonabsorbable drugs such as neomycin or colistin sulfate should be used for noninvasive organisms that produce enterotoxin.

In the context of a nursery outbreak of bacterial diarrhea, all nursery infants with enteropathogenic *E. coli* should be considered for treatment with neomycin or colistin sulfate administered orally, whether or not they are symptomatic. Neomycin is administered orally in a dosage of 100 mg/kg per day in three or four divided doses. Colistin sulfate is administered in a dosage of 15 to 17 mg/kg per day orally in four divided doses. The duration of therapy is 3 to 5 days.

All infants with *Salmonella* gastroenteritis should have blood cultures performed and be examined to determine whether the disease has developed at other sites, such as bones and joints. Newborn infants with symptomatic *Salmonella* infections should receive antimicrobial therapy if they are febrile or toxic or if their diarrhea is severe because there is greater potential for systemic infection in these patients.

Although shigellosis in the newborn infant is rare, it may be associated with high rates of morbidity and mortality. All newborns with symptomatic shigellosis should be treated with ampicillin in a dosage of 50 to 100 mg/kg per day, administered parenterally in two or three divided doses. The duration of therapy is approximately 5 days.

URINARY TRACT INFECTION

Most infants with significant bacteriuria are asymptomatic. The diagnosis of urinary tract infection is made by examination and culture of a properly obtained specimen of urine. At all ages, urinary tract infection may be present in the absence of leukocytes in the urine. The converse is also true. Leukocytes or round epithelial cells (easily confused with leukocytes) are often found in urine samples collected in a urine bag, particularly after circumcision, in the absence of urinary tract infection. For these reasons, culture (or, for rapid screening, Gram stain) of urine obtained by suprapubic bladder aspiration or sterile bladder catheterization is the only certain means to diagnose urinary tract infection. In newborns, in whom restriction of fluid intake is not appropriate, greater than 10,000 organisms/mm^3 of a single species (rather than greater than 100,000 as is often thought) is diagnostic if the specimen is obtained by bladder puncture or catheterization. Moreover, concern about whether an infection is in the upper or lower urinary tract is rarely justified in the newborn infant, because either one carries with it concerns about urinary tract anomalies and bacteremia.

In general, antimicrobial agents should initially be given parenterally because septicemia may occur in association with urinary tract infection, and antibiotic absorption after oral administration may be erratic in newborn infants. Ampicillin plus kanamycin or gentamicin should be administered to symptomatic infants with bacteriuria before the receipt of results of cultures and susceptibility studies. Final antibiotic selection is based on these studies.

A repeat urine culture taken 48 to 72 hours after initiation of appropriate therapy should be sterile or show a substantial reduction in the bacterial count. Infants with persistent bacteriuria should be evaluated for resistant organisms, obstruction, or possible abscess formation. In the patient without complications, therapy is usually continued for 10 to 14 days. Blood urea nitrogen and serum creatinine levels as well as blood pressure should be determined at the initiation and completion of therapy. If there is evidence of renal failure, dosage and frequency of administration of these drugs, particularly the aminoglycosides, may need to be altered. Approximately 1 week after discontinuing therapy, a repeat urine culture is obtained. If the culture is positive, therapy is reinstated and a thorough investigation of the urinary tract is made to exclude obstruction or abscess formation.

All infants with culture-documented urinary tract infections should have radiologic or ultrasonic evaluation of the urinary tract. The usefulness of DMSA renal scans in evaluation of culture-documented urinary tract infection has not been conclusively determined. An excretory urogram or renal ultrasound is obtained at the onset of therapy to rule out the possibility of gross congenital abnormalities of the urinary system. If obstruction is demonstrated, urologic procedures to ensure proper drainage are necessary if therapy is to be successful. Voiding cystourethrography can be obtained within 2 weeks of the end of antibiotic therapy if reflux is suspected. Results are affected by previous bladder inflammation.

It is the physician's responsibility to be certain that newborn infants with culture-documented urinary tract infections do not have congenital abnormalities of the urinary system. In such patients, recurrent urinary tract infections are common, and physical growth may be retarded until definitive surgery has been performed. One must conduct careful, long-term follow-up studies in every patient to detect recurrent infections, many of which are asymptomatic.

SEPTIC ARTHRITIS AND OSTEOMYELITIS

During the neonatal period and throughout infancy, the epiphyseal plate is traversed by multiple small transepiphyseal vessels that provide a direct communication between the articular space and the metaphysis of the long bones. Thus, infection of a metaphyseal site can spread across the growth plate to penetrate the epiphysis. Because these perforating vessels disappear at approximately 1 year of age, osteomyelitis is usually not associated with septic arthritis in older infants and children.

Group B streptococcus, *S. aureus*, and coliform bacteria are the most common etiologic agents. Prematurity, antecedent trauma (most commonly originating from a heel stick for blood sampling but also from infected cephalohematomas), umbilical vessel catheterization, respiratory tract disease, and femoral venipunctures have been implicated in the pathogenesis of these infections in some infants.

Initial signs and symptoms are usually nonspecific. Most infants are not brought to medical attention until local signs such as swelling, irritability, and decreased motion of an extremity become apparent. Fever may be observed, but normal temperature is found in most cases. Physical examination reveals swelling, localized pain on palpation, and resistance to movement of the affected extremity. These signs may be obscured in the term infant by subcutaneous fat and normal joint contractions soon after birth. Localized heat and fluctuation are late findings.

Although blood cultures are frequently positive, clinically the infants usually do not appear septic. An exception is group A beta-hemolytic streptococcal infection, in which the infant appears gravely ill.

Blood cultures should be obtained from all infants with suspected osteomyelitis or septic arthritis. Latex agglutination assays on urine or joint fluid for group B streptococcus or other pathogens should be obtained. In infants with septic arthritis, a percutaneous needle aspiration of intra-articular pus should be performed; in osteomyelitis, direct needle aspiration of the affected periosteum and bone is attempted. If pus is obtained, the material should be examined with Gram stain and cultured. Preliminary identification of the pathogen from stained smears is helpful in the selection of initial antimicrobial therapy.

In patients with suspected septic arthritis, radiographs may be normal or may show widening of the arterial space and capsular swelling. Later in the course of the disease, subluxation and destruction of the joint are common. Early in the course of osteomyelitis, the normal radiographic water markings of the deep tissues adjacent to the affected bone are obliterated, indicating inflammation. Lifting of the periosteum from the bone may also be observed, but cortical destruction is unusual before the 2nd week of illness, and new bone formation is a late finding. Resolution of bone changes is considerably slower than clinical improvement. Because of the multifocal nature of musculoskeletal sepsis in newborn infants, compulsory sequential examinations of other joints and bones must be undertaken in the affected child. Two types of bone scan may be useful, technetium phosphate and gallium scans. Technetium scans reveal areas of increased blood flow and new bone formation, whereas gallium scans identify areas of white blood cell accumulation.

Selection of initial antimicrobial therapy is based on results of the examination of stained smears of aspirated purulent material and on the presence of associated clinical findings such as furuncles or cellulitis. If gram-positive cocci are observed, the administration of oxacillin should be started. Either kanamycin or gentamicin is indicated if gram-negative organisms are noted. If no organisms are seen or if doubt exists regarding their identification, oxacillin plus gentamicin or kanamycin should be administered until results of the cultures are available. Direct instillation of an antibiotic into the joint space is unnecessary because most drugs penetrate the inflamed synovium, and adequate concentrations are achieved in purulent material. This also applies to treatment of osteomyelitis; direct instillation of antibiotics into acutely inflamed bone is unwarranted.

As a general rule, infection of the joint space and bone should be drained either by repeated aspiration or by surgery. Septic arthritis of the hip and shoulder is treated best with incision and drainage in order to prevent vascular compromise or extension of infection into the metaphysis. Orthopedic consultation should be obtained for all patients.

Parenteral antimicrobial therapy of neonatal musculoskeletal bacterial infections is continued for a minimum of 3 weeks. The use of oral antibiotics as a substitute for parenteral therapy during the 2nd and 3rd weeks of therapy is unwise because of the lack of experience with this route of administration in newborns. In general, systemic symptoms appear within several days of initiating therapy, although local signs such as heat, erythema, and swelling may persist for 4 to 7 days. The decision to discontinue therapy should be predicated on lack of systemic symptoms, sterile blood and joint fluid cultures, and improvement in the affected bone or joint. Full range of motion may not return to the involved limb for several months. Because of this problem, physical therapy should be instituted early in illness to prevent contractures. Complete resolution of the radiographic changes may take several months.

OPHTHALMIA NEONATORUM

High prevalence rates of sexually transmitted diseases among women in labor have been observed to correlate with a high incidence of gonococcal and chlamydial ophthalmia neonatorum. *Neisseria gonorrhoeae* is acquired during passage through the infected birth canal when the mucous membranes come in contact with infected secretions. Infection usually becomes apparent within the first 5 days of life and is initially characterized by a clear, watery discharge, which rapidly becomes purulent. This is associated with marked conjunctival hyperemia and chemosis. Both eyes are usually involved but not necessarily to the same degree. Untreated gonococcal ophthalmia may extend to involve the cornea (keratitis) and the anterior chamber of the eye. This extension may result in corneal perforation and blindness. Until the introduction of adequate prophylactic measures, ophthalmia neonatorum was the most frequent cause of acquired blindness in the United States. Any infant presenting with a conjunctival discharge should have the material stained and cultured for gonococcus and other bacterial agents. Demonstration of gram-negative intracellular diplococci on a stained smear is an indication for immediate antibiotic therapy before definitive laboratory diagnosis is made.

Common bacterial agents associated with conjunctivitis in newborns are *Haemophilus* species, *Chlamydia trachomatis, S. aureus, N. gonorrhoeae,* and *S. pneumoniae*. Study of a smear of the purulent material is helpful in differentiating these etiologic agents. However, the presence of bacteria on a Gram-stained smear of material is not necessarily related etiologically to the conjunctivitis. Normal inhabitants of the skin and mucous membranes, such as staphylococci, diphtheroids, and *Neisseria catarrhalis*, may be observed.

Conjunctivitis caused by *Chlamydia* (inclusion blennorrhea) is a venereally transmitted disease that is observed in infants 5 to 14 days of age. Clinical manifestations vary from mild conjunctivitis to intense inflammation and swelling of the lids associated with copious purulent discharge. Pseudomembrane formation and a diffuse "matte" injection of the tarsal conjunctiva are common. The cornea is rarely affected, and preauricular adenopathy is unusual. In the early stages of the disease, one eye may appear more swollen and infected than the other, but both eyes are almost invariably involved. Diagnosis is made by scraping the tarsal conjunctiva and culturing the material. In addition, the conjunctival scraping should also be examined for typical cytoplasmic inclusions within epithelial cells, using Giemsa stain. These inclusions are seen on smears of purulent discharge, and cultures of the discharge yield various bacteria that are not related etiologically to the clinical disease. Use of polymerase chain reaction with primers directed against the gene that encodes its major outer membrane protein and *C. trachomatis*–specific cryptic plasmid DNA has been shown to be equally specific and more sensitive than McCoy cell culture for detection of *C. trachomatis* from ocular specimens.

Ophthalmia neonatorum caused by *N. gonorrhoeae* should be treated with parenteral antimicrobial therapy. Because of the increased prevalence of penicillin-resistant *N. gonorrhoeae*, empiric therapy should include a penicillinase-resistant antimicrobial, for example, ceftriaxone (25 to 50 mg/kg per day intravenously or intramuscularly) given once. If hyperbilirubinemia is present, cefotaxime (50 to 100 mg/kg per day intravenously or intramuscularly in two divided doses) for 7 days is an alternative. If the infecting organism is penicillin sensitive, crystalline penicillin G should be administered intravenously or intramuscularly in a dose of 50,000 to 75,000 units/kg per day in two divided doses for infants younger than 1 week and in three divided doses for infants older than 1 week of age. The duration of parenteral therapy is 7 to 10 days. In addition to systemic antibiotic therapy, the eyes should be washed immediately and at frequent intervals with saline solution followed by topical administration of chloramphenicol or tetracycline. Initially, local saline irrigations are given every 1 to 2 hours, and gradually the interval is increased to every 6 to 12 hours as clinical improvement is noted. Patients with ophthalmia neonatorum should be isolated, and strict hand-washing techniques should be used because of the highly contagious nature of the exudate. Conjunctivitis caused by other bacterial agents should be treated parenterally with the single most appropriate agent as judged by susceptibility testing of the organism. Because the most likely source of ophthalmia neonatorum is the maternal genitourinary tract, detection of *N. gonorrhoeae* or *C. trachomatis* should prompt evaluation and treatment of the infant's mother and her sexual partners.

Inclusion blennorrhea is treated with the topical administration of 10% sulfacetamide or 1% tetracycline ointment applied every 3 to 4 hours for approximately 14 days. Marked reduction in swelling and discharge is observed within 24 hours of therapy.

Ophthalmia neonatorum is preventable. Recently, several studies have evaluated the relative effectiveness of 1% silver nitrate solution, 1% tetracycline ointment, 0.5% erythromycin ointment, and 2.5% solution of povidone-iodine for prevention of ophthalmia neonatorum. Although each of these interventions is effective, povidone-iodine has antiviral activity and elicits few toxic effects. None of these treatments should be irrigated with saline because this may reduce efficacy. Ophthalmic ointments containing chloramphenicol are also effective prophylactic agents.

CUTANEOUS INFECTIONS

The most common bacteria that cause skin infections during the neonatal period are *S. aureus* and groups A and B streptococci. Disease caused by *S. aureus* can assume several clinical forms, the most common of which are pustular lesions. These tend to concentrate in the periumbilical and diaper areas and rarely become invasive except when extensive areas are involved or when the use of monitoring devices, catheters, or other invasive procedures are necessary in gravely ill infants. The study of a stained smear and a culture of an intact lesion are usually helpful in identifying the pathogen. The organisms should be phage-typed (they usually belong to group I) so that if additional cases are encountered in the same nursery, these infants and others in the unit can be evaluated for the possibility of a nosocomial staphylococcal outbreak. If these infections are caused by the same phage type of staphylococci, prompt measures should be instituted to determine the source of infection and to prevent further colonization and disease.

Therapy of cutaneous staphylococcal disease depends on the extent of the lesions and the general clinical condition of the infant. The physician can manage small isolated pustules through local care using a mild cleansing agent or an antiseptic such as hexachlorophene or povidone-iodine. Infants with more extensive cutaneous involvement, systemic signs of infection, or both should be given parenteral antimicrobial agents. A penicillinase-resistant penicillin should be used initially; continuation of this drug depends on the results of sensitivity testing.

Group A and group B beta-hemolytic streptococci occasionally cause disease in the nursery. The most common manifestation is a low-grade omphalitis characterized by a wet, malodorous umbilical stump with minimal inflammation. Disseminated disease occurs secondary to invasion of the bloodstream or by direct extension to the peritoneal cavity by way of the umbilical vessels. Identification of one infant with group A streptococcal disease in a nursery necessitates surveillance by culture of the other infants and of the personnel in the unit. The organism is usually introduced into the nursery by personnel or parents who have an asymptomatic nasopharyngeal infection. When a nursery outbreak is suspected, specific M- and T-typing of the organism is useful in defining the source and spread of infection. Group B streptococci have been associated with cellulitis, impetiginous lesions, and small abscesses in a few newborn infants. Penicillin is the drug of choice for streptococcal infections.

Necrotizing fasciitis is an unusual disease of newborn infants. This disease is frequently associated with surgical procedures, birth trauma, or cutaneous infection. Staphylococci, either alone or associated with streptococci, are usually causative, but other bacteria, including gram-negative enteric bacilli, can be cultured. In this condition, subcutaneous tissues, including muscle layers, are invaded and the organism spreads along the fascial planes. Overlying skin may appear violaceous and is edematous, which imparts a thick "woody" sensation on palpation. The borders of the lesion are usually indistinct when compared with those seen with erysipelas, which are raised and easily palpated. Extensive surgery involving resection of destroyed tissue is imperative in treating necrotizing fasciitis. Blood and tissue cultures should be obtained, and oxacillin and gentamicin are the drugs of choice for initial therapy. Necrotic, fatty tissue may combine with calcium, resulting in tetany and convulsions.

Breast Abscess

Breast abscesses are most frequently encountered during the 2nd or 3rd weeks of life and occur more commonly in females. The disease does not occur in premature infants, presumably because of underdevelopment of the mammary gland in these infants. Bilateral disease is rare.

The major presentation of neonatal breast abscess is localized swelling with or without accompanying erythema and warmth. Systemic manifestations are uncommon, and only 25% of these infants have low-grade fever. *S. aureus* is the major pathogen; coliform bacteria and group B streptococci are also encountered. The diagnosis of breast abscess is best made by needle aspiration of the affected site. The single most important aspect of management is prompt incision and drainage by a skilled surgeon. Oxacillin should be administered for approximately 5 days during the period of drainage. Experience with this condition in Dallas indicates that antimicrobial therapy plays a secondary role to adequate drainage. Long-term follow-up studies suggest that some girls have diminished breast tissue on the affected side.

NOSOCOMIAL BACTERIAL INFECTIONS

Hospital-acquired (nosocomial) infections have become a significant problem in most hospitals and may affect 2% to 5% of all hospitalized patients. In nurseries, nosocomial bacterial infections are of particular importance because of the unusual susceptibility of small infants to severe illness. This applies both to routine, short-stay nurseries and to intensive care nurseries, in which babies are frequently incubated and placed on respirators and require monitoring or hyperalimentation by means of central catheters. In short-stay nurseries, problems are most frequently due to gram-positive organisms, such as *S. aureus* and streptococci (groups A and B). In intensive care nurseries, many organisms may pose a threat: *S. aureus*, especially strains that are resistant to several antibiotics, are important; *S. epidermidis* is the most frequently encountered organism; gram-negative enteric bacilli are frequently a hazard and are similarly often resistant to antibiotics. Fungi, particularly *Candida albicans*, and respiratory viruses, such as respiratory syncytial virus, are also seen.

In neonatal intensive care units, surveys have shown that as many as 15% of infants hospitalized over 48 hours acquire nosocomial infections from their environment, many of them more than once. In one such survey, surface conditions accounted for 40% of the total of nosocomial infections; pneumonia for 29%; bacteremia for 14%; and surgical, urinary tract, and central nervous system infections for many of the remainder. Staphylococci and gram-negative enteric bacilli were responsible for more than 90% of these infections.

Staphylococcal Infection

When staphylococcal disease occurs in a nursery, the extent of infection must first be determined.

Using molecular epidemiologic analysis and traditional methods to isolate infected patients and eradicate colonization from patients and staff, such outbreaks can be terminated. However, the importance of hand-washing between patients and attention to institution-specific practices are critical to containment and analytic strategies.

Personnel who are carriers in an epidemic situation and are implicated in spread should be treated. Bacitracin ointment is smeared on the mucosa of the anterior nares three times a day and hexachlorophene showers and shampoos should be taken daily for 3 days. If possible, carriers should be kept away from work until they are free of the organism.

In short-stay nurseries, staphylococcal infections are often clinically apparent only several days after the infants are discharged. For this reason, some reporting system that includes infants requiring care after discharge is essential.

It is often necessary for the physician to take certain precautionary measures before microbiologic and molecular characterization of the outbreak is available. Selection of one or several measures necessary to control a nursery epidemic must be individualized. The measures commonly used are as follows:

1. Isolation of all infants colonized with virulent *Staphylococcus*. It is advisable to form a cohort system in the nursery for exposed but as yet noncolonized infants and for all new admissions to the nursery. These separate cohorts are cared for by separate nursery staff and are maintained until discharge of the infants. Infected infants are removed from the cohort and placed in isolation.
2. Enforcement of infection control techniques, such as gowning, limited access to the unit, and thorough hand-washing before and after handling each patient.
3. Use of antimicrobial agents. Topical antimicrobial therapy may be used for minor skin infections (pustules); parenteral antistaphylococcal therapy should be used for systemic staphylococcal diseases.

4. Initiation of routine bathing with antistaphylococcal cleaning agents such as 3% hexachlorophene (diluted 1:2 to 1:5) or application of triple dye to the umbilicus of all new admissions to the nursery.
5. If all else fails, closing of the nursery to further admissions until the problem either has been solved or spontaneously disappears.

After an outbreak is controlled, it is sometimes helpful to monitor the activity of staphylococci for a limited period of time by routine culturing of umbilical stumps and noses of infants on discharge from the nursery. Surveillance for clinical infections after discharge by sending postcards to families of affected infants is also helpful.

Bacterial Diarrhea

Any nursery infant with diarrhea should be suspected of having a potentially communicable disease and be treated accordingly. Hand-washing and other routine infection control procedures should be strongly enforced, and bacterial stool cultures should be obtained. If a bacterial pathogen is isolated, the baby in whom it is found should be moved to a special isolation area, if one is available, and given appropriate antimicrobial therapy. If watery stools develop in other infants, they should be cultured, placed in the same isolation room as the index infant, and appropriately treated. Culturing of asymptomatic babies and personnel is not always indicated but is appropriate if it is clear that simple isolation and treatment of symptomatic cases is not controlling an outbreak. Tracing nosocomial transmission of gram-negative infections has been facilitated by molecular characterization of the organisms involved.

Group A Streptococcal Infection

Group A beta-hemolytic *Streptococcus* was a common cause of puerperal and neonatal sepsis in the 1930s and early 1940s. With the advent of penicillin and its frequent use in maternity and nursery units, neonatal infections caused by this organism have become relatively uncommon. The primary source of group A streptococci in nursery outbreaks is either an attendant (nurse or physician) working in the unit or the mother. Once group A streptococci are introduced into a nursery, many infants become colonized but few develop clinical disease. The most common clinical manifestation is a low-grade, granulating omphalitis that fails to heal despite the administration of therapy. However, more significant disease may occur, including extensive cellulitis, septicemia, and meningitis.

Identification of one newborn with group A streptococcal infection is enough to warrant epidemiologic investigations of the nursery. All infants in close contact with the index case, a random sampling of other infants, and all nursery personnel should be cultured. Nasopharyngeal and umbilical cultures from infants and nasopharyngeal and rectal cultures from personnel should be obtained. Because nursery and maternity personnel are frequently interchangeable, the epidemiologic workup should be coordinated with the obstetric service in the hospital.

Infants with streptococcal disease should be given aqueous or procaine penicillin G. During nosocomial outbreaks, all asymptomatic infants colonized with group A streptococci should receive penicillin. The prophylactic use of penicillin for all new admissions to the nursery may also be indicated. Benzathine penicillin G has been used effectively as prophylaxis against group A streptococcal infection in several nursery outbreaks.

Gram-Negative Infections

Since the early 1970s, a number of nursery outbreaks caused by specific gram-negative bacteria have been described, and virtually all have occurred in long-stay intensive care nurseries. Among the causative organisms were *K. pneumoniae, Flavobacterium meningosepticum, P. aeruginosa, Proteus mirabilis, Serratia marcescens*, and *E. coli*. A common feature of these outbreaks is that the majority of colonized infants are asymptomatic; those in whom disease develops usually have pneumonia, septicemia, or meningitis.

Infected fomites represent a common source of nursery outbreaks caused by gram-negative bacteria. Contaminated faucet aerators, sink traps and drains, suction equipment, bottled distilled water, cleansing solutions, humidification apparatus, and incubators have been incriminated. In addition, healthy colonized infants or nursery personnel may act as a source of infection because the organism is transmitted among infants by way of the hands or gowns of personnel. During epidemics, asymptomatic colonization of infants with the specific pathogen is variable, ranging from 0% to 90%.

TUBERCULOSIS

The risk of congenital tuberculosis has increased during the 1990s. The HIV/AIDS epidemic among reproductive age women has contributed to this increased risk. The staggering magnitude of the global tuberculosis problem (in 1990, tuberculosis developed in an estimated 8 million people, and 2.6 to 2.9 million people died) coupled with increasing travel, international adoption, and denial of nonemergency medical treatment to undocumented or illegal aliens has further increased the risk of congenital tuberculosis. Revised criteria for the diagnosis of congenital tuberculosis include proved tuberculous lesions and at least one of the following: (1) lesions in the first week of life, (2) a primary hepatic complex or caseating hepatic granulomas, (3) tuberculous infection of the placenta or the maternal genital tract, or (4) exclusion of the possibility of postnatal transmission by a thorough investigation of contacts, including the infant's hospital attendants, and by adherence to existing recommendations for treatment for infants exposed to tuberculosis.

Infants whose disease was acquired in utero may be ill at birth or may develop normally until fever, lethargy, hepatomegaly, and other signs or symptoms occur at several days to several weeks of life.

The infection may be sudden and overwhelming or insidious and prolonged. Symptoms are typically nonspecific: poor feeding, listlessness, fever, hepatosplenomegaly, lymphadenopathy, and later, respiratory distress, with a median age at presentation of 24 days (range 1 to 84). Because the liver is the primary site of bacterial replication, the chest radiograph is often normal until late in the disease course at which time the pattern of involvement is often miliary. Skin lesions (erythematous papules) may be seen.

Management of neonatal tuberculosis must begin with identification and treatment of the pregnant woman with tuberculosis. The first priority must be prevention of transmission to the fetus and newborn. All pregnant women with a history of tuberculosis or with a positive tuberculin skin test should be thoroughly evaluated. Household contacts should be evaluated.

Once cultures have been obtained, the pregnant woman with active tuberculosis should be started immediately on antituberculous chemotherapy, regardless of stage of pregnancy. The agents to be considered include isoniazid (INH), rifampin, and ethambutol. Although concern about fetal effects of the drugs restricted their use during pregnancy in the past, considerable experience currently suggests their safety. Women with adequately treated tuberculosis are unlikely to infect their infants; however, any clinical suggestion of active disease should prompt acquisition of smears and cultures and reinstitution of therapy. The infant should have a Mantoux test at 2 and 6 months of age.

Conversion of skin reactivity from negative to positive within the past 2 years should prompt initiation of chemotherapy. If the chest radiograph is normal, unchanged, or shows a healed primary complex, INH can be used alone. If the radiograph is abnormal or progressive disease is evident, INH plus ethambutol or rifampin should be started.

Women whose skin tests were positive in the distant past and who are younger than 35 years of age, are asymptomatic, and have never received antituberculous therapy should be given INH before delivery. Regardless of age, women who have a positive skin test, an abnormal chest radiograph (other than a healed Ghon complex or calcifications), or who have close contact with individuals who have active tuberculosis should receive INH preventive therapy.

If the mother has *miliary* disease, untreated in the last part of pregnancy, the infant is at greatest risk of having congenital tuberculosis. Such an infant deserves careful clinical evaluation, including a chest film, smear and culture of gastric washings and urine, examination and culture of the spinal fluid, and drug sensitivities determined on any organism recovered. The tuberculin test may not become positive for approximately 3 to 5 weeks or longer in such an infant, so reliance on a negative test is unwarranted. The necessity of separating the infant from the mother, who would be hospitalized, is obvious, and institution of INH, 10 mg/kg per day, is appropriate in the absence of manifest disease. The infant with manifest disease should receive INH (10 to 15 mg/kg per day), rifampin (10 to 20 mg/kg per day), pyrazinamide (15 to 30 mg/kg per day), and either streptomycin (20 to 30 mg/kg per day) or ethambutol (15 to 25 mg/kg per day) for the first 2 months, followed by INH and rifampin for 4 to 10 months depending on the severity of disease. If less than 4% of endemic *Mycobacterium tuberculosis* are resistant to INH, three-drug regimens are acceptable as initial treatment. Rifampin appears to have no unusual toxicities in this age group other than the well-recognized occasional problems of hepatotoxicity and allergy.

Prednisone at 1 mg/kg per day in infants with tuberculous meningitis for the first 30 days of illness is useful. Prednisone therapy should not be initiated until adequate blood levels of antituberculous drugs are achieved, presumably after approximately 48 hours of initiating treatment.

If the mother is sputum-positive for tuberculosis, the risk to the infant is greater than if the mother was on treatment for at least 2 weeks and is sputum-negative. It seems reasonable to separate the infant from the mother and other family contacts with active tuberculosis as long as they remain sputum-positive. Once the mother's sputum and sputum of family contacts have converted to negative and all are known to be taking medication regularly, separation from the infant is not necessary.

The possibility of relapse in the mother is greatest if her disease was arrested for less than 5 years. Since the risk to the infant of a mother with inactive tuberculosis depends on her likelihood of reactivation, careful and frequent examinations of the mother are essential. Indeed, a tuberculin test in all women during pregnancy and at the time of delivery is desirable. A postpartum chest film, one at 3 months, and another at 6 months are indicated in tuberculin-positive mothers. The infant should have a tuberculin test with 5 T.U. (0.1 mL intermediate PPD, or 0.0001 mg) at birth and a chest radiograph. The infant should receive INH prophylaxis until the Mantoux test is negative at 3 months of age and there are no clinical signs of disease. Two drugs (INH and rifampin) should be used if active disease is observed in the infant.

DIPTHERIA

Corynebacterium diphtheriae, generally of the gravis type, is the responsible organism. Its soluble toxin produces antitoxin in the host during the course of natural infection and may be used, modified to toxoid, as a potent antigen to stimulate the formation of antitoxin in inoculated persons. The antitoxic titer from either source persists for a variable number of years and is capable of being boosted by reinfection or by subsequent doses of toxoid. Many newborns receive no antitoxin from a mother whose natural or artificial antitoxin titer had diminished to the vanishing point over the course of years devoid of re-exposure either to *C. diphtheriae* or to stimulating injections. These infants are susceptible to diphtheria, and contact with an infected person or a healthy carrier may cause the disease. Prevention continues to be the best treatment: an exposed or unimmunized pregnant woman should receive two properly spaced disks of tetanus and diphtheria toxoids, preferably during the last two trimesters.

The diagnosis of diphtheria in the newborn differs in no respect from that in the older child. Faucial diphtheria is recognized by the characteristic membrane, nasal diphtheria by persistent discharge (often sanguineous), and the laryngeal form by slowly progressive hoarseness and aphonia and laryngotracheal obstruction. All are without sharp constitutional reaction. In all forms, diagnosis depends on bacteriologic identification of *C. diphtheriae*. Serodiagnosis by single serum antipertussis toxin antibody enzyme-linked immunosorbent assay has also been useful, but, in the neonatal period, concurrent assessment of maternal serologic status must be obtained. Complications, chiefly myocarditis and postdiphtheritic paralysis, have been similarly encountered in the newborn.

Diphtheria antitoxin must be given intravenously, when the condition appears serious, or intramuscularly, if the situation is less urgent. Doses of 20,000 to 50,000 units on 2 or 3 successive days is sufficient. Preliminary testing for sensitivity must be carried out. Because penicillin has a bactericidal effect on *C. diphtheriae*, it should be given in doses approximating 300,000 units every 8 to 12 hours. Erythromycin is also effective in the event of penicillin sensitivity. Treatment of complications is carried out as for that in older infants.

TETANUS NEONATORUM

The causative agent is the bacterium *Clostridium tetani*. This gram-positive, anaerobic spore bearer produces a protein neurotoxin (tetanospasmin) that is responsible for this paralysis. This protoplasmic protein is released after the cells of *C. tetani* autolyze. The protein is encoded within a plasmid not directly related to a bacteriophage. Like the botulinal toxins, tetanospasmin acts at myoneural junctions by inhibiting the release of acetylcholine. *C. tetani* usually gains entrance into the newborn's body by way of the stump of the umbilical cord that is cut by an unsterile instrument or covered with an unclean dressing. The organism is long-lived by virtue of its spore formation, is a normal inhabitant of the intestinal tract of many domestic animals, and hence abounds in the soil of many localities.

Immunity to tetanus depends on the presence in the blood of an adequate concentration of antibody to the toxin. Antibody is efficiently stimulated by immunization with toxoid. The blood of the newborn contains roughly the amount of tetanus antitoxin that is present in the mother's blood.

Signs appear between the 6th and 14th days after birth, most often at the beginning of the 2nd week. Restlessness, irritability, and difficulty in sucking are followed within a day or two by fever, muscle stiffness, and finally, convulsions. The temperature often elevates to between 40° C and 41° C (104° F and 106° F). Physical examination at this stage shows the characteristic trismus and risus sardonicus and the tenseness and rigidity of all muscles, including those of the abdomen. The fists are held tightly clenched and the toes rigidly fanned. Characteristic are the opisthotonic spasms plus clonic jerkings that follow sudden stimulation by touch or by loud noise.

Tetany of the newborn should never be confused with tetanus. Infants with tetany appear well between their convulsive episodes. The infant who is hypertonic from hypoxic-ischemic injury has usually shown evidence of brain injury from birth, before the first sign of tetanus could possibly appear. Extraocular palsies commonly are present and abdominal rigidity absent. Response to stimulation is depressed rather than increased.

The infant may die within a week after onset from respiratory arrest during a convulsive episode. If not, improvement becomes manifest within 3 to 7 days by gradual decline of temperature, decrease in the number of episodes of spasm, and slow resolution of rigidity. Complete disappearance of all signs of illness may take as long as 6 weeks.

The first requirement is for tetanus antitoxin to neutralize the circulating toxin not already bound to nerve tissue. Tetanus immune globulin (human) should be given intramuscularly, in a dose of 500 units. If this is not available, 10,000 units of equine or bovine tetanus antitoxin should be given intramuscularly. In addition, débridement of the infection site to remove devitalized tissue is imperative. Penicillin, which kills the vegetative form of the bacterium, should be given in a dose of 100,000 to 200,000 units/kg every 12 hours. Tetracycline may be of value as an alternative drug. Treatment with antibiotics and antitoxin should also be considered for infants whose umbilical cords have been cut with or exposed to surfaces that might bear *C. tetani*.

Every known sedative has been used to control spasm, and there is no general agreement as to which one should be chosen. Diazepam (Valium) has become the mainstay of treatment of older children with tetanus, and it is probably also of great value in newborns (1 to 2 mg/kg per day in divided doses). The ideal result is to control spasm without depressing respiration. Drug administration is important. When intensive care and respirators are available, neuromuscular blockade with pancuronium bromide (Pavulon), 0.05 to 0.1 mg/kg administered every 2 to 3 hours for the duration of the spasms (up to 6 weeks), has proved successful.

INFANT BOTULISM

Seven types (A, B, C, D, E, F, G) of *Clostridium botulinum*, a heterologous group of obligatory anaerobic, spore-forming, gram-positive, rod-shaped bacteria are distinguished by antigenically distinct toxins. Investigation of 81 cases by the CDC identified a potential source in opened jars of honey that had been added to baby food or used to coat pacifiers. Vacuum cleaner dust was found to contain spores of *C. botulinum* in the household of one infected infant. In a study from Utah, it was noted that digging or construction was common in the neighborhoods in which cases were reported. However, food exposures accounted for only a minority of the 68 infant botulism cases reviewed, and preexisting host factors, especially those related to intestinal flora, may be the most important risk indicators. Of the 121 cases reported to the CDC from 1975 to 1979, 65 (54%) involved *C. botulinum* type A, 55 (45%) type B, and one, type F. Three of the patients died.

Infant botulism has been described in patients as young as 1 week of age, but the peak incidence occurs at the usual time of weaning, from 6 weeks to 6 months of age. The infants have usually been born at term and described as normal. Constipation is frequently noted. The infants may seem lethargic and slow to feed. Some have a more acute onset of feeding difficulties, pooling of secretions, diminished gag reflex, loss of head control, and generalized weakness. If the diagnosis is not made and appropriate supportive treatment initiated, death from respiratory arrest may occur. Some infants diagnosed as victims of sudden infant death syndrome may have died from unrecognized botulism.

The diagnosis depends on recovery of *C. botulinum* with or without its toxin from the stool in the presence of a compatible clinical picture. Stool and serum specimens should be sent to a laboratory equipped to identify the organism and its toxin. Electromyography has been helpful in the clinical diagnosis. Brief small-amplitude motor reaction potentials have been described. Both *C. botulinum* and toxin have been found in the stools of normal infants.

Botulinal antitoxin has not been useful in infant botulism, perhaps because of the absence of demonstrable toxin in the serum. Ampicillin has been used, although its value in eliminating the organism is uncertain. Aminoglycoside antibiotics are contraindicated because of possible potentiation of neuromuscular weakness.

FUNGAL INFECTIONS

DISSEMINATED CANDIDIASIS

This once rare disease has become a common problem in many nurseries as a result of the intensive use of broad-spectrum antibiotics in premature (and more vulnerable) infants, and the increased use of intravascular catheters for hyperalimentation. While compulsive attention must be given to aseptic technique in the management of vascular catheters, it is not clear from currently available data whether these catheters cause infection, whether fluids administered through them (notably hyperalimentation fluid) causes infection, or whether they represent a marker for infants with increased susceptibility to candidiasis. *Candida albicans* grows in all alimentation solutions in use, but the rate depends on the composition and temperature. The organisms can reach densities of approximately 100,000/mL, and yet the solution appears clear to the eye; further infection from contaminated intravenous fluids produces an insidious infection. Several *Candida* species are known to cause disease in humans.

Peripheral blood cultures obtained by venipuncture are a reliable indicator of ongoing candidemia. In overwhelming infections, the organisms can be seen in stained smears of buffy coat preparations. Skin lesions can be seen that yield the organism on aspiration. Candidal ophthalmitis is an occasional complication of candidemia and can serve as a focus for continued candidemia. Every infant in whom the diagnosis of candidal sepsis is suspected should have indirect funduscopic examination. Among common presenting symptoms, usually at 1 to 2 months of age, are respiratory deterioration, hyperglycemia, and temperature instability. Fungal colonization represents a significant risk factor in infants weighing less than 1500 g. A substantial proportion of infants with persistent signs and symptoms of infection has central nervous system involvement. Other manifestations of candidal sepsis in newborn infants are osteomyelitis, meningitis, endocarditis, and arthritis.

Many examples of candidal infection acquired in utero have been reported. In these instances, ascending infection produces chorioamnionitis with dissemination to the fetus, which can lead to spontaneous abortion. In most instances, the severity of disseminated candidiasis acquired in utero is such that the infant dies before therapy can be considered.

On the one hand, cutaneous candidiasis, evident at the time of birth, can be seen in the absence of systemic involvement. Adverse outcome may also be avoided by accurate prenatal diagnostic procedures and prompt antifungal therapy in the neonatal period. On the other hand, cases of systemic candidiasis, probably acquired in utero, have been described in the absence of rash. The rash, when it does occur, evolves from maculopapular to vesicular to pustular. It thus appears that *Candida*, like bacteria, may infect the fetus by hematogenous dissemination from the umbilical vessels, leading to systemic infection, or may be limited to cutaneous candidiasis.

PROTOZOAL INFECTIONS

CONGENITAL TOXOPLASMOSIS

Congenital toxoplasmosis is caused by infestation with a protozoan, *Toxoplasma gondii*, so named because it was first isolated in 1909 from a North African rodent called the "gondi." The domestic cat is the only definitive host and is the reservoir of the infective oocysts that are passed in the feces. Maternal toxoplasma infection results primarily from ingestion of undercooked or raw meat, which contains tissue cysts, or ingestion of water or foodstuffs contaminated by oocysts that have been excreted in feces of infected cats. Congenital toxoplasmosis is caused by invasion of the fetal bloodstream by parasites during a stage of maternal parasitemia. It is likely that the parasitemia occurs only with initial infection and often in the absence of any maternal symptoms. Mothers whose infections become chronic and inapparent do not transmit the disease to subsequent fetuses. In 1974 Desmonts and Couvreur reported infection of the fetus in 33% of all maternal infections.

Toxoplasma is a crescent-shaped organism, 4 to 7 μm long, with a single, approximately central nucleus. In tissues it is intracellular, and small or large agglomerates are often seen. In later stages, the organism is often seen lying within a cystic space, especially in the brain and skeletal and heart muscle.

In the newborn, the principal locus of infection is the central nervous system. Lesions consist of areas of necrosis in which calcium is ultimately deposited and throughout which cysts or the naked parasite may be sparsely scattered. Similar lesions are less abundant in the liver, lungs, myocardium, skeletal muscle, spleen, and other tissues. There is little cellular inflammatory reaction, consisting mostly of lymphocytes, monocytes, and plasma cells. The pathologic picture is not specific unless organisms or cysts can be demonstrated.

Most of the infants with congenital toxoplasmosis (approximately 85%) have no symptoms or apparent abnormalities at birth. In Desmonts and Couvreur's series, there were two subclinical cases for each clinical one. In such infants, however, disease usually develops as they grow older. The natural history of the disease described by these authors may be different in the 1990s because of antenatal diagnosis, treatment, and the increasing proportion of reproductive-age women with HIV infection. Coinfection of the fetus with both HIV and *T. gondii* has also been observed. Recent reviews of the natural history of infants who are congenitally infected suggest that prenatal treatment and postnatal treatment for at least 1 year can significantly improve outcome, even in the presence of central nervous system calcifications or retinal changes.

The so-called classic triad of congenital toxoplasmosis is present in only a small proportion of symptomatic cases. Chorioretinitis, hydrocephalus, and intracranial calcifications were present in 86%, 20%, and 37%, respectively, of the large series of Eichenwald. Fever, hepatosplenomegaly, and jaundice are frequent signs, even in the absence of central nervous system or ocular findings. Rash and pneumonitis occasionally occur. The spinal fluid is often abnormal. Anemia is frequent, and thrombocytopenia and eosinophilia are occasionally seen. Cataracts, microphthalmia, and glaucoma, so common in rubella, are rare. Microcephaly is less common than hydrocephalus. Diarrhea is occasionally a prominent symptom.

Neurologic and ocular involvement frequently appear later if they are absent at birth. Convulsions, mental retardation, and spasticity are all common sequelae. A morphologically characteristic relapsing chorioretinitis is the most common sequela of congenital toxoplasmosis, although involvement of the anterior uveal tract also occurs. It is also clear that most, if not all cases of *Toxoplasma* chorioretinitis represent the sequelae of congenital infection. Treatment has significantly improved the rather grim prognosis of congenital disease.

Although some infants are highly symptomatic at birth, the disease may also be insidious in onset.

Because culture of the organism is tedious and expensive, laboratory diagnosis depends heavily on interpretation of various serologic tests. There are several valuable tests for antibody to *T. gondii*. Although the Sabin-Feldman dye test (lysis of *Toxoplasma* organisms by various dilutions of maternal or infant serum after incubation for 1 hour at 37° C) used to be the standard method, several newer tests easier to perform and of equal reliability have supplanted it in many laboratories, particularly the indirect fluorescent antibody (IFA) test and the enzyme-linked immunosorbent assay (ELISA). Both tests can be adapted to measure IgM antibody. As with other congenital infections, false-positive IgM antibody titers may be caused by rheumatoid factor. Complement fixation and indirect hemagglutination tests may also be performed but are somewhat more difficult to interpret. Detection of IgA antibodies against P30, a major surface protein of *T. gondii*, has recently been reported to be more sensitive than detection of anti-P30 IgM antibodies in identification of congenitally infected infants. All eight congenitally infected infants from 26 mothers infected during pregnancy were identified by the presence of anti-P30 IgA antibodies, and anti-P30 IgM antibodies were found in three of the eight infected infants.

Antibody develops during acute infection in the mother and remains high or decreases slowly over a year's time. A single high antibody titer implies, but does not prove, recent infection. A serologic diagnosis of acute infection requires an increase in antibody titer in serial samples obtained at least 3 weeks apart and tested in parallel in the same laboratory. In the infant, the titer at birth equals or exceeds the mother's, regardless of whether the baby is congenitally infected. Over the 1st year in the uninfected infant, the titer decreases with a half-life of approximately 30 days. In the infected infant, although the titer may decrease somewhat for the first few months, it increases again to a high level by the first birthday. IgM anti-*Toxoplasma* antibody may be present at birth or at any time for the next few months. A negative *Toxoplasma* antibody titer in the infant's serum at 6 months to 1 year of age essentially excludes the diagnosis.

Maternal treatment for women who acquire *Toxoplasma* infection during pregnancy reduces the likelihood of congenital transmission by as much as 70%. Because 85% to 95% of women of childbearing age in the United States are at risk and only 10% of immunocompetent women are symptomatic if infected, serologic screening before or early in pregnancy should be strongly considered to identify women at risk for infection. Seroconversion should prompt institution of maternal therapy (spiramycin, 3 g per day). This treatment should be continued throughout pregnancy. If fetal infection is diagnosed, 3 weeks of spiramycin therapy should be alternated with 3 weeks of pyrimethamine, 50 mg per day, and sulfadiazine, 3 g per day after the 24th week of gestation. Careful hematologic monitoring should be performed along with concurrent treatment with folinic acid. Because of the lack of data, it is currently impossible to estimate the teratogenic and toxic risks to the fetus from antenatal therapy with pyrimethamine and sulfadiazine. Before initiation of therapy, fetal diagnosis should be attempted to permit evaluation of risk and benefit of these drugs.

Treatment is recommended for all cases of congenital toxoplasmosis or congenital *Toxoplasma* infection. Future treatment may involve more direct fetal therapy by intra-amniotic infusion of drugs.

After confirmation of fetal infection, therapeutic abortion is a treatment option that needs to be considered. In one study, 53 of 241 pregnant women (22%) diagnosed serologically with *Toxoplasma* infection between 1988 and 1993 elected to terminate their pregnancies.

It has been known for some time that the prognosis in untreated infants with overt disease at birth is poor. Cerebral calcifications were thought to be a particularly ominous finding. Prospective follow-up studies in the 1960s and 1970s of congenitally infected infants asymptomatic at birth have shown that, even in this group, chorioretinitis is frequent and central nervous system involvement is not uncommon. In 1980, Wilson and coworkers found that, in 11 of 13 such infants, chorioretinitis developed and that, in one, seizures and severe psychomotor retardation also developed. In the same study, 11 other children were identified and followed up because they presented with symptoms. All 11 had been asymptomatic at birth. In this group, major neurologic sequelae developed in three, five were blind in both eyes, and three were blind in one eye. Ocular involvement may not begin until the end of the first decade. More recently, the impact of antenatal diagnosis, antenatal treatment, and treatment during infancy has decreased the frequency of major neurologic sequelae.

CONGENITAL MALARIA

The incidence of malaria in the United States and North America increased during the 1980s and 1990s because of increasing overseas travel, immigration, and the spread of drug-resistant parasites. Infections have involved all four species of *Plasmodium* infecting humans. The incidence in endemic areas has been estimated to be 0.3%, with disease more likely when a mother acquires malaria for the first time during pregnancy and in primigravidas. The risk of transfusion-acquired malaria in the United States from 1972 to 1981 was 0.25 per million donor units. Transfusion has been infrequently associated with malaria infection in neonatal intensive care units.

The mother may or may not have symptomatic malaria during pregnancy, and cases have been described in which maternal disease was acquired not in an endemic area but through intravenous drug use or transfusion. In most instances, however, the history of exposure to malaria is clear. The child is usually normal at birth. Symptoms appear at 3 to 12 weeks of age. Fever is followed by hepatosplenomegaly, loss of appetite, listlessness, progressive hemolytic anemia, diarrhea, and jaundice.

The diagnosis is normally confirmed by demonstration of characteristic parasites on a thin or thick blood smear, and the particular species is determined by the morphologic appearance of the stained forms. Serologic studies can be used to confirm the diagnosis. If intrauterine transmission occurred, IgM antibody may be present in cord blood.

Congenital malaria, like transfusion-acquired malaria, has no exoerythrocytic (liver) stage. When the organism is chloroquine sensitive, therefore, chloroquine alone (5 mg/kg of base by mouth or gavage daily for 5 days) is adequate for treatment, and primaquine is not required. Chloroquine pharmacokinetics has been studied in children, and the drug can be used in infants who do not tolerate enteral treatment. Parenteral chloroquine (0.83 mg of base per kg per hour for 30 hours intravenously, or 3.5 mg/kg every 6 hours by intramuscular or subcutaneous injection) provided there is an acceptable therapeutic ratio. When chloroquine resistance is suspected, multiple drugs may be necessary, including parenteral quinidine gluconate or alternatively, exchange transfusion.

Not every child of every mother with malaria requires treatment at birth, because most will not acquire the disease. When maternal malaria is recognized at parturition, the infant should be followed up carefully, and treatment instituted, if necessary. Blood transfusion is frequently necessary in affected children, and, in areas with a high frequency of HIV infection, these transfusions put congenitally infected children at increased risk for HIV infection. In a recent comparison of 260 children born to HIV-seropositive women with 327 children born to seronegative mothers over a 13-month period, there was no evidence that malaria was more frequent or more severe in children with progressive HIV infection, and malaria did not appear to accelerate the progression of HIV disease.

Follow-up blood smears should confirm that treatment has been successful. In such instances, the prognosis is excellent.

Prevention of malaria during pregnancy represents a high priority for travelers from nonendemic areas as well as women from endemic areas. Even though no chemoprophylactic regimen is completely effective because of differences in drug resistance, timing of infection during pregnancy, and other currently incompletely understood factors, chloroquine is a safe, well-tolerated, and effective drug for chemoprophylaxis. Travel to areas in which chloroquine-resistant *Plasmodium falciparum* malaria is endemic should be avoided.

SPIROCHETAL INFECTIONS

CONGENITAL SYPHILIS

The organism responsible for syphilis is *Treponema pallidum*. This delicate, corkscrew-shaped, flagellated, highly motile spirochete is almost identical in appearance to *Treponema pertenue*, which causes yaws. These two diseases, like smallpox and cowpox, produce a cross-immunity for one another. This fact was established for Alexander Schaffer, the first editor of this textbook, when, after having spent 2 years on yaws-infested Fiji without encountering one case of syphilis, he was transferred to yaws-free India, where syphilis became one of his main medical preoccupations.

Syphilis can be acquired by introduction of *Treponema* through an abrasion in the skin or mucous membrane or by transplacental transmission. Whereas adults and some children become infected percutaneously, young infants almost invariably receive the organism from their mothers via the placenta and the umbilical vein. Transplacental transmission may take place at any time during gestation but ordinarily occurs during the second half of pregnancy. Fetuses infected early may die in utero or are at high risk for significant neurodevelopmental morbidity. The impact of the current epidemic on potentially preventable fetal deaths has not been evaluated. The usual outcome of a third-trimester infection is the birth of an apparently normal infant who becomes ill within the first few weeks of life. Whereas virtually all infants born to women with primary or secondary infection have congenital infection, only 50% are clinically symptomatic. Because of increasing pressure from managed care organizations for early discharge of new mothers, which has occurred during the current epidemic, identification of congenitally infected, asymptomatic infants whose maternal infections occurred late in the third trimester and whose syphilis serologic tests are not yet positive at the time of delivery has presented an unusually difficult problem for tracking and treatment. It is critical that all infants undergo serologic testing for syphilis at the time of delivery. Early latent infection results in a 40% infant infection rate, and late latent infection results in a 6% to 14% infant infection rate.

Because *Treponema* enters the fetal bloodstream directly, the primary stage of infection is completely bypassed. There is no chancre and no local lymphadenopathy. Instead, the liver, the immediate target of the invasion, is flooded with organisms, which then penetrate all the other organs and tissues of the body to a lesser degree. Exactly where they take root and arouse local pathologic response, which in turn produces the presenting signs and symptoms, is unpredictable. Principal sites of predilection are the liver, skin, mucous membranes of the lips and anus, bones, and the central nervous system. If fetal invasion has taken place early, the lungs may be heavily involved in a characteristic *pneumonia alba*, but this condition is seldom compatible with life. *Treponema* may be found in almost any other organ or tissue of the body but seldom causes inflammatory and destructive changes in loci other than the ones named previously.

The earliest sign of congenital syphilis may be snuffles. The nose becomes obstructed and begins to discharge clear fluid at first, then purulent or even sanguineous material later. Cutaneous lesions appear at any time from the 2nd week on. They are sparse or numerous and are copper-colored, round, oval, iris-shaped, circinate, or desquamative. Even more characteristic than their appearance is their distribution, which most frequently includes perioral, perinasal, and diaper regions. Palms and soles are also involved, but the rash is soon replaced there by diffuse reddening, thickening, and wrinkling. In heavily infected infants, the rash may become generalized. Mucocutaneous junctions become involved in typical fashion. The lips become thickened and roughened and tend to weep. Radial cracks appear that traverse the vermilion zone up to and a bit beyond the mucocutaneous margins of the lips. These are the beginnings of the radiating scars that may persist for many years as rhagades. Similar mucocutaneous lesions involve the anus and vulva, but in these locations, the white, flat, moist, raised plaques known as "condylomata" are also encountered, although less frequently.

Radiographs of the bones reveal characteristic osteochondritis and periostitis in 80% to 90% of infants with symptomatic congenital syphilis. In most, the bone lesions are asymptomatic, but in a few, they are severe enough to lead to subepiphyseal fracture and epiphyseal dislocation, and extremely painful pseudoparalysis of one or more extremities may supervene. In a recent study by Brion and coworkers, 12 of 59 asymptomatic, congenitally infected infants had metaphyseal changes consistent with congenital syphilis. Radiographic alterations include an unusually dense band at the epiphyseal ends, below which is a band of translucency whose margins are at first sharp but which later become serrated, jagged, and irregular. The shafts become generally more opaque, but spotty areas of translucency throughout them may give them a moth-eaten look. The periosteum of the long bones becomes more and more thickened. Epiphyses separate because the dense end plate breaks away from the shaft by fracture through the subepiphyseal zone of decalcification. This is exactly what happens in the pseudoparalysis of scurvy, although the reason for the weakening of the subepiphyseal bone is different. In syphilis, pseudoparalysis appears within the first 3 months of life; in scurvy, it seldom presents before 5 months of life.

Signs of visceral involvement include hepatomegaly, splenomegaly, and general glandular enlargement. Palpable epitrochlear nodes are not pathognomonic but are highly suggestive of congenital syphilis. The liver may be greatly enlarged, firm, and nontender. Associated with this may be jaundice, which appears in the 2nd or 3rd week of life, is seldom intense, and does not persist for many days. Anemia, probably indicative of bone marrow infection and hematopoietic suppression, may become severe. Lesions in the gastrointestinal tract and pancreas may occur and produce distention and delay in passage of meconium.

Clinical signs of central nervous system involvement seldom appear in the newborn infant, even though one third to one half of those infected suffer such involvement. This is demonstrated by cerebrospinal fluid changes of increased protein content, by a mononuclear pleocytosis of up to 200 or 300 cells/mm^3, or by positive Venereal Disease Research Laboratories (VDRL) test. Additional diagnoses associated with congenital syphilis are non-immune hydrops, nephrosis, and myocarditis.

Diagnosis is confirmed by dark-field visualization of *Treponema* in scrapings from any lesion or from any body fluid, by characteristic bone changes on radiographs, and by positive serologic tests for syphilis. These tests must be interpreted with caution, however. Because the IgG portion of reagin is transmitted across the placenta, its finding in the baby's serum means no more than that the mother has or has had syphilis. She may have been cured during pregnancy and yet still have quantities of reagin in her blood or she may not have received treatment at all and still not have passed the disease on to her fetus. A higher titer in the infant's blood than in the mother's is not evidence of fetal infection, nor is an elevated concentration of total IgM in the cord serum.

The most helpful specific test is a positive finding in the newborn's blood of IgM antibody against

TABLE 5–2
Recommended Treatment of Pregnant Patients with Syphilis

Stages of Syphilis	Drug	Dose
Early (<1 yr duration)	*Recommended*	
Primary, secondary, or early latent		
HIV antibody negative	Benzathine penicillin G°	2.4 million units IM single dose; possibly repeat in 1 week
	Procaine penicillin G	600,000 units IM daily × 10–15 days
HIV antibody positive	Procaine penicillin G	1.2 million units IM daily × 15 days
	Aqueous penicillin G	4 million units every 4 hr × 15 days
	Alternative	
	Erythromycin°	500 mg qid × 15 days orally
	Penicillin desensitization†	

Latent (>1 yr duration)

Recommended

Benzathine penicillin G   2.4 million units IM weekly × 3 weeks
Procaine penicillin G   600,000 units IM daily × 15 days

Alternative

Erythromycin‡   500 mg qid × 30 days orally
Penicillin desensitization†

---

*Use currently discouraged; offspring should be given penicillin.
†For details, see Centers for Disease Control and Prevention: Guidelines for the prevention and control of congenital syphilis. MMWR Morb Mortal Wkly Rep 37:S1, 1988.
‡After neurosyphilis is excluded.
HIV, human immunodeficiency virus; IM, intramuscularly.
From Ingall D, Dobson RM, Musher D: Syphilis. In Remington JS, Klein JO (Eds): Infectious Diseases of the Fetus and Newborn Infant. Philadelphia, WB Saunders, 1990, p 387.

TABLE 5–3
Recommended Treatment of the Newborn with Syphilis

Maternal Rx	Clinical Findings	Drug (Penicillin G)	Dose (50,000 units/kg)
None or inadequate	Present or absent	Aqueous or procaine	IM or IV daily × 10 days in 2 divided doses IM daily × 10 days
Adequate	Absent	Benzathine (only if follow-up cannot be ensured)	IM single dose

IM, intramuscularly; IV, intravenously.
From Ingall D, Dobson SRM, Musher D. Syphilis. *In* Remington JS, Klein JO (Eds): Infectious Diseases of the Fetus and Newborn Infant. Philadelphia, WB Saunders, 1990, p 388.

T. pallidum, IgM-FTA-ABS (fluorescent treponemal antibody absorption). This is fluorescent *Treponema* antibody from which antibodies from treponemes other than *T. pallidum* have been removed by absorption. If positive, this finding is usually an indicator of congenital syphilis, although in the presence of rheumatoid factor, false-positive tests are occasionally seen. However, this test is not always positive at first, even when infection is present in the infant, possibly because, if the infection is acquired late in pregnancy, specific antibodies do not have time to form.

Thus, when an infant's blood VDRL is positive at birth, the diagnosis of congenital syphilis is not justified unless pathognomonic signs are also present. If they are not, serial determinations of reagin titer must be performed. If antibodies are passively acquired, the titer decreases to zero within 4 to 12 weeks; it increases if the disease is actually present. If the IgM-FTA-ABS test is also positive at birth, treatment may be initiated. If the test is negative, however, it should be repeated several times at 3- or 4-week intervals.

Treatment is recommended for all pregnant women regardless of the stage of pregnancy (Table 5–2). Recommendations from the CDC for treatment of symptomatic or asymptomatic infants are listed in Table 5–3.

CHAPTER 6

Respiratory System

CONTROL OF BREATHING

APNEA OF PREMATURITY

Apneic spells usually seen in infants are episodic and random. Episodes prolonged for 20 seconds or more or those accompanied by bradycardia or color change are considered significant. Infants with significant apnea of prematurity do not perform as well on neurodevelopmental follow-up as similar premature infants without recurrent apneas. The diagnosis of apnea of prematurity can be made only after exclusion of all other causes of recurrent apnea. The incidence of apneic spells is inversely related to gestational age. Although commonly stated otherwise, apneic episodes frequently start on the 1st day of life. In some infants, only bradycardia is recognized, but polygraphic recordings indicate that bradycardia is nearly always preceded by apnea. It is thought that 40% of the episodes are central or diaphragmatic, 10% are obstructive, and 50% are mixed, which may indicate either obstructive followed by central apnea or central followed by obstructive apnea. In an individual infant, one type tends to dominate. Central apneas tend to be shorter, whereas obstruction tends to prolong the episode and accelerate the onset of bradycardia. Obstructive apneas are particularly common on the 1st day of life in premature infants.

It was once thought that bradycardia was not related to hypoxemia but rather had a central brain stem origin or was a reflex response to the cessation of lung inflation. However, investigators have now concluded that episodes of bradycardia are associated with oxygen desaturation. Bradycardia is likely a peripheral chemoreceptor response to hypoxemia.

A number of theories have been considered for central, diaphragmatic, and obstructive apnea. The neurons of the central pattern generator are poorly myelinated and have a reduced number of dendrites and synaptic connections, thus impairing the capability for sustained ventilatory drive. Prolonged auditory conduction times have been demonstrated in infants with apnea, a problem assumed to reflect the function of the medulla in general. Along similar lines, because infants with apnea of prematurity have a deficiency of catecholamine excretion in the urine, others have suggested a neurotransmitter deficiency. Infants with apnea of prematurity have a decreased ventilatory response to CO_2 inhalation in comparison with premature infants of the same gestation without apnea of prematurity.

The chest wall of premature infants is highly compliant, so considerably more work is performed to generate adequate tidal ventilation. This results in substrate depletion and diaphragmatic failure from fatigue. Evidence for fatigue has been shown by examination of the diaphragmatic electromyogram.

There is some evidence that the diaphragm may activate before the upper airway abductors, which would predispose to upper airway closure during inspiration. The same problem may occur if abductor activation is insufficient. Because airway obstruction imposes a load on the inspiratory muscles, the ability to load-compensate is important. It has been shown that load compensation is poor in small premature infants and increases as term is approached. The poor load compensation is due to the highly compliant chest wall and the presence of an intercostal phrenic inhibitory reflex, which is activated by chest distortion and which shortens the duration of inspiration. This problem predisposes to obstructive apnea, especially under conditions of excessive neck flexion, when the upper airway tends to narrow, and in the supine position, when the tongue falls backward.

Relation to Sleep State

Most apneas occur during active sleep and are less common during states of quiet sleep or wakefulness. During active sleep, there is a low-voltage electrocortical state, decreased arousal from sleep, decreased muscular tone, absence of upper airway adductor activity, decreased respiratory drive, irregular breathing, and inspiratory chest wall distortion. The loss of chest wall muscle tone and airway adductor activity causes a 30% reduction in lung volume and a decreased arterial Po_2. Reduced ventilatory drive causes a slight elevation in arterial Pco_2. The ventilatory response to hypoxia is depressed during active sleep, much more than in quiet sleep. The ventilatory sensitivity to CO_2 is also thought to be more depressed in active sleep. The newborn and premature infant is asleep 80% of the time, compared with the adult who is asleep for 30% of the time. More than 50% of sleep is active in the small premature infant, and the mature amount of 20% is not reached until 6 months of age.

Treatment

All infants at risk for apnea should have a heart rate monitor, which should be continued until the infant is at least 34 weeks' postconceptional age or after that time until the infant has been free of bradycardia for 1 week. Heart rate monitors are preferred because apnea without bradycardia is not significant apnea, obstructive apnea with bradycardia is detected reliably, and false alarms are infrequent. Most monitors in the neonatal intensive care unit also include an apnea monitor; the principal objections to the apnea monitor alone are that it misses obstructive apnea and may confuse bradycardia with breathing. It has become common to monitor with pulse oximetry because of the importance of both oxygen desaturation and heart rate.

Because respiratory center output is dependent on general neuronal traffic, cutaneous stimulation is effective. It is reasonable to maintain the patient in the prone position because in this position there is a significant reduction in the duration of episodes of desaturation and bradycardia. Even in larger premature infants near hospital discharge, there may be advantages to the prone position in the form of improved oxygenation and a better ventilatory response to hypercarbia. However, by discharge we train the mothers to have babies subsequently sleep on their backs to reduce risk of the sudden infant death syndrome. Because diaphragmatic fatigue has been implicated, it is essential to maintain the circulation and a general state of good nutrition; the infusion of amino acids may increase the ventilatory response to hypoxia and hypercarbia.

If the patient is hypoxemic, oxygen supplementation is essential, but there is no evidence that significant apnea is reduced if the patient is hyperoxygenated, and harm to the immature retina may be inflicted with such a strategy. Pulse oximeters vary in their ability to detect hyperoxemia ($PaO_2 > 90$ mm Hg), but in one commonly used instrument, Adams and coworkers (1994) found that setting the upper limit at 95% detected nearly all instances of hyperoxemia. If the infant must be given occasional bag-mask ventilation, it is important to ensure that the oxygen concentration remains stable and is not increased. Because an oxygen hood interferes with access to the infant, many centers prefer to use nasal cannulas to administer oxygen, usually at a flow of 1 to 2 L per minute and with blended humidified oxygen to maintain the pulse oximeter reading in the range of 92% to 95% saturation. Some evidence suggests that nasal cannula therapy may cause improvement in chest wall distortion, less asynchrony between chest and abdomen, and therefore a more efficient breathing strategy.

Most infants are treated with methylxanthines, which have been demonstrated to be effective in controlled trials. Because caffeine produces less tachycardia, has a more favorable therapeutic index, and produces less erratic blood level fluctuations, it may be preferred over theophylline. Either drug may be given for 2 weeks and then stopped to observe whether apnea has ceased, or it may be continued until 32 to 34 weeks' postconceptional age, by which time the problem of apnea has frequently resolved. Methylxanthines may increase

CO_2 sensitivity, decrease diaphragmatic fatigue, and improve load compensation. Methylxanthines reduce the ventilatory depression following hypoxia by blocking adenosine receptors. Others have suggested that theophylline increases the activity of the peripheral chemoreceptors in term infants.

The other mainstay of treatment is nasal continuous positive airway pressure (CPAP). Although the effect of 5 cm H_2O should be tried, frequently as much as 8 to 10 cm H_2O is necessary for satisfactory control; this may be because many of these infants have chest cage insufficiency and a low lung volume. Infants may be fed by continuous gastric infusion during this procedure. The chest radiograph should be reviewed periodically to avoid overdistending the lungs. It has been postulated that CPAP provides increased ventilatory drive by directly stimulating the pulmonary stretch receptors, but this hypothesis could not be confirmed in premature infants.

Cyanotic Spells Without Apnea in Preterm Infants ($\dot{V}/\dot{Q}$ Spells)

About 15% of premature infants have episodes of bradycardia, which are associated with appropriate nasal air flow but significant oxygen desaturation. The rate at which oxygen desaturation develops is even more rapid than during apnea. The likely cause of this phenomenon is sudden $\dot{V}/\dot{Q}$ mismatching secondary to peripheral airway dysfunction. The latter may respond to CPAP therapy or increased positive end-expiratory pressure (PEEP) if the infant is on a ventilator, but this is not proven. Investigators have described episodes of severe oxygen desaturation without bradycardia, without apnea, and without squirming motions, but they were not sure of the cause; they suggested that premature infants less than 32 weeks' gestation should be monitored with pulse oximeters until at least 36 weeks' postconceptional age.

Bolivar and coworkers (1995) described episodes of oxygen desaturation in premature infants on mechanical ventilation; these episodes were preceded by increased esophageal pressure as a result of active expiratory efforts, produced, it was thought, during efforts at crying. The presence of an endotracheal tube prevented the larynx from closing and allowed the lung volume to decrease suddenly, causing a decrease in lung compliance and an increase in airways resistance; then continued mechanical ventilation or spontaneous breathing was relatively ineffective during a period of severe oxygen desaturation. Bolivar and coworkers suggested that increased PEEP might be effective, that further sedation might prevent the attempts at crying, or that extubation would allow the larynx to function properly to maintain the lung volume.

SYMPTOMATIC RECURRENT APNEA

Apnea is a frequent manifestation of general problems in newborn and premature infants. The more common ones are as follows: (1) local infection such as a scalp abscess; (2) bacteremia or septicemia; (3) necrotizing enterocolitis; (4) hypoxic-ischemic encephalopathy; (5) intracranial hemorrhage, posthemorrhagic hydrocephalus, and periventricular leukomalacia; (6) patent ductus arteriosus with a large left-to-right shunt; (7) gastroesophageal reflux; (8) hypoglycemia; (9) hypocalcemia; (10) anemia; (11) drugs or anesthesia; (12) environmental overheating; (13) any condition causing hypoxemia or hypovolemia; and (14) upper airway obstructions such as nasal stenosis, choanal atresia, or vocal cord paralysis. These should be excluded and appropriately treated before a diagnosis of apnea of prematurity is made.

CONGENITAL HYPOVENTILATION SYNDROME

Although this uncommon condition is more frequently described in older infants, the severe form occurs in newborns and may need attention in the delivery room or the newborn nursery. These infants have significant hypoventilation with small tidal volumes and prolonged apneas while asleep but tend to have more normal ventilation while awake. There is little evidence of a response to asphyxia, so severe oxygen desaturation and hypercarbia develop without signs of an increased effort to breathe. Because the arousal responses may be present but the ventilatory responses to hypoxia and hypercarbia are absent, it is thought that this condition is caused by a failure to integrate signals from the central and peripheral chemoreceptors into the respiratory centers. The head sonogram, the head computed tomography scan, and the head magnetic resonance imaging scan are usually normal; the auditory brain stem responses may be abnormal. No respiratory stimulant drugs have been found effective, at least in the severe newborn type, and most infants must be treated by prolonged home mechanical ventilation with a tracheostomy. Phrenic nerve pacemakers may be useful sometimes, but because the upper airway muscles are not activated by the phrenic nerve, a tracheostomy is still necessary. Initially the ventilator may be needed for much of the day, but there may be some improvement at about the age of 6 months, after which the infant may need the ventilator only at night while sleeping. Some of these infants may have Hirschsprung disease, a dysautonomia syndrome, or a neuroblastoma, suggesting a more widespread problem. Seizure disorder, mild cerebral atrophy, and developmental delay may occur, possibly as a result of multiple asphyxial episodes. Many families cope with these children surprisingly well, and some of the children may even go to school.

APNEA OF INFANCY

Isolated apneas of 5 to 15 seconds, with or without periodic breathing, occur commonly in term infants during the first 6 months of life. There is no associated bradycardia or color change, and the episodes resolve spontaneously. Certain infants have significant apneas, usually more than 20 seconds' duration but sometimes shorter and associated with bradycardia or color change. These too usually resolve spontaneously. The diagnosis of apnea of infancy is reserved for those with onset after 38 weeks' gestation, to distinguish them from infants with apnea of prematurity persisting until 42 weeks' postconceptional age.

Usually after discharge from the nursery, some infants with apnea of infancy have an acute life-threatening event (ALTE), requiring resuscitation by vigorous stimulation or positive-pressure ventilation. Apnea of infancy is just one cause of an ALTE, perhaps representing 50% of the cases. Other causes include (1) gastroesophageal reflux, (2) pharyngeal incoordination, (3) convulsions, (4) infection, (5) heart disease, (6) breath-holding spells, (7) central hypoventilation syndrome, (8) central nervous system abnormality, and (9) accidental or intentional smothering by the mother. Many infants with an ALTE, after appropriate investigation to exclude other causes, are considered to have *near-miss sudden infant death syndrome*. Investigation of these infants, by a 24-hour recording of their breathing, reveals that they have an increased incidence of periodic breathing, brief apneas and prolonged apneas, when compared with control infants. It is not clear if the infants had the same abnormalities before their ALTE. Nevertheless, a significant number of these infants later die suddenly.

SUDDEN INFANT DEATH SYNDROME

Sudden infant death syndrome (SIDS) describes the sudden death of an infant, which is unexplained by history, by a thorough death scene investigation, and by an adequate autopsy. Death occurs during sleep, most commonly during the night. The incidence in the United States is generally 2 per 1000 live births. It is a major cause of infant mortality, with a peak incidence between 2 to 4 months. One hypothesis has been that these infants die from obstructive apnea and that they have apnea of infancy before their demise.

In fact, infants with apnea of infancy, diagnosed by pneumogram, have only a slightly increased risk of SIDS over that in the general population, except if they experience an ALTE, when the risk increases to 4%. If they have several ALTEs, the risk is enormous. Only 7% of infants with SIDS, however, have a preceding ALTE. Nonselected infants destined to die of SIDS do not have a breathing pattern, based on 24-hour recordings, that is significantly different from the breathing pattern of closely matched infants who do not die of SIDS. Infants with SIDS seldom have a prior diagnosis of apnea of infancy or persistent apnea of prematurity. It seems reasonable to conclude that the apnea hypothesis for SIDS remains unproved and that SIDS and apnea of infancy should be considered separate problems.

HOME APNEA MONITORING PROGRAMS

There remains some controversy about whether some infants should have apnea monitoring at home. Parents must be skilled in the use of the monitor, in the interpretation of frequent false alarms, and in cardiopulmonary resuscitation. There is no evidence that home apnea monitoring reduces the number of deaths, and the incidence of SIDS remains unchanged despite the use of home monitors.

Barrington and associates (1996) performed a pneumogram on small premature infants believed to be ready for discharge from intensive care. In a few with worrisome apneas, discharge was delayed until the recordings improved, but in the end most infants had less worrisome apneas recorded just prior to discharge, and all infants were sent home without a home apnea monitor. During 6 months follow-up, only 3 of 176 infants had an ALTE, and the predischarge pneumogram could not distinguish these 3 from the others without an ALTE. The only justification for the predischarge pneumogram is that it may detect undiagnosed apneas; however, the significance of such apneas is currently unknown.

A national survey showed that the home apnea monitor is not the standard of care, and there is no evidence that the home apnea monitor strategy prevents any deaths; it may, however, be cost-effective in comparison with continued hospitalization, and it may be unwise to alienate an anxious and insistent family.

PRONE SLEEPING POSITION

There is evidence that the prone sleeping position is associated with an increased incidence of SIDS. An American Academy of Pediatrics Task Force on sleeping position and SIDS recommended that infants should sleep in the supine or lateral position. The relative risk of SIDS in the prone position ranges from 3.5 to 9.3 in seven reported studies; no study has reported a relative risk of less than 1.0. Critical review of reports from several countries has shown that previously observed large reductions in the SIDS rate with supine or lateral positioning were sustained over time and that further reductions in the incidence of prone positioning were accompanied by further reductions in the incidence of SIDS. It was concluded that the supine position was not associated with an increase in complications such as upper airway obstruction or aspiration pneumonia.

The decreased incidence of SIDS is more marked with supine than with lateral positioning. While asleep, the infant placed in the side position may roll into the prone position. The American Academy of Pediatrics recommendations may or may not be appropriate for premature infants, those with significant gastroesophageal reflux, or those with craniofacial abnormalities such as the Pierre Robin syndrome or laryngomalacia.

Infants in the normal newborn nursery should be placed in the supine or lateral position. Premature infants should be encouraged to lie in this position before being discharged, unless they are still having significant apnea of prematurity. Mothers should be appropriately advised of the advantages of the supine position.

No consensus on the cause of the problem with prone positioning has been developed. Chiodini and Thach (1993) showed that the prone position may be associated with rebreathing and hypoxia; this is especially true when the infant assumes a persistent face-down position, a not uncommon occurrence, and when the infant sleeps on soft bedding rather than on a firm mattress; the same authors could find little evidence for the development of any airway obstruction, however. Kahn and coworkers (1993) demonstrated that the prone position was associated with a longer duration of sleep, a larger amount of deep sleep, and significantly fewer and shorter arousals from sleep; it seems possible that arousal from sleep may be an important protective mechanism against SIDS, which always occurs during sleep.

RESPIRATORY DISTRESS IN THE NEWBORN

HYALINE MEMBRANE DISEASE

Hyaline membrane disease (HMD), frequently referred to as *respiratory distress syndrome* (RDS), occurs after the onset of breathing in infants with insufficiency of the pulmonary surfactant system.

There are an estimated 40,000 cases of HMD annually in the United States, about 14% of all low-birth-weight infants. The incidence is 60% at 29 weeks' gestation but declines with maturation to near 0 by 39 weeks. The condition is more common in male than in female infants; it is more common in white than in nonwhite infants. At each level of gestational age, RDS is less common in black infants, and this phenomenon is not explained by other factors that may influence lung maturity. At any given gestational age, the incidence is higher for cesarean section without labor than for vaginal delivery. There is a significantly increased risk if elective cesarean section is performed before completion of 39 weeks' gestation.

When corrected for the important effect of gestational age, the occurrence of HMD is significantly increased in gestational diabetes and in insulin-dependent mothers without vascular disease. Most such infants of diabetic mothers are large for gestational age, and similar overnourished infants in the absence of maternal diabetes are also at increased risk. Evidence suggests that the incidence of RDS in infants of diabetic mothers is now much less, almost certainly because of improved medical control of diabetes.

Early reports in comparatively large infants suggested that the risk is decreased in infants who are small for gestational age; however, in much less mature infants seen, comparisons of appropriate-for-gestational-age and small-for-gestational-age infants, both weight matched and gestation matched, suggest that immature small-for-gestational-age infants do not have this advantage. In fact, there is some evidence that the risk of RDS at constant gestational age may be increased in small-for-gestational-age infants and that the mortality may be higher. Maternal conditions that compromise fetal growth and may produce decreased risk include pregnancy-induced hypertension, chronic hypertension, subacute placental abruption, narcotic addiction, and maternal smoking.

Suggestions that birth asphyxia predisposes to HMD are based on lower Apgar scores in human infants with RDS and some experimental evidence in lambs. In an examination of umbilical artery blood at birth, however, it was found that infants with RDS are not more acidemic at birth and that lower Apgar scores associated with RDS are better explained by relative immaturity and defective lung function.

The gross findings at autopsy in infants dying without mechanical ventilation include diffuse lung atelectasis, congestion, and edema. If the lungs are inflated at postmortem examination, distensibility is greatly reduced, and the lungs collapse more readily with deflation. On histologic examination, the peripheral air spaces are collapsed, but more proximal respiratory, bronchioles, lined with necrotic epithelium and hyaline membranes, have an overdistended appearance. There is obvious pulmonary edema with congested capillaries, and the lymphatic and interstitial spaces are distended with fluid. The epithelial damage appears within 30 minutes of the onset of breathing, and the hyaline membranes, composed of plasma exudation products and associated with damaged capillaries, appear within 3 hours of birth. In experimental animals, the bronchiolar lesions may be completely prevented and the leakage of protein may be considerably reduced by the administration of surfactant at birth. This finding has led to the conclusion that the bronchiolar lesions are secondary to atelectasis in terminal air spaces and to disruptive overdistention of more proximal airways.

In HMD, the respiratory rate is elevated, so despite a reduction in each tidal volume, the minute ventilation initially is increased. The functional residual capacity, analyzed by nitrogen washout, is reduced; the greater the need for oxygen, the smaller is the measured value for functional residual capacity. In keeping with the reduced static lung compliance found at autopsy, the static lung compliance measured by multiple airway occlusions during exhalation is also markedly reduced, the average value being only 0.5 mL/cm H_2O/kg. As a result, the work of breathing is greatly increased. Measurements of airway resistance suggest values in the normal range, but there is a tendency toward an increase. Edberg and coworkers found decreased compliance, increased resistance, decreased lung volume, and reduced gas mixing efficiency in very-low-birth-weight infants with RDS. From these data, it can be approximated that the overall time constant in HMD would be less than 0.05 second. Because the patency of small peripheral airways depends on proximal spread of surfactant, in some regions of lung the local time constants may be more prolonged.

The Aa-DO_2 and right-to-left shunt while breathing 100% oxygen are greatly increased, many infants having values for shunt in the range of 50% to 90% of cardiac output. Because there is no evidence for a diffusion limitation, it is commonly stated that large shunts at the foramen ovale and ductus arteriosus and in atelectatic lung constitute the only cause of severe hypoxemia in HMD. If this were true and the shunt were 50%, changing inspired oxygen would have little effect on arterial oxygen pressure, and oxygen therapy would be relatively ineffective. In fact, precipitous falls in arterial oxygen tension occur if inspired oxygen is reduced. This phenomenon indicates the presence of an open, poorly ventilated lung compartment with extremely low $\dot{V}/\dot{Q}$, representing a significant portion of the lung and producing variable hypoxic vasoconstriction and alterations in right-to-left shunt as the inspired oxygen changes. Therefore, in infants with HMD, the severity of arterial hypoxemia is directly related to the size of the open, poorly ventilated compartment. The relationship among $\dot{V}/\dot{Q}$, alveolar oxygen tension, and changing inspired oxygen indicates how oxygen as high as 90% is required before the oxygen pressure in low $\dot{V}/\dot{Q}$ units rises significantly. Because perfusion of the open, extremely low $\dot{V}/\dot{Q}$ compartment is greatly reduced by hypoxic vasoconstriction, it makes only a small contribution to cardiac output, and measurements of aA-DN_2 are not greatly increased in HMD. It should not be overlooked that this lung compartment makes a significant contribution to the oxygenation defect in HMD.

Measurements of aA-DCO_2 and alveolar dead space are markedly increased in HMD. Although minute ventilation is increased, the alveolar ventilation is actually decreased, as reflected by the elevated values for arterial CO_2 tension. Because a large part of the lung is collapsed or poorly ventilated, most alveolar ventilation is diverted to a relatively small part of the lung, represented by the reduced functional residual capacity. Because this compartment is small, it is relatively overventilated, so the $\dot{V}/\dot{Q}$ and the measured aA-DCO_2 are high. Measurements of pulmonary blood flow, using the disappearance of gases that enter ventilated parts of the lung, confirm that perfusion of ventilated lung is low. Therefore, in HMD three lung compartments are prominent: shunt, open low $\dot{V}/\dot{Q}$, and high $\dot{V}/\dot{Q}$. Under conditions of changed inspired oxygen and changed levels of CPAP, there is a close correspondence between predicted and measured values for aA-DCO_2, suggesting the validity of this model.

In infants with RDS undergoing treatment in a neonatal intensive care unit, the pulmonary artery pressure declines more slowly after birth than in preterm infants without RDS. The systemic artery pressure is maintained similar to that in controls and tends to rise slowly with time; by 24 hours, the systemic artery pressure is well above the pulmonary artery pressure. Extrapulmonary right-to-left shunting at the foramen ovale or the ductus arteriosus disappears by 24 hours, and left-to-right shunting at the ductus arteriosus is common by age 24 hours. As the pulmonary artery pressure continues to fall with time, the ductal shunt assumes greater importance. In preterm infants without RDS, the ductus arteriosus tends to close within 4 days of birth, whereas in RDS the ductus tends to remain open and may become a significant problem by 3 to 4 days of age or sooner after surfactant treatment.

The infant with HMD is almost always premature. There is rapid or labored breathing, beginning at or immediately after birth. Infants usually have a characteristic grunt during expiration, caused by closure of the glottis, the effect of which is to maintain lung volume and gas exchange during exhalation. Frequently the unventilated infant requires 40% to 50% oxygen after birth but then develops an increasing oxygen requirement over 24 to 48 hours; this may reach as high as 100%. In other infants, the oxygen requirement transiently decreases as acidosis or hypothermia is corrected or fetal lung fluid is cleared; the oxygen requirement begins to increase only after 3 to 6 hours. More severely affected infants have an immediate high oxygen requirement that progresses rapidly to 100% and without mechanical ventilation, they may die within 24 hours. Another group of larger infants needs less oxygen initially and manifests a slowly progressive course of generalized atelectasis over 48 to 72 hours. The urine output is low for the first 24 to 48 hours, but soon after this time a diuresis ensues. If HMD is uncomplicated, recovery starts after 48 hours. The decline in oxygen requirement is relatively rapid after 72 hours, and usually oxygen can be discontinued after 1 week. The very-low-birth-weight infant (< 1500 g) usually requires mechanical ventilation and has a more prolonged course. A few infants with RDS (often the more mature premature infants with a greater than 1500-g birth weight) have persistent pulmonary hypertension of the newborn (PPHN); they are easy to ventilate, especially after exogenous surfactant, but are difficult to oxygenate.

Infants with HMD have a moderate to severe oxygenation defect, significant hypercarbia, and a mild metabolic acidosis with elevation of blood lactate. The lecithin/sphingomyelin (L/S) ratio and phosphatidylglycerol (PG) remain low in serial tracheal aspirate samples for 48 hours, then increase with recovery; the saturated phosphatidylcholine (PC) levels remain low in RDS and reach normal levels after 4 to 7 days; the surfactant protein A (SP-A)/saturated PC (SPC) ratio is low in RDS and is even lower in infants destined to develop bronchopulmonary dysplasia (BPD). SP-A in tracheal aspirate samples is low in infants with RDS, remains low for 3 to 4 days, and then rises in survivors but remains low in nonsurvivors.

Diffuse, fine granular densities that develop during the first 6 hours of life are seen on the chest radiograph; these densities are influenced by size of the infant, severity of disease, and degree of ventilatory support. The appearance may be more marked at the lung bases than at the apices. The lung volume may appear normal early, especially if the infant is strong enough to overdistend less affected regions, but ultimately the lung volume is decreased. Positive airway pressure frequently obliterates these diagnostic findings. Other conditions, such as pneumonia or pulmonary edema, may have a similar appearance.

HMD is primarily a developmental deficiency in the amount of surface-active material at the air-liquid interface of the lung, as demonstrated by pressure-volume curves with air and saline in infants who died from HMD. Saline extracts of minced lung have higher surface tension than do controls as described in a classic paper by Avery and Mead in 1959. Infants with HMD may synthesize adequate amounts of SPC but cannot package and export it to the alveolar surface in a way that makes it function as surfactant. In infants who die, deMello and associates have demonstrated the complete absence of tubular myelin and a modest deficiency of lamellar bodies in type 2 cells in comparison with controls.

Infants who die with RDS have a deficiency of immunostained SP-A in the endoplasmic reticulum and lamellar bodies of the type 2 cells. It is not established that infants with RDS have a deficiency of surfactant protein B (SP-B), but infants with genetic SP-B deficiency have severe RDS that differs from classic RDS in that it is accompanied by an alveolar proteinosis–like chest radiograph (see SP-B Deficiency).

Surfactant function in infants with HMD is inhibited by a variety of proteins and other factors that leak into the respiratory bronchioles at the sites of overdistention and epithelial damage. Fibrinogen, hemoglobin, and albumin are potent inhibitors of surfactant. It is of critical importance to the lungs to have adequate surfactant at the gas-liquid interface from the earliest possible moment after birth; otherwise, acute lung injury and surfactant inhibition supervene rapidly and contribute to a cycle of worsening disease. Thus, RDS is associated with a developmental deficiency of surfactant at birth, but associated lung injury results in surfactant dysfunction as well.

While studies of surfactant in infants with HMD have shown its importance, other features of lung immaturity may contribute to the disease, especially in the more immature premature infants, for example, incomplete alveolarization; underdeveloped capillary bed; small compliant airways; increased interstitial space; and decreased clearance of alveolar fluid.

Because HMD is a problem of insufficient lung maturity, the best way to prevent it is to prevent premature birth; for this purpose, the effective strategies are thought to be cervical cerclage, discovery and treatment of bacteriuria, and liberal use of tocolytics. At present, however, the two major approaches to the problem are (1) prediction of the risk for HMD by antenatal testing of amniotic fluid samples and (2) antenatal treatment of women in preterm labor with glucocorticoid hormones to accelerate fetal lung maturation.

Before birth, the surfactant system can be assessed in amniotic fluid because some fetal lung fluid enters the amniotic cavity. The most common material measured is lecithin or PC, in particular, SPC. Because changes in amniotic fluid volume may alter the concentration of SPC, it is standardized to the concentration of sphingomyelin, which remains relatively constant throughout gestation; it is expressed as the L/S ratio.

In normal pregnancy, the L/S ratio displays a remarkably stable pattern, increasing slowly to 1 at 32 weeks, rising more rapidly to 2 at 35 weeks, and accelerating rapidly thereafter. In abnormal pregnancy, there is much wider scatter, reflecting conditions that accelerate or decelerate lung maturation. The ratio may reach 2 as early as 28 weeks or remain at 1 until close to term. The incidence of HMD is only 0.5% for an L/S ratio of 2 or more but 100% for an L/S ratio less than 1; between 1 and 2, the risk of HMD decreases progressively. Elective cesarean section delivery of infants having an unrecognized low L/S ratio carries an unnecessary risk of HMD.

The appearance time of PG may be accelerated or delayed in the same way as the L/S ratio. The presence of PG at 1% of total phospholipid indicates a remarkably low risk for HMD, less than 0.5%. If a patient has both an L/S ratio of less than 2 and a PG of less than 1%, the risk for HMD is greater than 80%. Besides an L/S ratio below 1, this combination is the best predictor of HMD available to the clinician. In certain pregnancies characterized by diabetes and Rh isoimmunization, the L/S ratio has proved less reliable, the risk of HMD at a value between 2 and 3 still being approximately 13%. In those with both an L/S ratio above 2 and PG of 1% or more, however, the risk has been reduced to 0. There are other factors to be considered in the interpretation of the L/S ratio: A low L/S ratio carries a much smaller risk at a more advanced gestation, and in black infants the risk of RDS is low with an L/S ratio of more than 1.2.

A rapid test for the evaluation of amniotic fluid

samples is the foam stability test, in which samples of variable dilution are shaken with 95% alcohol and the tubes examined for stable foam. A modification of this shake test is the stable microbubble test, in which stable bubbles are counted under the microscope; fewer than 5 stable microbubbles/mm^2 is considered positive for RDS. This test has been found to have a positive test predictive value of 95% to 100% and a negative test predictive value of 85% to 90%. This test is rapid and inexpensive and may be adapted to tracheal aspirate samples after birth.

A vast literature on the usefulness of corticosteroid hormones on lung and surfactant maturation has accumulated. Since 1972, when Liggins and Howie described decreased mortality, decreased incidence of RDS, and less severe RDS in a prospective blinded study done in New Zealand, more than 23 clinical studies have been published worldwide. Not all of these studies have been of appropriate size, and not all have been of sufficient quality to exclude the problems of bias and error; this has resulted in widespread misinterpretation of the results and a regrettable underuse of glucocorticoid therapy.

Meta-analyses of all trials indicate that maternal steroid therapy significantly reduced the incidence of RDS, intraventricular hemorrhage, necrotizing enterocolitis, and neonatal death; in addition, they concluded that the duration and costs of hospital care for the newborn infant were greatly decreased. The benefits applied to all infants at a gestational age of 24 to 34 weeks, and this was not affected by race or gender or by the presence of prelabor rupture of amniotic membranes.

Recommendations of a National Institutes of Health (NIH) panel are as follows: (1) All fetuses between 24 and 34 weeks' gestation are candidates for this therapy; (2) the decision should not be influenced by race, gender, premature rupture of membranes, or anticipated surfactant therapy; (3) all patients eligible for tocolytic therapy should receive steroids; (4) because therapy for less than 24 hours is effective, all patients should be treated unless immediate delivery is anticipated; (5) patients of less than 30 weeks' gestation should be treated because of the reduction in intraventricular hemorrhage; (6) treatment may be withheld in the presence of overt amnionitis; (7) treatment consists of betamethasone, 12 mg every 24 hours for two doses, or dexamethasone, 6 mg every 12 hours for four doses.

Prenatal glucocorticoids appear to have several other beneficial effects in the small preterm infant. Some investigators have found a lowered incidence of intraventricular hemorrhage. A significant reduction in the incidence of clinically significant patent ductus arteriosus occurs with prenatal betamethasone therapy. The incidence of BPD is reduced in preterm infants exposed to prenatal corticosteroids. This appears logical in view of the evidence relating RDS, especially severe RDS, to the occurrence of BPD. Other effects observed in animal models include decreased pulmonary protein leaks, induction of rat lung antioxidant enzymes, and acceleration of renal function in the fetal lamb.

The results for prenatal steroid therapy can be further improved; the effects of prenatal steroid and exogenous surfactant therapy proved to be additive. The effect of prenatal steroids has been retrospectively analyzed in the large number of infants enrolled in the many large controlled trials of exogenous surfactant performed in the last 10 years. The beneficial effects of steroids are clearly apparent in populations that have also been treated with exogenous surfactant.

Treatment

Because secretion of surfactant is improved by expansion of the lungs at birth, many believe that it is appropriate to intubate all infants weighing less than 1000 g at birth and to initiate mechanical ventilation with PEEP (Positive End-Expiratory Pressure) in the delivery room. Similar treatment may be used for larger premature infants if they have respiratory distress or are not vigorous in the delivery room.

Infants less than 1000 g birth weight should be treated prophylactically with exogenous surfactant within 15 to 30 minutes of birth after adequate stabilization. Larger infants should be treated as early as possible, preferably before the age of 2 hours and certainly before the age of 6 hours. A mammalian surfactant is currently preferred. The dose should be 100 mg/kg, the interval between doses should be 12 hours, and two to three doses should be given but omitted when the inspired oxygen decreases below 30%. The dose should be given as rapidly as possible followed by bag-tube ventilation to ensure even distribution, but it should not be given so rapidly as to obstruct the airways and promote hypercarbia; the number of aliquots for each dose does not matter, 2 aliquots being as good as 4 aliquots. Although widely practiced, there is little evidence to support rotation and tilting of the patient during the procedure. After surfactant instillation, it is customary to maintain the patient on conventional mechanical ventilation, but Verder and coworkers have demonstrated that larger infants may be extubated to nasal CPAP (Continuous Positive Airway Pressure) and the need for endotracheal intubation and conventional mechanical ventilation reduced.

Infants with HMD require monitoring of blood pressure, blood gases, electrolytes, calcium, and glucose. Blood samples may be obtained from an umbilical arterial catheter.

Oxygen therapy is beneficial, despite the presence of large right-to-left shunts. Increased inspired oxygen produces (1) a rise of alveolar oxygen pressure in open low $\dot{V}/\dot{Q}$ units, (2) relief of regional hypoxic vasoconstriction in this compartment, (3) a reduction in true right-to-left shunt, and (4) an increase of arterial oxygen saturation.

Because HMD is characterized by high surface tension pulmonary edema and high permeability pulmonary edema, fluid restriction is indicated for many infants with HMD for the first 48 hours or until the onset of diuresis. Close attention should be paid to fluid intake, urine output, urine concentration, and serum electrolytes. Premature infants have an excess of extracellular fluid and are expected to lose at least 10% of body weight by the end of the 1st week of life. It is not necessary or beneficial to administer sodium in the first day of life. Potassium should also be restricted because hyperkalemia may be troublesome. In the very immature infant (24 to 26 weeks' gestation) with extremely permeable skin, there may be excessive evaporative losses, and much higher amounts of fluid may be required. If the serum sodium rises sharply (greater than 140 mEq/L) it can be assumed that insensible water losses through the skin are excessive, and the fluid intake should be liberalized accordingly. To minimize insensible water losses, it is useful to manage the infant in a humidified incubator; alternatively, if the infant is on an open warmer, it is useful to place a transparent plastic cover across the infant and across the sides of the bassinet and to run a gentle flow of heated mist into the infant's microenvironment.

Manipulations, such as heel sticks, tracheal suctioning, diaper changes, and even weighing, should be kept to a minimum because these procedures have been shown to reduce arterial oxygen tension; they probably also increase oxygen consumption and may contribute to the genesis of cerebral hemorrhage by rapidly raising arterial blood pressure to excessive levels. It is not appropriate to give enteral feedings to infants with HMD because this condition is usually accompanied by poor intestinal motility. Many centers now insert an umbilical vein catheter as well as an arterial catheter and use the venous catheter to infuse glucose and the arterial catheter to infuse saline.

Premature infants with RDS frequently have a low arterial blood pressure in the first 12 hours of life, as defined by normative data. Many extremely-low-birth-weight infants with RDS probably have a low blood pressure for many days after birth, and this may predispose them to brain injury. In small premature infants without intraventricular hemorrhage, the normal mean blood pressure is more than 30 mm Hg during the 1st week of life. Intraventricular hemorrhage is more common in those who have a mean blood pressure less than 30 mm Hg, and a mean blood pressure less than 30 mm Hg is more common in those who develop an intraventricular hemorrhage.

Adequate oxygenation may be difficult in the

presence of hypotension and reduced pulmonary blood flow. In infants with a low hematocrit, poor peripheral perfusion, and metabolic acidosis, the hypotension is often due to hypovolemia and responds to a cautious infusion of 10 or 20 mL/kg of saline, human plasma protein fraction (Plasmanate), or blood. Only a few infants have obvious signs of hypovolemia, however, and echocardiographic studies in small premature infants have shown that many have decreased cardiac contractility, which is reflected in a poor cardiac output and significant hypotension. If there are no signs of hypovolemia, the infusion of dopamine at 5 to 10 μg/kg per minute is usually effective at increasing the mean blood pressure. A randomized, controlled trial of Plasmanate versus dopamine in hypotensive preterm infants showed that only 45% responded to Plasmanate, whereas 89% responded to dopamine. Others have suggested that dopamine is superior to dobutamine for the correction of hypotension in small premature infants.

Many small preterm infants with RDS have low cortisol levels, and their hypotension is corrected with hydrocortisone. Dexamethasone often corrects the low blood pressure in these infants after an interval of 6 to 12 hours. One of the many benefits of prenatal corticosteroid therapy is that the mean blood pressure is higher in treated infants.

Severe metabolic acidosis may increase pulmonary vascular resistance, impair surfactant synthesis, reduce cardiac output, and ultimately reduce ventilation. An early trial showed that continuous infusion of glucose-bicarbonate solutions reduced the mortality of HMD. With the introduction of better methods for oxygenating infants, however, bicarbonate therapy no longer appears to have much benefit, and it may be harmful by increasing risk of intracranial hemorrhage.

CPAP may be administered by endotracheal tube, endopharyngeal tube, nasal prongs, face mask, or head box, or it may be administered by negative pressure applied around the body with the airway at atmospheric pressure. Since it was first described, CPAP has been shown to reduce mortality in infants who weigh more than 1500 g and to reduce the requirements for oxygen and mechanical ventilation in all infants with RDS.

Nasal prong CPAP of 5 cm H_2O may be started early for any signs of RDS; this approach is used in many hospitals, even for the tiniest infants, with the expectation that some infants will avoid intubation, mechanical ventilation, lung injury, and perhaps chronic lung disease. There may be some evidence for this approach, in that these hospitals may have a lower incidence of BPD than other hospitals. It may be possible to improve this strategy; some centers that use nasal CPAP in this way have suggested that in larger infants it is reasonable to intubate for surfactant administration and to mechanically ventilate briefly, while surfactant distribution is completed, and then to extubate the infant and continue with nasal CPAP. In a controlled trial, it was shown that the subsequent requirement for intubation and mechanical ventilation was significantly reduced with the addition of exogenous surfactant to the early nasal CPAP strategy.

Because CPAP may overdistend the lung and impair the pulmonary circulation, attempts have been made to identify optimal levels. As CPAP is increased and approaches optimum, the aA-D_{CO_2} falls significantly, but as the optimal level is exceeded, both the aA-D_{CO_2} and the arterial P_{CO_2} rise significantly. Under clinical conditions, increased hypercarbia may indicate excessive CPAP, which should be recognized and corrected before oxygenation deteriorates.

Infants with HMD who weigh less than 1500 g and infants treated with exogenous surfactant usually require mechanical ventilation. Otherwise the standard indications are (1) significant apnea, (2) hypercarbia with pH less than 7.20, and (3) arterial oxygen pressure under 50 mm Hg in 80% to 100% oxygen. There is no agreement on the settings for rate, peak pressure, inspiratory time, or PEEP, but the principles should not be in doubt. The aim is to correct the blood gas abnormalities with as little lung injury and circulatory compromise as possible. Because the time constant in RDS is short, long inspiration times are not necessary and may be associated with pulmonary air leaks. Oxygenation is dependent on the level of mean airway pressure; in a condition characterized by low lung volume and low lung compliance, it is efficient to use generous levels of PEEP. Many clinicians allow modest hypercarbia to avoid excessive peak pressures and tidal volumes; it is high tidal volumes that injure the lung, not high peak pressures. Under isocarbic conditions, smaller tidal volumes can be used if the rate is higher. If the infant's breathing is asynchronous, especially if the blood pressure is low, it is common to find that the blood pressure wave fluctuates.

Especially in infants less than 1000 g birth weight, a patent ductus arteriosus may contribute significantly to the overall problem during recovery from RDS and may predispose the infant to the development of BPD. If the ductus is demonstrated to be patent at the age of 3 to 4 days by two-dimensional echocardiography and pulsed Doppler ultrasonography, the evidence suggests that it is unlikely to close spontaneously within a reasonable time, and therefore it should be closed, either with indomethacin therapy or with surgery. In infants under 1000 g, many neonatologists start indomethacin within 12 hours of birth for intraventricular prophylaxis as well as for its effects on ductal closure.

The chances of survival in HMD are directly related to birth weight and gestational age and are affected by prenatal treatment with glucocorticoids, by surfactant replacement therapy, and by the severity and complications of the disease.

TRANSIENT TACHYPNEA OF THE NEWBORN

Transient tachypnea of the newborn (TTN) is also known as *delayed clearance of fetal lung fluid*. In 1966, Avery and coworkers reported on eight near-term infants with early onset of respiratory distress whose chest radiographs showed hyperaeration of the lungs, prominent pulmonary vascular markings, and mild cardiomegaly. The respiratory symptoms were transient and relatively mild, and most infants improved within 2 to 5 days. The investigators named the disorder *transient tachypnea of the newborn* and speculated that it was the result of delayed clearance of fetal lung liquid.

Most authors agree with Avery and coworkers that TTN represents a transient pulmonary edema resulting from delayed clearance of fetal lung liquid. Clearance of the fetal lung liquid actually begins before birth (during the last few days of gestation and during labor). During the first step of this process, secretion of lung liquid is inhibited by increased concentrations of catecholamines and other hormones. Then reabsorption occurs: passively, secondary to differences in oncotic pressure between the air spaces, the interstitium, and blood vessels, and actively, secondary to active transport of sodium out of the air space. Infants born prematurely or those born without labor do not have the opportunity for early lung liquid clearance, and they begin their extrauterine life with excess water in the lungs. After birth, water in the air spaces moves rapidly to the extra-alveolar interstitium, where it pools in perivascular cuffs of tissue and in the interlobar fissures. It is then cleared gradually from the lung by the lymphatics or by absorption directly into the small blood vessels. Infants with TTN, however, are often hypoproteinemic, and decreased plasma oncotic pressure may delay the direct absorption of water into the blood vessels. In addition, these infants can have elevated pulmonary vascular pressures and ventricular dysfunction, which increase central venous pressure and impair thoracic duct function and the removal of interstitial water by the lymphatics. This is especially true in infants who receive a large transfusion of blood from the placenta as a result of delayed cord clamping or milking of the cord.

The symptoms of TTN may result from compression of the compliant airways by water that has accumulated in the perivascular cuffs of the extra-alveolar interstitium. This compression results in airway obstruction and hyperaeration of the lungs secondary to gas trapping. Hypoxia results from the continued perfusion of poorly ventilated lung units; hypercarbia results from mechanical interference with alveolar ventilation and from central nervous system depression. Lung function measurements in infants with TTN are compatible with airway obstruction and gas trapping. The functional residual capacity measured by gas dilution is normal or reduced, whereas measurements of thoracic gas volume by plethysmography are increased, suggesting that some of the gas in the lungs is not in communication with the airways.

It was initially thought that TTN was limited to term or larger preterm infants, but it is now clear that small infants also may present with pulmonary edema from retained fetal lung liquid. This may complicate their surfactant deficiency and account for some of their need for supplemental oxygen and ventilation. There is often a history of heavy maternal sedation, maternal diabetes, or delivery by elective cesarean section. Affected infants may be mildly depressed at birth, and this may mask many of their early symptoms. They are often tachypneic with respiratory rates ranging from 60 to 120 breaths/min and may have hyperinflation with grunting, chest wall retractions, and nasal flaring.

Arterial blood gas tensions often reveal a respiratory acidosis, which resolves within 8 to 24 hours, and mild to moderate hypoxemia. These infants seldom require more than 40% oxygen to maintain an adequate PaO_2 and usually are in room air by 24 hours of age. They have no evidence to indicate right-to-left shunting of blood at the ductus arteriosus or foramen ovale.

Chest radiographs reveal hyperaeration, which is often accompanied by mild cardiomegaly. Water contained in the perivascular cuffs produces prominent vascular markings in a *sunburst pattern* emanating from the hilum. The interlobar fissures are widened, and pleural effusions may be present. Occasionally, coarse, fluffy densities may be present, indicating alveolar edema. The radiographic abnormalities resolve over the first 2 to 3 days after birth.

As its name implies, TTN is a benign, self-limited disease. The infant's need for supplemental oxygen is usually highest at the onset of the disease then progressively decreases. Infants with uncomplicated disease usually recover rapidly without any residual pulmonary disability. Although the symptoms of

TTN relate to pulmonary edema, one controlled trial that assessed therapy with diuretics found no evidence for their efficacy; however, many infants respond to nasal CPAP.

PERSISTENT PULMONARY HYPERTENSION OF THE NEWBORN

Successful transition from intrauterine to extrauterine life requires that the pulmonary vascular resistance decrease precipitously at birth. In infants with persistent pulmonary hypertension of the newborn (PPHN), this decrease does not occur: Pulmonary arterial pressure remains elevated, and blood is shunted right to left across the ductus arteriosus and foramen ovale. In addition, the persistently high pulmonary vascular resistance increases right ventricular afterload and oxygen demand and impairs oxygen delivery to the right ventricle, the posterior wall of the left ventricle, and the subendocardial regions of the right ventricle. Ischemic damage resulting from this reduction in oxygen delivery may cause both right and left ventricular failure, papillary muscle necrosis, and tricuspid insufficiency. Finally, increased right ventricular afterload results in displacement of the septum into the left ventricle, impaired left ventricular filling, and reduced cardiac output.

Active constriction of pulmonary vessels can complicate the course of bacterial sepsis, meconium or bacterial pneumonia, or RDS in the newborn. Experiments in animals show that this increase in pulmonary vascular resistance is temporally related to increased plasma thromboxane concentrations; it can be blocked by the administration of inhibitors of prostaglandin synthesis.

Anatomic abnormalities of the pulmonary vascular bed fall into two general categories: those associated with underdevelopment of the lung and those that result from maldevelopment of the vessels. In the case of pulmonary hypoplasia, lung mass is reduced, yet cardiac output is appropriate for body size. As a result, the volume of blood flowing through the existing pulmonary vessels is relatively high, pulmonary arterial pressures are high, and relative pulmonary vascular resistance is increased. In addition to this anatomic impediment to flow, infants with pulmonary hypoplasia are likely to have maldevelopment of the pulmonary vessels and an increased pulmonary vascular resistance from anatomic obstruction of existing vessels.

Premature closure of the ductus arteriosus secondary to maternal ingestion of inhibitors of prostaglandin synthesis has been associated with PPHN. In two groups of infants with idiopathic PPHN, those without ductal level shunting had higher salicylate levels than those with ductal level shunting. Experiments in animals show that premature closure of the ductus results in maldevelopment of pulmonary vessels, presumably by forcing a greater portion of the combined ventricular output through the lungs at a significantly higher pressure.

One of the more important functions of the vascular endothelium is to produce the vasodilator nitric oxide (NO). NO is produced in endothelial cells from L-arginine by the enzyme NO synthase. It diffuses rapidly into smooth muscle cells where it stimulates production of cyclic guanosine monophosphate (GMP) and smooth muscle relaxation. NO production by endothelial cells is responsible for the vasodilation that occurs in response to substances such as acetylcholine and bradykinin. As a result, these mediators are called *endothelial cell–dependent vasodilators*. Because NO is such a potent pulmonary vasodilator, it is tempting to speculate that impaired NO synthesis contributes to PPHN. In support of this speculation, investigators have shown that infants with PPHN have lower urinary nitrite and nitrate concentrations than do infants without pulmonary disease, suggesting that their ability to produce NO may be impaired.

In addition to production of the vasodilator NO, endothelial cells also produce endothelin 1, which may act as a pulmonary vasoconstrictor in the newborn. Infants with PPHN have increased concentrations of endothelin 1 in arterial blood. These concentrations correlate with the severity of the pulmonary hypertension.

Affected infants are usually delivered at term or

post-term and frequently are born through meconium-stained fluid. They are often thought to be normal after brief distress at birth. Then within the first 12 hours after birth, they are recognized as having cyanosis and tachypnea without apnea and retractions or grunting. They frequently have a cardiac murmur that is compatible with tricuspid insufficiency, but systemic blood pressure is normal. Hypoglycemia frequently complicates many of the associated conditions, such as sepsis and meconium aspiration; hypocalcemia also occurs often. Arterial blood gas tensions reveal severe arterial oxygen desaturation with relatively normal CO_2 tensions. In infants with significant ductal level shunting, the oxygen saturation measured from the right brachial or radial artery is greater than that obtained from the umbilical artery. Chest radiographs may reveal cardiomegaly. For infants with idiopathic PPHN, the lung fields are clear and appear undervascularized. For the remainder of the associated entities, chest radiographs reflect the underlying parenchymal disease. Electrocardiograms reveal ventricular hypertrophy appropriate for age; in more severe cases, they also reveal ST segment depression in the precordial leads, suggestive of ischemia. All infants suspected of having PPHN should undergo ultrasound examination of the heart to rule out cyanotic congenital heart disease, to document right-to-left shunting of blood at the foramen ovale and ductus arteriosus, and to measure systolic time intervals. Prolonged systolic time intervals support a diagnosis of pulmonary hypertension, but they are not definitive because they also can be prolonged by right ventricular dysfunction. Infants in whom cyanotic congenital heart disease cannot be ruled out by echocardiogram should undergo cardiac catheterization. At some point in the course of the disease, most infants with PPHN increase SaO_2, at least transiently, in response to some therapeutic intervention. Infants who can never be oxygenated should be considered for cardiac catheterization.

The objectives for therapy for infants with PPHN are to lower the pulmonary vascular resistance, to maintain the systemic blood pressure, to reverse the right-to-left shunts, and to improve arterial oxygen saturation and oxygen delivery to the tissues. Based on results from several centers suggesting that conservative medical management of infants with PPHN may reduce the need for extracorporeal membrane oxygenation and improve outcome, the authors have adopted an approach to therapy that seeks to reduce oxygen demand while maximizing oxygen delivery.

All of these infants should be nursed in a neutral thermal environment. Cold stress raises the metabolic rate, increases oxygen consumption, and causes the infant to release norepinephrine, which is a pulmonary vasoconstrictor. Fluids should be restricted and hypoglycemia and hypocalcemia corrected. Systemic hypotension and acidosis should be corrected by judicious use of blood and alkali. Calcium, blood products, and hyperosmolar solutions are potentially vasoactive and should be infused with caution in this group of infants. Infusion of dopamine at low doses (2 to 10 μg/kg/min) may increase cardiac output without affecting systemic or pulmonary vascular resistance. At higher doses, dopamine exhibits considerable α-adrenergic activity and may result in systemic vasoconstriction and increased blood pressure along with an actual reduction in cardiac output. In addition, higher doses of dopamine can constrict pulmonary as well as systemic vessels. If the central hematocrit is greater than 60% to 65%, a partial exchange transfusion should be performed to lower the hematocrit and to reduce the effects of hyperviscosity on the pulmonary artery pressure.

In infants with PPHN, the pulmonary circulation seems to be exceptionally sensitive to changes in oxygen tension. Therefore, it is advisable to try to maintain the PaO_2 between 80 and 100 mm Hg if possible. There is no evidence to suggest that maintaining PaO_2 in excess of 100 mm Hg improves the outcome of the infant with PPHN, and prolonged exposure to excessively high PaO_2 can injure other organs, such as the brain and the eye. Furthermore, in patients with severe PPHN, attempts to maintain PaO_2 between 80 and 100 mm Hg may result in unacceptable complications of therapy. Therefore, many centers now tolerate much lower values for PaO_2 ($\geq$40 mm Hg) in infants with severe PPHN and use repeated measurements of blood lactate and pH to provide insurance of adequate tissue oxygenation.

Oxygen should be given by hood, up to 100% if necessary. If oxygen alone does not lower the pulmonary vascular resistance and improve arterial oxygen saturation, the next step is to induce alkalosis. Although several studies in animals have shown that both respiratory and metabolic alkalosis effectively lower pulmonary vascular resistance, only respiratory alkalosis has been studied in infants. The use of neuromuscular blockers such as pancuronium bromide in these infants is controversial and should probably be reserved for infants requiring extremely high inspiratory pressures. Because these infants are extremely sensitive to external stimuli, they should be sedated with either morphine or fentanyl and handled as little as possible. To avoid alveolar overdistention, the inspiratory time is kept short (0.15 to 0.20 second). The lungs of infants with PPHN frequently have normal to prolonged expiratory time constants, so expiratory time must be kept relatively long to prevent gas trapping. Therefore, the respirator rate is set at 60 to 80 breaths/min. Inspiratory pressure is adjusted to control the $PaCO_2$. PEEP is useful only in patients with parenchymal lung disease. If the pulmonary hypertension is severe, however, the infant frequently develops surfactant deficiency and pulmonary edema and consequently may respond to end-expiratory pressure later in the course of the disease.

After 3 days of ventilation with high concentrations of oxygen and high airway pressures, infants with PPHN develop pulmonary parenchymal abnormalities that are characterized by decreased lung compliance and infiltrates on chest radiograph compatible with pulmonary edema. At this point, the pulmonary vascular bed is no longer sensitive to changes in pH and much less sensitive to changes in FIO_2. This probably is in part the result of vascular remodeling that occurs in these infants.

Both high-frequency jet ventilation and high-frequency oscillator ventilation are highly effective in controlling $PaCO_2$. As a result, several groups have postulated that these ventilatory modalities may be effective in improving oxygenation in infants with PPHN when associated with parenchymal disease. High-frequency jet ventilation results in a reduction in both $Paco_2$ and ventilator pressures in infants with PPHN but has no effect on ultimate outcome. In a single randomized trial, high-frequency oscillator ventilation was more successful than conventional ventilation in reducing the need for extracorporeal membrane oxygenation in this patient population.

Data suggest that surfactant deficiency may play a role in several of the diseases associated with PPHN. Meconium aspiration pneumonia and bacterial pneumonia are both associated with surfactant inactivation, and surfactant replacement therapy improves gas exchange in these infants. Infants with congenital diaphragmatic hernia appear to have delayed maturation of the pathways for surfactant synthesis. Preliminary data from studies in lambs with diaphragmatic hernia suggest that administration of exogenous surfactant may improve outcome.

Several studies have shown that inhalation of NO in concentrations ranging from 5 to 80 ppm selectively dilates pulmonary vessels and improves oxygenation in infants with PPHN. As discussed previously, NO is an important regulator of vascular tone, and an inability to generate NO or respond to NO may underly some of the conditions associated with PPHN.

Tolazoline was at one time the drug most commonly used to try to dilate the pulmonary vascular bed. It is an α-adrenergic blocker with some mild cholinergic properties and is also a potent releaser of histamine, which, in the newborn, is a pulmonary, vasodilator. Its effects are not specific for the lung. In one study, complications referable to tolazoline therapy occurred in 70% of the patients: 42% had increased gastrointestinal secretions, 31% had gastrointestinal bleeding, and 32% developed hypotension. As a result, tolazoline is seldom used to treat infants with PPHN.

In the past, the mortality for infants with PPHN ranged from 20% to 40%, and the incidence of neurologic handicap ranged from 12% to 25%.

In most centers, extracorporeal membrane oxygenation (ECMO) has further reduced mortality from severe PPHN. Data from the ECMO Registry shows that for infants requiring extracorporeal membrane oxygenation because of meconium aspiration pneumonia, sepsis, or idiopathic PPHN, the survival rates are now 93%, 76%, and 83%. The improvement for infants with diaphragmatic hernia has not been as dramatic, and survival is still only 58% for those that require extracorporeal membrane oxygenation. Overall, neurologic morbidity for infants with PPHN requiring extracorporeal membrane oxygenation remains high, nearly 20%.

MECONIUM ASPIRATION PNEUMONIA

Meconium, an odorless, thick, blackish green material, is first demonstrable in the fetal intestine during the 3rd month of gestation. It is an accumulation of debris that consists of desquamated cells from the alimentary tract and skin, lanugo hairs, fatty material from the vernix caseosa, amniotic fluid, and various intestinal secretions. Meconium is biochemically composed of a mucopolysaccharide of high blood group specificity, a small amount of lipid, and a small amount of protein that decreases throughout gestation. Its blackish green color is the result of bile pigments.

Meconium staining of amniotic fluid (MSAF) occurs in roughly 10% to 26% of all deliveries. The risk of MSAF is strongly correlated with gestational age. Before 37 weeks' gestation, the risk of MSAF is less than 2%, whereas the risk after 42 weeks' gestation is nearly 44%.

The cause of MSAF is controversial. At one time, the passage of meconium in utero was thought to be synonymous with fetal asphyxia. At present, however, the correlation between MSAF and fetal asphyxia is not clearly understood. Many studies have failed to show any consistent effects of MSAF on Apgar score, fetal scalp pH, or incidence of fetal heart rate abnormalities. Several studies have suggested that the presence of meconium, especially thick meconium, increases the risk of fetal acidosis and an adverse neonatal outcome. The strong correlation between MSAF and gestational age indicates that: (1) It is possible that the passage of meconium in utero is the result of transient parasympathetic stimulation from cord compression in a neurologically mature fetus. (2) Passage of meconium in utero is a natural phenomenon that reflects the maturity of the gastrointestinal tract. Despite these theories, most physicians agree that MSAF in connection with fetal heart rate abnormalities is a marker for fetal distress and is associated with an increased perinatal morbidity.

Meconium may enter the trachea and airways in utero. In one study, meconium was recovered from the tracheas of 56% of meconium-stained infants in the delivery room. It is likely that meconium is aspirated into the tracheobronchial tree when the fetus begins to gasp deeply in response to hypoxia and acidosis. Data showing that cord arterial pH is lower in meconium-stained infants with meconium in their tracheas at delivery support this hypothesis.

If meconium is not removed from the trachea after delivery, with the onset of respiration it migrates from the central airways to the periphery of the lung. Initially, particles of meconium produce mechanical obstruction of the small airways that results in hyperinflation with patchy atelectasis. Later, small airway obstruction is the result of chemical pneumonitis and interstitial edema. During this later stage, hyperinflation persists, and areas of atelectasis become more extensive. In addition, there is infiltration of the alveolar septa by neutrophils, necrosis of alveolar and airway epithelia, and accumulation of proteinaceous debris within the alveolus.

Infants who die of meconium aspiration pneumonia (MAP) complicated by pulmonary hypertension frequently have evidence of injury to the vascular bed of the lung. In these infants, vascular smooth muscle extends into the walls of normally nonmuscular intra-acinar arterioles and reduces their luminal diameter, which subsequently interferes with the normal postnatal drop in pulmonary vascular resistance. In addition, these infants may demonstrate plugs of platelets in their small vessels that reduce the overall cross-sectional area of the pulmonary vascular bed.

Airway resistance is increased in newborn infants with MAP. In addition, dynamic lung compliance is reduced while static lung compliance is unchanged, suggesting that airway obstruction is patchy and located in peripheral airways. Functional residual capacity is increased in animals with MAP but not in humans.

The effects of meconium on surfactant function have been studied in a number of animal models of meconium aspiration. Meconium inactivates surfactant. Furthermore, several investigators have shown that surfactant replacement improves gas exchange in human newborns with MAP. Hypoxia is the result of continued perfusion of poorly ventilated lung units, whereas hypercarbia is the result of a decrease in minute ventilation and increase in respiratory dead space. Many infants with MAP have concomitant hypertension and right-to-left shunt.

Infants with MAP are often postmature and have visible meconium staining of the nails, the skin, and the umbilical cord. Many infants with MAP have been asphyxiated, and much of the early distress may relate more to asphyxia and retained fetal lung fluid complicated by elevated pulmonary vascular resistance than to the presence of meconium in the airways. Infants with MAP have clinical evidence of lung overinflation, with a barrel chest. Auscultation of the chest reveals diffuse rales and rhonchi. The chest radiograph shows patchy areas of atelectasis and areas of overinflation. Pneumothorax and pneumomediastinum are common. The clinical symptoms progress over 12 to 24 hours as meconium migrates to the periphery of the lung. Because meconium must ultimately be removed by phagocytes, respiratory distress and requirements for supplemental oxygen may persist for days or even weeks after birth. Infants who present with a shorter course and with rapid resolution of symptoms are more likely to have had retained fetal lung fluid than MAP.

Symptomatic infants with meconium suctioned from their tracheas should be given chest physiotherapy and warmed humidified oxygen to breathe.

Lung lavage may result in deterioration of lung function. Because of the high incidence of air leaks, positive-pressure ventilation should be avoided, if possible. Judicious use of nasal or endotracheal CPAP (4 to 7 cm H_2O) may improve oxygenation in the patient who is unresponsive to oxygen administration alone. This improvement in oxygenation is achieved presumably by stabilizing the small airways and improving the ventilation of poorly ventilated lung units. High airway pressures may impair oxygenation by impeding blood flow to well-ventilated lung units. Mechanical ventilation should be reserved for infants with apnea from birth asphyxia or for those who cannot maintain their PaO_2 greater than 50 mm Hg in 100% oxygen. These infants are often large and vigorous and tend to fight mechanical ventilation, which makes oxygenation difficult and increases the chances of air leak. If this occurs, the patient may require neuromuscular blockade. Because MAP is an obstructive lung disease, the time constant for expiration is prolonged in severely involved areas of the lung. Careful attention must be paid to expiratory time (ventilatory rate) to prevent inadvertent PEEP, further gas trapping, and alveolar rupture.

The role of antibiotics in the treatment of MAP is controversial. Meconium enhances bacterial growth by reducing host resistance, and the risk of intra-amniotic infection is increased in the presence of MSAF. No studies have shown that infection plays a role in the pathogenesis of MAP. Because of the difficulty in distinguishing MAP from bacterial pneumonia, the authors routinely treat infants with presumed MAP with antibiotics pending negative cultures.

The use of corticosteroids for treatment of MAP is not recommended at this time. The time for weaning to room air is prolonged by corticosteroids in infants with MAP, and the mortality of rabbits with experimental MAP is increased by treatment with corticosteroids. More recent studies are revisiting whether steroid treatment is of some use in this disease.

As discussed earlier, there is some evidence that

infants with MAP have surfactant inactivation. A recent controlled trial studied the effects of surfactant replacement (up to 4 doses of 150 mg/kg of beractant every 6 hours) on infants that were being mechanically ventilated for MAP. They found that surfactant replacement therapy, if started within 6 hours after birth, improved oxygenation and reduced the incidence of air leaks, severity of pulmonary morbidity, and duration of hospitalization. Other therapies for the infant with MAP and PPHN include the use of high-frequency ventilation, NO, and extracorporeal membrane oxygenation.

In the past, MAP carried a risk of pneumothorax and pneumomediastinum of between 10% and 20%. This risk increased to as high as 50% if the infant required mechanical ventilation. Now with improved approaches to the management of PPHN and the availability of extracorporeal membrane oxygenation, the mortality for infants with MAP is lower. The mortality for infants with MAP requiring extracorporeal membrane oxygenation is less than 7% in most centers and approaches 0 in some units.

The American Heart Association and the American Academy of Pediatrics have recommended a combined obstetric and pediatric approach to the infant with MSAF. For infants born through thin watery meconium, no special management is necessary. For infants born through thick particulate or *pea soup* meconium, they recommend the following steps:

1. When the infant's head is delivered, the mouth, pharynx, and nose should be thoroughly suctioned by the obstetrician using a 10 French or larger suction catheter.
2. As soon as the infant has been placed on the radiant warmer and before drying, the hypopharynx should be visualized and residual meconium removed by suctioning. Then the trachea should be intubated and meconium suctioned from the lower airway. Tracheal suctioning should be performed using an appropriately sized endotracheal tube and a large-bore meconium aspirator. In the presence of

severe asphyxia, it may not be possible to clear the trachea of all meconium, and clinical judgment must be used to determine the amount of suctioning. Intubation and suction is required even when meconium is not visible in the posterior pharynx. Studies have found that 7% to 10% of meconium-stained infants had meconium in their tracheas even when there was not any meconium visible at the vocal cords. A free flow of oxygen should be provided via oxygen tubing to minimize hypoxia during suctioning. After tracheal suctioning, the stomach should be emptied to prevent aspiration of swallowed meconium.

A more recent study questioned the need for intubation and suctioning of *nondistressed* term infants who were born with thick meconium in the amniotic fluid. This study suggested that in the absence of neonatal depression these infants were unlikely to have significant amounts of meconium in their tracheas and that intubation was of no benefit in reducing risk of MAP.

A number of investigators have tried to prevent meconium aspiration by infusing saline into the amniotic cavity of mothers with thick MSAF. Several randomized trials have shown that amnioinfusion decreases the risk of meconium below the vocal cords, and a meta-analysis of five controlled trials found that amnioinfusion decreased the risk of meconium below the vocal cords and the risk of MAP. One large retrospective study and a randomized, controlled trial found no benefit to a policy of routine amnioinfusion.

RESPIRATORY DISTRESS SYNDROME IN TERM INFANTS

It is apparent that a small but significant number of term infants have a severe lung disease, which cannot be described under any of the preceding conditions discussed. It is likely that they represent a heterogeneous group, but they all appear to have a condition characterized by the radiographic appearance of pulmonary edema, they may or may not have experienced clinical asphyxia during the delivery process, and they may or may not have evidence of myocardial failure. Because of the last-mentioned, these conditions may be described under names that emphasize the heart as the primary problem. The infants are usually full-term infants of 38 weeks or more, they may have severe respiratory failure, and they are sometimes candidates for high-frequency oscillator ventilation or extracorporeal membrane oxygenation. There is no evidence for tracheal aspiration of meconium, and bacterial cultures are invariably negative. It is often not possible to be sure of the diagnosis, and clinicians may differ in the diagnosis they assign, but the following conditions represent some of the possibilities.

Postasphyxial Pulmonary Edema

Pulmonary edema in newborn lambs following asphyxia from umbilical cord occlusion was described by Adamson and colleagues (1970). The lambs showed transudation of fluid from the circulation into the lungs in the presence of elevated lung capillary pressures. Infants with this condition are often depressed in the delivery room and require mechanical ventilation immediately or soon after birth. In other infants breathing unassisted, there may be severe respiratory distress because of pulmonary edema, transient cardiomegaly, and cerebral irritation; Strang called this condition *postasphyxial lung edema*. In many infants, there is postnatal evidence of neurologic depression, and there may be seizures, consistent with a background of intrapartum asphyxia. The radiographic appearance of the lungs is that of pulmonary congestion or pulmonary edema with diffuse coarse densities, and in some reports this may be called pneumonia. The heart may be enlarged on the chest radiograph with evidence of mitral or tricuspid valve insufficiency, hypotension, hepatomegaly, poor perfusion, and reduced urine output. On the echocardiogram, there may be evidence of poor myocardial contractability and low cardiac output. Some infants have ischemic changes on the electrocardiogram, and they may have elevated creatine phosphokinase and liver transaminase levels in the blood.

SP-B Deficiency

Several families have been described in which full-term infants developed prolonged and eventually fatal RDS; detailed tissue analysis suggested that they had surfactant protein B (SP-B) deficiency. The parents give no history of neonatal RDS, and many siblings are not affected; the mode of inheritance is autosomal recessive. The condition is now known to be associated with a number of mutations in the SP-B gene; the most commonly described mutation (121 ins 2) involves a 2 base-pair insertion at position 375 in codon 121 of the cDNA; the additional two bases produce a frameshift signal for termination of translation after codon 214. There is no detectable mRNA for SP-B.

The chest radiograph shows the granular pattern characteristic of HMD in preterm infants, and hence these infants may initially resemble other term infants with RDS. There is frequently evidence for severe pulmonary hypertension. The alveolar spaces are packed with a proteinaceous material rich in SP-A and surfactant protein C (SP-C) but poor in surfactant phospholipids; there is no normal tubular myelin because of the SP-B deficiency, and surfactant function assessed by pulsating surfactometer is abnormal. The lamellar bodies in granular pneumocytes are poorly formed, and there may be basal, rather than apical, secretion, indicating defective transport protein signaling within the type 2 epithelial cells.

Oxygen, mechanical ventilation, repeated administrations of bovine surfactant containing relatively high levels of SP-B, and eventually extracorporeal membrane oxygenation have not been successful in changing the outcome. A few infants have survived for several months on mechanical ventilation. More recently, several infants have undergone lung transplantation with apparent success.

PNEUMOTHORAX AND OTHER AIR LEAK PROBLEMS

PULMONARY INTERSTITIAL EMPHYSEMA

Pulmonary interstitial emphysema (PIE) is the result of alveolar rupture from overdistention of alveoli abutting against nonalveolar structures and marginal alveoli. It occurs most commonly in preterm or term infants undergoing mechanical ventilation for some form of parenchymal lung disease. In these infants, distribution of inspired gas is nonuniform, with the bulk of each breath being distributed to the more normal lung units. As a result, these lung units may become overdistended and rupture. Gas trapping from an insufficient expiratory time can also result in alveolar overdistention and rupture. Once alveolar rupture occurs, air is forced from the alveolus into the loose connective tissue sheaths surrounding airways and pulmonary arterioles and into the interlobular septa containing pulmonary veins. The air follows a track along these sheaths to the hilum of the lung, producing the characteristic radiographic appearance of PIE.

PIE increases the volume of gas within the lung parenchyma and splints the lung in full inflation, thereby decreasing lung compliance. Air trapped within the interstitial cuffs compresses airways and increases airway resistance. In addition, air in the interstitial space impairs lymphatic function, allowing fluid to accumulate in the interstitial cuffs and in alveoli. $PaCO_2$ increases, and PaO_2 decreases. The increase in $PaCO_2$ occurs early and is the result of increased respiratory dead space and reduced minute ventilation. The decrease in PaO_2 results in part from reduction in alveolar ventilation and in part from ventilation-perfusion mismatch secondary to mechanical obstruction of airways by interstitial air and edema fluid. It also results from compression of pulmonary arterioles by air in the perivascular cuffs with increased pulmonary vascular resistance and right-to-left shunting of blood.

Once interstitial air reaches the hilum of the lung, it coalesces to form large hilar blebs, or it tracks beneath the visceral pleura to form large subpleural pockets of air. In both instances, these accumulations of air can be large enough to compress normal lung and impair ventilation or cause circulatory embarrassment by encroaching on mediastinal structures.

The cause of PIE is alveolar overdistention and rupture. Therefore, ventilatory techniques that minimize alveolar overdistention would be expected to reduce the risk of PIE. Previous data have shown that increases in inspiratory time are associated with pulmonary air leaks, and controlled trials have shown that techniques for ventilation that rely on shorter inspiratory times decrease the incidence of PIE.

Because the site of the air leak behaves like a check valve, gas trapping occurs and results in further alveolar overdistention and rupture. Therefore, the first step in treatment must be to interrupt this cycle by putting the more severely involved areas in the lung to rest. If PIE is unilateral, this can be done by positioning the infant with the involved side down or by selectively intubating the main stem bronchus on the uninvolved side. If PIE is bilateral, the involved areas can be put to rest by taking advantage of regional differences in time constants in the lung. Areas with PIE have airway compression and long time constants for inspiration and expiration. Mechanical ventilation using short inspiratory times (0.1 second), low inflation pressures, and small tidal volumes are ineffective in inflating these areas of the lung and should not contribute to further gas trapping. Over time, these areas deflate and collapse. It may be difficult to maintain oxygenation and ventilation while selectively underventilating the areas of the lung with PIE. If this happens, it may be necessary to increase the respirator rate to 80 to 100 breaths/min. The advantage of rapid-rate ventilation is that it makes maximal use of the less severely involved lung units and may compensate for the respiratory deterioration associated with selective underventilation of areas with extensive PIE. A multicenter controlled trial found that high-frequency jet ventilation allowed the use of lower peak and mean airway pressures in the treatment of infants with PIE than did rapid-rate conventional ventilation. Furthermore, high-frequency jet ventilation led to more frequent and rapid improvement in PIE than did rapid-rate conventional ventilation.

PIE is a serious complication of mechanical ventilation. Infants who develop PIE have a significantly increased mortality and risk of developing chronic lung disease. In fact, for infants who develop PIE on days 0 or 1 after birth, the gestational age–adjusted odds ratio for risk of dying is nearly 10 to 1 and for developing chronic lung disease is 3 to 1.

PNEUMOMEDIASTINUM AND PNEUMOTHORAX

The incidence of spontaneous pneumomediastinum and pneumothorax in term infants is 1% to 2%, presumably because high transpulmonary pressures exerted at birth, when coupled with some degree of ventilation inhomogeneity, result in alveolar overdistention and rupture. In the presence of underlying lung disease, the incidence of pneumothorax increases dramatically. Ten percent of infants with retained fetal lung fluid develop pneumothorax, as do 5% to 10% of spontaneously breathing infants with hyaline membrane disease. Continuous positive airway pressure does not appear to increase the incidence of pneumothorax in infants with hyaline membrane disease, but positive-pressure ventilation does produce an increase (incidence between 20% and 50% of ventilated infants). Positive-pressure ventilation of term infants with meconium aspiration pneumonia or persistent pulmonary hypertension is associated with an incidence of pneumothorax of roughly 40%.

Pneumomediastinum occurs when air that has tracked through the perivascular and peribronchial cuffs to the hilum ruptures into the mediastinum. From there air can rupture through the mediastinum into the pleural space and produce tension pneumothorax. Available evidence suggests that air in the mediastinum seldom achieves enough tension to cause circulatory embarrassment because as the tension increases, air can dissect into the soft tissues of the neck to produce subcutaneous emphysema or rupture into the intrapleural space. Tension pneumothorax can result in high pressures within the pleural space, collapsing the lung on the involved side and resulting in immediate hypoxia and hypercapnia. In addition, by compressing mediastinal structures and impeding venous return, pneumothorax may result in circulatory collapse.

Pneumomediastinum is usually asymptomatic or associated with mild tachypnea. In the spontaneously breathing infant, however, pneumothorax usually results in clinically significant tachypnea, grunting, irritability, pallor, and cyanosis. The cardiac point of maximal impulse may be shifted away from the pneumothorax, and often the affected hemithorax appears to bulge. Differential breath sounds are unreliable markers of pneumothorax in the infant. Arterial pressure tracings may reveal a reduction in pulse pressure. In the infant on the mechanical ventilator, signs may be more dramatic with sudden onset of hypoxemia and cardiovascular collapse. Transillumination of the chest is increased over the affected side. Pneumothorax should be confirmed by chest radiograph, if at all possible. Needle aspiration of the chest to diagnose pneumothorax relieves acute distress but should be discouraged. If needle aspiration is performed, it should ordinarily be followed by tube thoracostomy.

Asymptomatic or mildly symptomatic spontaneously breathing infants may simply be observed closely until spontaneous resolution occurs. Although allowing infants to breathe 100% oxygen hastens reabsorption of intrapleural air, the risk associated with prolonged hyperoxia limits usefulness of this therapy in preterm infants. Infants with moderate to severe symptoms and all infants receiving positive-pressure ventilation must be treated with tube thoracostomy. Because most mechanically ventilated infants are nursed supine and because gas rises, the tube is usually placed in the second intercostal space in the midclavicular line and directed toward the diaphragm so that the tip lies between the lung and the anterior chest wall. Alternatively, the tube may be inserted at the midaxillary line and directed anteriorly. When placing the tube, one must take care to avoid impaling the lung, especially if a trocar is used to direct the tube rather than curved hemostats. Care must also be taken to avoid placing the tube too far into the chest and compressing mediastinal structures. The thoracostomy tube usually is connected to water seal with 10 to 20 cm H_2O negative pressure and is left in place until it ceases to drain. The negative pressure should be discontinued, and the tube should be left under the water seal for 12 to 24 hours before removal. Infant chest tubes should never be clamped.

Pneumopericardium results from direct tracking of interstitial air along the great vessels into the pericardial sac. Gas under tension in the pericardium impairs atrial and ventricular filling, decreases stroke volume, and ultimately decreases cardiac output and systemic blood pressure. Infants present with increasing cyanosis, muffled heart sounds, and decreased systemic blood pressure. The chest radiograph is diagnostic. Needle aspiration alleviates the acute symptoms, but because recurrence rate is high (53%), continuous tube drainage is frequently necessary. The mortality rate associated with pneumopericardium has been reported to be as high as 75%.

Pneumoperitoneum results from dissection of air from the mediastinum along the sheaths of the aorta and vena cava, with subsequent rupture into the peritoneal cavity. Infants with this condition present with sudden abdominal distention and a typical abdominal radiograph. Occasionally the pneumoperitoneum may be large enough to cause respiratory embarrassment by compromising descent of the diaphragm and may require drainage. A more common problem, however, is the difficulty of distinguishing this cause of peritoneal air from a primary gastrointestinal catastrophe, such as perforated ulcer or necrotizing enterocolitis. Obtaining more than 0.5 mL of green or brown fluid on paracentesis is suggestive of primary bowel disease, especially if bacteria are present on Gram stain. Measurement of the Po_2 of the gas aspirated from the abdomen may also be of some help because it is likely to be high if the gas is of pulmonary origin. A careful upper gastrointestinal series performed with water-soluble contrast material may be of use in distinguishing the cause of intraperitoneal air.

Intravascular air results from air being pumped directly into the pulmonary venous system and occurs only when airway pressure is extremely high (70 cm H_2O). It results in immediate cardiovascular collapse and is often diagnosed when air is withdrawn from the umbilical arterial catheter. Although intravascular air is usually fatal, placing the infant head down on the left side may favor displacement of cerebral emboli.

CHRONIC LUNG DISEASE

BRONCHOPULMONARY DYSPLASIA

The spectrum of patients affected by chronic lung disease (CLD) includes tiny preterm infants who require ventilatory support because of pulmonary structural immaturity as well as infants with severe initial surfactant deficiency. For purposes of uniform reporting, however, the definition of CLD has been changed to *respiratory sequelae in an infant requiring oxygen at more than 28 days after birth or supplemental oxygen at 36 weeks post-conceptual age.*

The incidence of bronchopulmonary dysplasia (BPD) is clearly highest in very-low-birth-weight (VLBW) infants who require mechanical ventilation for severe respiratory distress. The incidence is inversely related to birth weight (75% for survivors weighing 700 to 800 g and 13% for those weighing 1250 to 1500 g). Based on expected survival and estimating that full resolution takes 3 years, one would expect that there are at least 3000 infants with BPD in the United States at any given time. Since the advent of surfactant therapy (1990), more very premature infants are surviving but their chronic lung disease appears less severe.

With the survival of an increasing number of infants of 24 to 26 weeks' gestation, the number of infants with significant BPD has also risen markedly.

Multiple factors predispose to BPD. Even for infants of early gestational age, there is clearly a difference in the maturational level of the lung in infants of certain families compared with those of others. It is also clear that a familial history of asthma and reactive airway disease puts the infant at an additional disadvantage.

Immaturity is clearly a major etiologic factor, whether it is surfactant deficiency that leads to severe hyaline membrane disease or immaturity of the parenchymal structure of the lung or chest wall that contributes to chronic pulmonary insufficiency of prematurity. There is a strong clinical association between BPD and exposure to high concentrations of oxygen. An association between oxygen exposure and lung damage in ventilated and nonventilated infants suggests that even prolonged exposure to 60% oxygen can be toxic to the lungs of newborn infants.

The lung is equipped with antioxidant enzymes to protect it from injury by reactive oxygen. Superoxide dismutases (SODs), located in the mitochondria (Mn SOD), cytosol (Cu Zn SOD), and outside the cells (extracellular SOD), catalyze the conversion of superoxide anion to hydrogen peroxide. H_2O_2 concentrations are kept low by catalase, located in the peroxisomes, and by glutathione peroxidase, located in the cytosol and the mitochondria. Glutathione peroxidase converts H_2O_2 to water in a reaction with glutathione, and is the predominant mitochondrial defense against H_2O_2. Because of its lipid solubility and ability to donate hydrogen atoms, vitamin E is important in stopping the chain reaction of lipid peroxidation in cell membranes. These defense mechanisms develop roughly in parallel with the surfactant system and may be inadequate at birth in preterm infants, especially those with hyaline membrane disease. In particular, recent data suggest that preterm infants may be glutathione deficient at birth and more susceptible to injury by reactive oxygen, even in relatively low oxygen

285

environments. The glutathione content of lung epithelial cells is up to 100 times greater than in the plasma, and this is reflected in high levels in alveolar epithelial lining fluid.

Augmentation of the lung antioxidants by inducing the enzyme systems, or by direct supplementation, may offer some protection from oxygen toxicity. Transgenic mice that overexpress Mn SOD are resistant to oxygen-induced lung injury.

BPD is a disease that made its appearance only after the introduction of positive-pressure mechanical ventilation for premature infants with RDS. Taghizadeh and Reynolds concluded that BPD was due to overdistention of terminal airways by high inflation pressures at a time when the terminal air spaces could not be inflated easily because of surfactant deficiency.

Barotrauma, particularly that associated with high inspiratory pressures, is a major factor in the evolution of lung injury, independent of any injury produced by oxygen. It is characterized by epithelial disruption in the conducting airways and increased capillary permeability to proteinaceous fluid. It is not high pressure alone that causes lung injury but rather high tidal volumes associated with overdistention; for when chest expansion is physically restricted during mechanical ventilation in experimental animals, the inflation pressures remain high, but lung injury is remarkably reduced or absent. It would be more correct to speak of *volutrauma*. Several clinical studies have found an association between hypocarbia and an increased incidence of BPD, suggesting that the peak inflation pressure was too high in relation to the lung compliance. There is a strong association between the occurrence of pneumothorax and pulmonary interstitial emphysema, always associated with lung overdistention, and an increased incidence of BPD. In a multivariate analysis of autopsy data, investigators have found a strong association between the occurrence of pulmonary interstitial emphysema in the first week of life and the occurrence of interstitial cell proliferation/lung fibrosis in BPD infants surviving more than 28 days.

In response to a primary form of injury, oxygen

toxicity or volutrauma, there is an inflammatory response that is reflected in increased numbers of neutrophils in the bronchial lavage samples as early as the second day of life. The bronchial lavage sample neutrophil count peaks on the fourth day of life and then declines rapidly to normal by the end of the first week in those who recover from respiratory distress syndrome (RDS) but declines much more slowly and persists in those who go on to develop BPD. The neutrophils are of neonatal, not maternal, origin, and surfactant therapy does not induce any change in the neutrophil profile during the first week of life.

More specifically, there is the appearance of increasing high levels of neutrophil elastase during the first few days of life in RDS. The neutrophil elastase levels follow the same course as the neutrophils, peaking at 4 days, declining to normal by 1 week in those who recover, and persisting in those who go on to develop BPD. In the bronchial lavage samples during the first week, there are also elevated levels of mediators and cytokines, such as leukotrienes, platelet-activating factor, fibronectin, fibroblast-activating factors, and others; there are elevated levels of interleukins and adhesion molecules; and in one of the earliest responses to injury, there are markedly elevated levels of interleukin 6 in bronchial lavage samples on the first day of life in those destined to develop BPD.

In patients with RDS who recover without BPD, there is a compensatory increase in proteinase inhibitor in the bronchial lavage samples, whereas in RDS which progresses to BPD, there is no such change, and the ratio of elastase to proteinase inhibitor becomes, and continues to be, unfavorable. It is believed that the lung is subjected to elastase and mediator attacks and that this further injury plays an important role in the genesis of BPD.

Later, between 1 and 4 weeks of age, the bronchial lavage samples contain increased levels of additional factors, such as fibronectin, platelet-derived growth factor, tumor necrosis factor, histamine, and others. This is the time when BPD is developing and there is persistent inflammation and persistent high permeability pulmonary edema, aggravated by mediators, chemoattractants, and cytokines. Premature infants with early BPD have higher levels of neutrophils, complement fragments, leukotrienes, and interleukins in the bronchial lavage samples, and increased levels of albumin, which reflect the capillary injury typical of BPD. In addition, the levels of fibronectin in tracheal aspirate samples are elevated in infants with early BPD, and this would favor the development of pulmonary fibrosis, seen in the later stages of BPD.

Some studies have stressed the importance of pulmonary edema, owing to excessive fluid administration, in the genesis of BPD. A controlled trial of fluid restriction in the management of RDS has established that reduced fluid administration is associated with a decreased incidence of BPD. There was a significant reduction in the number of deaths and in the incidence of BPD by radiologic criteria in the fluid-restricted group. In an analysis of three Harvard NICUs in 1992, it was concluded that a major cause of BPD was excessive fluid and colloid administration.

Patent ductus arteriosus (PDA) makes a major contribution to the genesis of BPD by favoring the development of pulmonary edema. Dudell and Gersony showed, in a population of small premature infants with RDS, that if the ductus closed spontaneously at the age of 3 days, then the incidence of BPD was low (22%), but if it remained open at the age of 3 days, the incidence of BPD was significantly higher (68%). However, for therapeutic closure of the PDA, the data are not so convincing. If the ductus was surgically closed at the age of about 1 week, the duration of intubation and hospitalization was greatly shortened. Although there was no documentation that the incidence of BPD was reduced, this study has been widely interpreted to mean that it was. Some studies, in which the ductus was closed with indomethacin given at the age of 3 days, have suggested that the incidence of BPD was reduced, but not all studies have confirmed this.

During the past 10 years, reports have appeared suggesting that organisms such as *Ureaplasma, Chlamydia*, or cytomegalovirus may produce chronic infection and thereby contribute to the pathogenesis of BPD. Cassell and colleagues have claimed that *Ureaplasma* pneumonia is responsible for many cases of BPD, but other studies have not supported this hypothesis. A recent meta-analysis of multiple studies of this problem has suggested that colonization alone with *Ureaplasma* may nearly double the risk for developing BPD. This controversy can be settled only by large prospective therapeutic trials with effective antibiotics.

There is some evidence that premature infants are deficient in vitamin A as a result of too early delivery, that vitamin A is important in the process of epithelial repair in the injured lung, that infants with BPD have more evidence of vitamin A deficiency than infants without BPD, and that attempts to supplement vitamin A are hampered by vitamin A degradation in the intravenous tubing used for parenteral nutrition. In a controlled trial of vitamin A supplementation, Shenai and colleagues found a significant reduction in the incidence of BPD in the treated infants. In a major multi-center controlled trial sponsored by the National Institutes of Health, infants who were given vitamin A supplementation (5000 IU three times a week for 4 weeks by intramuscular injection) had a 7% reduction in death or BPD ($p = 0.03$) (Tyson et al. 1999).

Another factor under consideration is that premature infants may be deficient in selenium, with low levels of selenium-dependent glutathione peroxidase in red blood cells and possibly in the lung. Darlow and associates found a significant inverse relationship between plasma selenium levels at the age of 28 days and the number of days of oxygen therapy in premature infants, but they could not discern whether this was cause or effect. No trials of selenium supplementation in premature infants have appeared at this time.

Stage 4 BPD is a type of chronic obstructive lung disease. The infants have a barrel chest, prolonged expiration time, expiratory wheezing, and evidence of lung overinflation on chest radiograph. Pulmonary function tests demonstrate increased airway resistance and functional residual capacity and decreased tidal volume. Increased airway resistance is in part the result of damage and destruction of airways, in part the result of increased airway reactivity, and in part a manifestation of the interstitial edema that invariably accompanies BPD. Infants with BPD have bronchial smooth muscle hypertrophy, and cold air provocation tests and trials of bronchodilators have demonstrated that bronchospasm may contribute to their increased airway resistance, even when they are as young as 14 days. In addition, infants with BPD have radiographic and clinical evidence of pulmonary edema. Presumably, the loss of arterioles and capillaries in the lung along with some vascular remodeling results in increased blood flow through remaining vessels and increased filtration of fluid from these vessels. In infants with cor pulmonale, systemic venous pressure is high and the ability of the lymphatics to clear this filtered fluid is impaired. Fluid in perivascular cuffs compresses airways and increases airway resistance.

In infants with BPD, static lung compliance is usually decreased but may be increased if damage to the lung is sufficient to result in loss of elastic recoil. Dynamic compliance is invariably decreased and nitrogen washout is delayed, indicating a severe maldistribution of ventilation. Maldistribution of ventilation results in mismatch of ventilation and perfusion, which leads to hypoxemia. Although the respiratory rate is usually increased, physiologic dead space is also increased so that alveolar ventilation is decreased and arterial P_{CO_2} is increased.

Obliteration of arterioles and capillaries results in a reduction in available surface area for gas exchange and may contribute to arterial hypoxemia, especially during exercise. The loss of vessels, coupled with smooth muscle hypertrophy from chronic alveolar hypoxia, may also result in pulmonary hypertension and cor pulmonale. With cor pulmonale, cardiac output falls and oxygen delivery may be impaired.

Since infants with BPD usually outgrow their CLD, a major aim of therapy is provision of adequate nutritional support for growth and prevention of complications. Nutritional support is complicated by an increased resting metabolic rate with a caloric need for as much as 140 to 160 kcal/kg per day in the face of a relative inability to tolerate fluid loads. Thus, these infants must often be fed high-caloric-density formulas supplemented with calcium and potassium to replace losses resulting from concomitant diuretic therapy.

Supplemental oxygen should be administered to maintain the infant's arterial P_{O_2} between 55 and 70 mm Hg and the pulse oximeter reading above 95% to prevent alveolar hypoxia. Reduced alveolar oxygen levels may cause airway constriction and pulmonary hypertension; oxygen must be given in sufficient amounts to prevent cor pulmonale. This approach may require prolonged mechanical ventilation initially, but eventually patients can be managed with administration of oxygen by nasal continuous positive airway pressure (CPAP), Oxy-Hood, or nasal cannula. In the past, chronic oxygen administration usually required prolonged hospitalization; however, several neonatal programs have reported successful management of these infants at home.

Booster transfusions of blood to maintain the hematocrit above 40% have been shown to reduce resting oxygen consumption and to increase systemic oxygen transport in infants with BPD and some programs also administer erythropoietin and iron to minimize transfusion.

Fluid restriction may reduce interstitial edema in the lung and improve pulmonary function; therefore, these infants are usually fed with concentrated formulas. It has been shown in a controlled trial that furosemide facilitates extubation from mechanical ventilation in BPD. Furosemide alone and chlorothiazide in combination with spironolactone, has been shown to be effective in improving lung mechanics and gas exchange, thus reducing the oxygen requirements in infants with BPD; however, the effects last only so long as the drugs are continued. Chronic diuretic therapy may result in excessive urinary losses of calcium, potassium, sodium, and chloride. Calcium loss may compromise bone mineralization and exacerbate osteopenia of prematurity. In addition, prolonged administration of furosemide has been associated with nephrocalcinosis in infants with BPD and also with cholelithiasis. Although it has been suggested that substitution of chlorothiazide for furosemide may reduce calcium wasting, a recent study has questioned this effect; and Engelhardt and associates were unable to demonstrate improvement in lung mechanics with chlorothiazide-spironolactone treatment. In addition, chloride loss can result in metabolic alkalosis, decreased ventilatory drive, and hypercarbia; this may contribute to an erroneous conclusion that furosemide therapy is ineffective. These infants must be supplemented with potassium chloride and occasionally sodium chloride to prevent the bicarbonate concentration from reaching 30 mEq/L. Alternate-day furosemide therapy has proved effective while minimizing the electrolyte disturbances.

Infants with BPD often have a family history of asthma and frequently have very high levels of urinary leukotrienes, comparable to those seen in asthma. Episodes of acute deterioration in infants with BPD resemble acute asthmatic attacks and are often attributed to bronchospasm. Furthermore, increased airway resistance secondary to bronchoconstriction is believed to play a role in prolonging ventilator requirements in this population of infants. Multiple authors have shown that administration of a variety of beta-adrenergic agents to infants with BPD results in improvements in lung compliance, airway resistance, and gas exchange.

Management of acute episodes of bronchoconstriction is best accomplished by the use of beta-adrenergic agents. For ventilated infants, albuterol may be delivered by metered-dose inhaler, using a spacer placed between the ventilator circuit connector and endotracheal tube connector. This technique allows more precise control of the delivered dose than techniques of in-line nebulization. In one study a dose of 100 µg of albuterol by metered-dose inhaler significantly increased respiratory system compliance and decreased resistance in 65% of patients, and 200 µg was effective in the remainder. These changes lasted 3 hours and were accompanied by increased oxygen saturation by pulse oximetry and an increased heart rate. Beta-adrenergic agents may also be administered by nebulization into the ventilator circuit or into a face mask. The usual medication is albuterol (1 mg/kg) repeated every 4 to 6 hours; the large dose is a reflection of the inefficiency of this method of administration. In some instances it may be useful to assess the response to a single dose of terbutaline (5 to 10 µg/kg) administered subcutaneously and then to continue bronchodilator therapy only if a significant improvement in lung function is observed. Both terbutaline and albuterol produce some tachycardia, which is well tolerated, and in some patients there is hyperglycemia, hypertension, or tremor. In rare situations terbutaline may be administered as a continuous intravenous infusion (0.25 to 0.50 µg/kg per minute) in very ill ventilator-dependent patients with evidence of severe bronchoconstriction.

Inhaled beta-adrenergic agents are also useful in the chronic management of infants with BPD and increased airway reactivity. In addition, administration of theophylline has been shown to relieve bronchoconstriction and in some centers is used in combination with a selective beta$_2$-adrenergic agonist. As it is very poorly absorbed from the respiratory tract, it does not produce significant systemic effects. One further medication, which works differently, is cromolyn sodium; it is a mast cell stabilizer and inhibits the release of histamine and leukotrienes, which may play a role in producing bronchoconstriction. It has been tried in infants with severe BPD and may be effective.

The Collaborative Dexamethasone Trial Group in Europe performed a large controlled trial of corticosteroids in ventilator-dependent premature infants with BPD enrolled at the age of 30 days and found that a 7-day course of dexamethasone, repeated in some cases, significantly reduced the time to extubation from a median of 18 days in the control group to a median of 11 days in the treated group. The median time on oxygen was decreased by 19 days, but the length of hospitalization was not shortened by dexamethasone treatment. This trial also showed some benefits in extubated infants on oxygen therapy. In another important trial, it was shown that a 3-day dexamethasone course, at the age of 30 days in infants with BPD, significantly reduced the oxygen requirements, significantly increased the static lung compliance, and significantly reduced neutrophils, neutrophil elastase, fibronectin, and albumin in tracheal aspirate samples. These authors concluded that steroids suppressed lung inflammation and improved the permeability of lung capillaries and that dexamethasone exerted its favorable effects within 3 days.

The side effects of dexamethasone include hyperglycemia, hypertension, neutrophilia, infection, and reduced growth and in the animal model disturbed myelinization and neurodevelopment. Some infants have developed concentric hypertrophic cardiomyopathy, especially with prolonged treatment, which resolves with time after discontinuation of the drug. Other infants treated with dexamethasone have developed systemic candidiasis, which is a worrisome complication associated also with extreme prematurity and vaginal delivery. Although long courses of dexamethasone may suppress adrenal function, it does not appear that a 5- to 7-day course of dexamethasone at 0.5 mg/kg per day significantly suppresses function of the adrenal gland.

There have been few studies of inhaled steroids in the treatment of this condition. In a controlled trial, it was found that beclomethasone by metered-dose inhaler produced improved airway resistance and improved dynamic lung compliance after treatment for 2 weeks in comparison with controls. In a small controlled trial of nebulized flunisolide for 28 days in ventilator-dependent infants with BPD, improvements were found in oxygen requirements, lung mechanics, and time to extubation in comparison with control groups. Konig and coworkers have described the use of nebulized flunisolide in older infants with BPD. In another small controlled trial of nebulized dexamethasone for 10 days in ventilator-dependent preterm infants, the dynamic lung compliance was markedly improved and airway resistance was modestly improved, whereas no such improvements occurred in the control subjects. Rozycki and associates have described an excellent method for administering medication using a metered-dose inhaler with a spacer and a ventilation bag.

Prevention of preterm birth is, of course, the

most effective means of preventing BPD; if we could recognize premature labor and delay delivery until 30 weeks' gestation, more than 75% of BPD cases would not occur. Short of that possibility, acceleration of lung maturation with prenatal glucocorticoid treatment is the optimal approach. It is known that prenatal steroids induce the development of antioxidant enzymes in the lung, as well as surfactant synthesis enzymes, and have a beneficial effect on lung structure as well. There is some evidence that the addition of thyrotropin-releasing hormone to betamethasone for antenatal prophylaxis against RDS may be effective in further reducing the incidence of BPD.

Preventive management of the newborn includes administration of exogenous surfactant at birth. In institutions that routinely use nasal CPAP initially after birth, there may be a reduced use of mechanical ventilation and a reduced incidence of BPD; however, there are no controlled trials to confirm this idea. Maintenance of low inspired oxygen concentrations is believed to be important in preventing oxygen toxicity. It is recommended that the arterial PO_2 be maintained at 50 to 70 mm Hg and not higher. Reduced inspired oxygen can be accomplished to some degree by the use of continuous distending pressure. Mechanical ventilation with a strategy of reduced inflation pressures and acceptance of relatively high levels of arterial PCO_2 may reduce the incidence of BPD; but again, this hypothesis for permissive hypercarbia has never been adequately tested in clinical trials.

The mortality rate among infants with BPD after discharge from the hospital is roughly 10%. Survivors have an increased incidence of lower respiratory tract infections and of increased airway reactivity in the first year after discharge. Later, although pulmonary function studies may indicate increased small airway resistance among children with BPD, the exercise tolerance of these children is comparable to that of their normal peers. Growth may be delayed initially, but catch-up growth occurs with resolution of the pulmonary abnormalities.

In general, when discharged to a good home, and when provided with appropriate nutrition and oxygen supplementation, these infants achieve a reasonable neurodevelopmental status if they have not sustained a significant intracranial insult. Gray and colleagues examined a large cohort of premature infants at the age of 2 years and compared infants with BPD and birth-weight matched control subjects. They found an increased incidence of neurodevelopmental disabilities in those with BPD, but the problems were related to periventricular hemorrhage,cerebral ventricular dilation, and sepsis; BPD was not an independent risk factor for neurologic disability.

CHRONIC PULMONARY INSUFFICIENCY OF PREMATURITY

Chronic pulmonary insufficiency of prematurity (CPIP), which occurs usually in premature infants weighing less than 1200 g at birth, is also known as *late-onset respiratory distress* and is characterized by the development of serious respiratory difficulty and recurrent apnea after the first few days of life. During the first month, these infants exhibit a substantially reduced lung volume that is manifested clinically by an oxygen requirement of 25% to 40%, the presence of modest hypercarbia, and poorly defined, diffuse lung densities without cystic changes on the chest radiograph. The $Aa\text{-}DO_2$, $aA\text{-}DCO_2$, and $aA\text{-}DN_2$ all are increased.

The very compliant chest wall of these infants probably contributes to the atelectasis associated with this condition; small premature infants have more flexible ribs and less intercostal muscle mass than larger more mature infants. Heldt has measured the volume displacement of the diaphragm during inspiration in small premature infants and related it to the volume of each breath; he found that the volume displacement of the diaphragm was much greater than the lung volume change in small infants and attributed the difference to chest wall distortion or collapse during inspiration; the difference decreased with increasing maturity, as the chest wall became less compliant and chest wall distortion decreased. This phenomenon is believed to be almost universal in small premature infants but is likely more prominent in those who develop the signs of CPIP. It means that the diaphragm is less effective in producing a normal lung minute volume and that diaphragmatic work is greatly increased.

Apnea and bradycardia spells are common, but the relationship between apnea and CPIP is not firmly established; most authors believe that apnea of prematurity is related to deficiencies in respiratory drive, but diaphragmatic fatigue related to chest wall distortion may also be important. Both conditions appear to respond well to prolonged management with low concentrations of oxygen administered by nasal CPAP or by nasal cannula therapy. Clinical recovery in CPIP generally occurs during the second month of life, but apnea and bradycardia may persist in some infants for a longer period. The best interpretation of the data is that CPIP aggravates apnea of prematurity by producing diaphragmatic fatigue.

WILSON-MIKITY SYNDROME

Wilson-Mikity syndrome is an eponym for a form of late-developing respiratory distress in small premature infants, which was described in 1960 by Wilson and Mikity. It may, in fact, represent one end of the spectrum of CPIP. It is characterized by the onset of tachypnea, chest retractions, and cyanosis at 1 to 4 weeks of age in infants who were free of RDS at birth. Some of these infants have mechanical ventilation for other reasons, such as apnea, but they need low pressures and low oxygen concentrations. Their respiratory distress progresses for about 2 months and then slowly regresses until recovery is achieved over a period of 1 to 2 years. As the condition develops, the chest radiograph shows that the lung has a "bubbly" appearance, with diffuse streaks of infiltrate and widespread cystic change; during the recovery phase, hyperinflation is present at the lung bases, with flattening of the diaphragm, and streaky atelectasis at the apices.

The cause of Wilson-Mikity syndrome is unknown. The airways of premature infants are extremely compliant, and if compliance values are unevenly distributed, this might cause airway closure and gas trapping in certain regions of the lung, and adjacent compression atelectasis in other regions. In Burnard's experience, this condition was rarely diagnosed following the advent of CPAP treatment; it is possible that higher mean airway pressures stabilized the peripheral airways and prevented widespread closure.

CHAPTER 7

Cardiovascular System

PATENT DUCTUS ARTERIOSUS IN THE PREMATURE INFANT

The ductus arteriosus represents a persistence of the terminal portion of the left pulmonary or sixth branchial arch. More muscular than the elastic pulmonary artery and aorta at either end, the ductus arteriosus also has a looser structure with increased amounts of acid mucopolysaccharide in the muscle media. During fetal life, it serves to divert blood away from the fluid-filled lungs toward the descending aorta and placenta. Obliteration of the ductus arteriosus takes place after birth. In the full-term animal or human neonate, the ductus begins to constrict rapidly after delivery with initiation of air breathing. In addition to both circumferential and longitudinal vasoconstriction, the media indents into the lumen and the intima increases in size, forming intimal mounds that help to occlude the lumen.

Many investigators have demonstrated that oxygen is responsible for constricting the ductus arteriosus after birth. However, the biochemical basis for the oxygen response has never been fully explained. Although neural and hormonal factors possibly contribute to ductus closure under physiologic conditions, they do not mediate oxygen-induced vessel closure.

Oxygen has a greater constrictor effect in the ductus from near-term versus immature fetuses. The increased effectiveness of oxygen in the mature ductus arteriosus is due to a developmental alteration in the sensitivity of the vessel to locally produced vasodilators. Isolated ductus arteriosus, from preterm animals, is much more sensitive to the dilating action of prostaglandin E_2 (PGE_2) and nitric oxide (NO) than are those from animals near term. In addition to being much more sensitive to the vasodilators PGE_2 and NO, the ductus from extremely immature fetuses (< 0.7 gestation) also has decreased contractile capacity. These factors probably account for the higher incidence of persistent patent ductus arteriosus (PDA) in preterm infants. Inhibitors of prostaglandin production such as indomethacin, ibuprofen, and mefenamic acid have proven themselves to be effective agents in promoting ductus closure.

In normal full-term animals, loss of responsiveness to PGE_2 shortly after birth prevents the ductus arteriosus from reopening once it has constricted. Loss of ductus arteriosus responsiveness is directly related to the degree of prior ductus arteriosus constriction because constriction causes loss of luminal blood flow and ischemia of the inner vessel wall. This appears to be the first step in permanent closure of the ductus. In contrast to full-term infants, premature infants are more likely to have a ductus arteriosus that continues to dilate in response to PGE_2 and NO. This occurs even after complete obliteration of ductus luminal blood flow. Consequently, once the ductus arteriosus has closed in the premature infant (either spontaneously or as a result of indomethacin), it may reopen at a later date, with recurrence of the left-to-right shunt. The incidence of ductus arteriosus reopening is inversely related to gestational age: in 33% of infants delivered before 26 weeks' gestation, the ductus arteriosus reopens after initial closure (demonstrated by echocardiography), whereas in only 5% of infants delivered after 26 weeks' gestation, the ductus arteriosus reopens.

Virtually all shunting through the ductus in the preterm infant is left to right. Only in larger infants with persistent pulmonary hypertension does right-to-left shunting become a problem.

Very-low-birth-weight infants with a PDA have been found to have increased flow in the ascending aorta and decreased flow in the descending aorta, with an associated metabolic acidosis. Such alterations in cardiac output distribution have been implicated in the high incidence of intracranial hemorrhage and necrotizing enterocolitis associated with PDA. Significant aortic backflow has been observed over large distances in some infants with PDA, consistent with a "diastolic steal" of blood from the abdominal organs to the pulmonary artery. The continuous distention of the pulmonary vessels during diastole may be important in the production of pulmonary vascular disease and bronchopulmonary dysplasia.

The decreased ability of the preterm infant to maintain active pulmonary vasoconstriction may be responsible in part for the earlier presentation of a "large" left-to-right PDA shunt in the most immature infants. In addition, therapeutic maneuvers (e.g., surfactant replacement) that lead to decreased pulmonary vascular resistance can exacerbate the amount of left-to-right shunt in preterm infants with respiratory distress syndrome (RDS). Two recent meta-analyses of the surfactant therapy trials have demonstrated an increased incidence of both clinically symptomatic PDAs and pulmonary hemorrhages in the infants receiving prophylactic surfactant.

The combination of two-dimensional echocardiographic visualization of the ductus with either pulsed, continuous wave, or color Doppler measurements are not only sensitive but also specific for identifying ductus patency. This combination may also be useful in determining pressure gradients across the ductus. Determining the size of the lumen of the ductus arteriosus and the magnitude of the Doppler signal from the shunt give only qualitative measures of the size of the shunt.

Although the magnitude of shunt flow plays a significant role in creating neonatal morbidity, equally important factors are the duration of exposure to the shunt and the infant's ability to compensate for the shunt. For example, the same magnitude left-to-right PDA shunt may be clinically "silent" when present within the first 24 hours after delivery, whereas it may be associated with signs of congestive failure if it persists for 7 to 10 days. Even though echocardiographic findings can predict in which infants clinical symptoms eventually will develop, it does not automatically follow that treatment of the PDA should begin when these signs are first present.

Clinical signs of a PDA usually appear later than echocardiographic signs. Certain signs, such as continuous murmur or hyperactive left ventricular impulse, are specific for a PDA but lack sensitivity; conversely, ventilatory support criteria are sensitive but lack specificity. On the other hand, the appearance of three or more of these clinical signs (systolic murmur, hyperdynamic precordial impulse, full pulses, widened pulse pressure, or worsening respiratory status) correlates well with the subsequent development of PDA-related morbidity.

Pulsed Doppler echocardiographic assessments of full-term infants indicate that functional closure of the ductus has occurred in almost 50% of all full-term newborns by 24 hours, in 90% by 48 hours, and in all by 72 hours. The rate of ductus closure is delayed in preterm infants; however, essentially all healthy preterm infants of 30 weeks' gestation or greater will have a closed ductus by the 4th day after birth. RDS also delays ductus closure; however, in most infants who are 30 weeks' gestation or greater, the actual impact of RDS on ductal shunting may be less than commonly assumed. On the other hand, preterm infants of less than 30 weeks' gestation with severe respiratory distress have a high incidence of persistent PDA.

The introduction of exogenous surfactant therapy has altered both the incidence and the presentation of the PDA. Although surfactant has no effect on the contractile behavior of the ductus, its effects on pulmonary vascular resistance lead to an earlier clinical presentation of the left-to-right shunt in preterm animals and infants. A recent meta-analysis of the surfactant trials has found that there is an increased risk for development of a clinically symptomatic PDA following surfactant therapy; this risk is highest among infants who have received prophylactic treatment with surfactant.

Various treatments are effective for PDA. The addition of positive end-expiratory pressure has been found useful. When end-expiratory pressure is added, the amount of left-to-right shunt through the ductus arteriosus decreases; as a result, effective systemic blood flow increases. A low hematocrit has been shown to aggravate left-to-right shunting by lowering the resistance to blood flow through the pulmonary vascular bed. Higher hematocrits diminish excessive shunting through the PDA and help ensure systemic oxygen delivery when perfusion is limited. Similarly, demands on left ventricular output should be minimized in infants with PDA by maintaining adequate oxygenation and by keeping the patient in a neutral thermal environment. Nevertheless, such therapies usually only delay, rather than prevent, the ultimate need for PDA closure. Cotton and colleagues demonstrated that failure to close the ductus after significant clinical symptoms of cardiovascular compromise have developed (approximately 7 to 10 days after birth) significantly increases neonatal morbidity.

Indomethacin appears to be an effective alternative to surgery for treatment of a PDA. Its efficacy and toxicity have been explored extensively, and it appears comparable to surgical ligation in preventing the complications associated with a PDA: bronchopulmonary dysplasia (BPD), necrotizing enterocolitis (NEC), intracranial hemorrhage (ICH), and intolerance of enteral feedings. In most intensive care nurseries, indomethacin has replaced surgery as the preferred therapy for a persistent PDA, probably because the most frequently occurring risks associated with ligation (increased incidence of cicatricial retinopathy of prematurity and need for thoracotomy) seem more serious than those associated with indomethacin (decreased urine output and increased bleeding other than ICH). Even though there may be general consensus on the efficacy of indomethacin for treatment of a PDA, questions about proper dosage, treatment duration, and optimal timing of treatment remain controversial.

I recommend an initial dose of 0.2 mg/kg of lyophilized indomethacin, by intravenous (never intra-arterial) administration over 20 to 30 minutes when treating a clinically symptomatic PDA in infants weighing more than 1250 g or older than 7 days. A second and third dose of 0.2 mg/kg are given 12 and 36 hours after the first dose. Infants who weigh less than 1250 g at birth are given only

0.1 mg/kg for the second and third dose (unless they are older than 7 days).

Prostaglandin production is only transiently suppressed following indomethacin therapy. Within 6 to 7 days after completion of therapy, circulating PGE_2 concentrations return to the normal range. This interval may not allow enough time for anatomic remodeling of the ductus in the most immature infants. A prolonged maintenance course of low-dose indomethacin (0.1 mg/kg every 24 hours for 5 to 7 days) appears to both increase the success of the initial closure rate and decrease the relapse rate when compared with a shorter course (2 to 3 doses over 24 hours). This dosage regimen still needs further evaluation because, in some reports, a higher mortality rate was observed in the infants receiving prolonged maintenance indomethacin.

In addition to its effects on the ductus, indomethacin also is associated with vasoconstriction of other vascular beds (e.g., cerebral, mesenteric, renal). Prolonging the rate of indomethacin infusion (20 to 30 minutes) alleviates some of the decrease in organ blood flow; a continuous indomethacin infusion, of the same total daily dose, appears to decrease the detrimental effects of indomethacin even further.

Indomethacin treatment may be most effective in the first 24 to 48 hours after delivery, but is that necessarily the best time to administer it? Ninety percent of infants with severe respiratory distress have echocardiographic evidence of a PDA during the first 24 hours; however, in only 40% do symptoms subsequently develop of a hemodynamically large left-to-right shunt that will require intervention with indomethacin or surgery. In addition, in most infants, symptoms of cardiovascular compromise do not develop before 7 days. Therefore, treatment given within the first 24 to 48 hours implies that, in approximately 60% of such infants, symptoms of cardiovascular compromise would never have developed.

A recently reported meta-analysis of more than 25 randomized, controlled trials examined the relative merits of the different timing strategies that have been used to treat the PDA. In each of the trials, a backup treatment (either indomethacin or surgical ligation) was included to close the PDA, if the initial study treatment failed. As was demonstrated previously, clinical signs of a PDA frequently develop in premature infants within the first 2 to 3 days of life (early symptomatic PDA); however, it may not be until 7 to 10 days after birth that signs of congestive failure develop (late symptomatic PDA). The initial treatment trials (late symptomatic treatment versus later backup treatment) were designed to evaluate the effectiveness of indomethacin in closing the late symptomatic PDA. Infants were randomized to receive indomethacin or no additional therapy when signs of congestive failure developed (age 7 to 10 days). If the infant's condition did not improve within 2 to 6 days after initial randomization, then backup treatment was started. The early symptomatic treatment versus late symptomatic treatment trials were designed to evaluate whether the early treatment of a symptomatic PDA, when clinical signs first appeared (age 1 to 3 days), would decrease PDA-related morbidity below that of a backup treatment strategy that was not initiated until signs of congestive failure appeared (age 7 to 12 days). The prophylactic treatment versus early symptomatic treatment trials were designed to evaluate whether administration of indomethacin, before the appearance of any PDA clinical signs (usually within the first 24 hours after birth), would reduce morbidity to less than that associated with a strategy wherein no treatment was given until signs of an early symptomatic PDA appeared (age 3 to 4 days). All three treatment strategies prevented either the development or the need for backup treatment of a symptomatic PDA.

EVALUATION OF NEWBORNS WITH POSSIBLE CARDIAC PROBLEMS

Early diagnosis remains the key to minimizing morbidity and mortality among symptomatic newborn infants, whether term or preterm. Separating cardiovascular from pulmonary problems in symptomatic newborns can be difficult for even experienced diagnosticians. Further, not infrequently cardiovascular and pulmonary problems coexist, even in premature infants. In fact, in virtually every infant with respiratory distress syndrome (RDS), patent ductus arteriosus (PDA) is also present because maturations of the surfactant system and ductal tissue are both incomplete. Left-to-right ductal shunts in infants with RDS compromise pulmonary compliance. Serial evaluation is equally important in the management of symptomatic newborn infants. Serial evaluation is essential in confirming initial diagnoses, in assessing the stage and progress of the normal postnatal respiratory and circulatory transition to air breathing and serial circulation, and in assessing the impact of therapeutic interventions.

In evaluating the symptomatic newborn, at least two issues must be addressed simultaneously. The most important issue is how sick the infant is now and how much sicker the infant is likely to become without intervention over the next few hours. This judgment drives decisions about the urgency of possible transport to a major center, about the performance of further diagnostic testing at the local hospital (such as arterial blood gases, blood cultures, chest radiographs, or echocardiograms), and about the possibly immediate institution of therapeutic measures. Such measures, which might include supplemental oxygen, endotracheal intubation, antibiotics, pressors, transfusion, surfactant, or prostaglandin E_1 (PGE_1) (depending on the working diagnosis), must sometimes be instituted even before the arrival of a team for neonatal stabilization and transport. As in the rest of medicine, better than 9 times out of 10 a single diagnosis accounts for all symptoms in a given newborn.

The second major issue is the seemingly simple, but too often difficult, distinction between heart disease and lung or systemic disease. Accurately making this fundamental distinction is useful in stabilizing symptomatic newborns. Infants with virtually any form of congenital heart disease that causes symptoms in the first 48 hours after birth can be stabilized by initiation of PGE_1. Mechanical ventilation and antibiotics can at least temporarily stabilize the great majority of infants with respiratory failure or sepsis (or both). In reaching the preliminary clinical judgment as to whether heart or lungs or systemic problems are causing symptoms, all information available from the history, physical examinations, laboratory tests, and any therapeutic trials (such as supplemental oxygen) must be considered quickly but carefully.

Much useful information can be garnered from the history of the pregnancy. Length of pregnancy is the single most important fact available from the maternal history because typically quite different diseases afflict term and premature infants. Symptomatic term infants suffer from a wide spectrum of heart, lung, and systemic diseases, whereas symptomatic premature infants typically have lung disease complicated by left to right ductal shunting. Other important information includes (1) the presence or absence of maternal or gestational diabetes because the incidences of RDS, congenital heart disease, cardiomyopathy, and hypoglycemia are all higher in diabetic pregnancies; (2) results of amniocentesis and fetal ultrasonography because the incidence of congenital heart disease is high in chromosomal disorders and in a variety of syndromes that can be diagnosed prenatally, such as VACTERL (*v*ertebral, *a*nal, *c*ardiac, *t*racheal, *e*sophageal, *r*enal, and *l*imb) syndrome; (3) the length of rupture of membranes because the incidence of infection increases with the duration of rupture and because prolonged leakage of amniotic fluid is strongly associated with pulmonary hypoplasia; (4) evidence of maternal infection, including fever, uterine tenderness, or purulent vaginal discharge, any of which raises the risk of fetal/neonatal infection; (5) maternal use of over-the-counter or prescription medications, such as ibuprofen (which can close the ductus in utero and cause postnatal pulmonary hypertension), phenytoin (Dilantin) (associated with fetal Dilantin sydrome, characterized by cleft palate, muscular ventricular septal defect [VSD], and hypoplastic nails), and lithium (associated with Ebstein anomaly); and (6) identification of fetal dysrhythmias, such as complete heart block or supraventricular tachycardia.

The events of labor are also important in the assessment of the symptomatic newborn. Infants delivered before the spontaneous onset of labor are at higher risk of RDS. Infants born with meconium staining are at risk for meconium aspiration pneumonia. Infants born after fetal distress are at risk for the consequences of asphyxia, such as shock lung and myocardial dysfunction.

A history of shoulder dystocia or nuchal cord can be a clue to underlying asphyxia despite seemingly normal Apgar scores. Delivery by cesarean section is associated with transient tachypnea of the newborn in term and near-term infants. Apgar scores at 1 and 5 minutes provide insight into the infant's uteroplacental reserve during labor and delivery.

In the neonatal period the single most important piece of information is the presence or absence of a symptom-free interval after birth. Infants who are symptomatic from birth almost always have parenchymal lung disease of one kind or another.

Infants with ductal dependent congenital heart disease usually present in one of three patterns: cyanosis, shock with congestive heart failure, or shock without congestive heart failure. Further, each pattern has a typical age of presentation.

Infants whose lives depend on ductal patency for pulmonary blood flow (e.g., pulmonary atresia, critical pulmonary stenosis, severe tetralogy of Fallot [TOF], some forms of tricuspid atresia) present in the first few hours of life (almost always before 4 hours of age) with cyanosis despite good air exchange. Even modest constriction of the pulmonary end of the ductus precipitates worsening cyanosis in such infants, and constriction of the pulmonary end of the ductus normally begins shortly after birth. Such infants can be cyanotic in the delivery room, and sometimes they end up incubated and mechanically ventilated as a result. More frequently, infants with pulmonary atresia and the like are assigned Apgar scores of 9 and 9 (one off for color) and are sent to the normal nursery initially. There progressive cyanosis and tachypnea result in transfer to intensive care. In the neonatal intensive care unit, administration of oxygen has no effect on the cyanosis, and the possibility of congenital heart disease arises. Reopening the pulmonary end of the ductus with PGE_1 in deeply cyanotic infants with hypoplasia of the right heart is a lifesaving measure.

Infants with transposition of the great vessels (TGV) and intact ventricular septum are also made more cyanotic by ductal closure, but in such infants ductal closure reduces mixing of the two circulations rather than pulmonary blood flow. Similar to infants with hypoplasia of the right heart, infants with uncomplicated TGV also present by 4 hours of age in the great majority of cases.

Infants whose lives depend on ductal patency for systemic blood flow (e.g., interrupted aortic arch, hypoplastic left heart syndrome [HLHS], critical aortic coarctation) almost always present after 4 hours of age with poor perfusion and hyperpnea. Cyanosis is not part of the presentation. Time of presentation, cause of hyperpnea, and presence or absence of congestive heart failure usually vary with underlying cardiovascular anatomy.

When the entire systemic cardiac output is dependent on ductal patency (e.g., aortic or mitral atresia), affected infants usually present early (4 to 24 hours of age) with pulmonary congestion, decreased lung compliance, and signs of shock. In such infants, normal postnatal ductal constriction of the pulmonary end of the ductus compromises coronary blood flow as well as lower body blood flow, impairs ventricular function, and also forces more blood flow into the lungs. The end result is typical left-sided congestive heart failure characterized by pulmonary edema, reduced lung compliance, and poor systemic perfusion. The progressive impairment of cardiac function caused by ductal closure in such infants culminates in obvious shock with cool, gray extremities; hypotension; tachycardia; and metabolic acidosis.

In contrast, when only perfusion of the lower body is dependent on ductal patency (e.g., interrupted aortic arch, critical aortic coarctation), coronary flow is supplied normally from antegrade flow through the aorta, and constriction of the pulmonary end of the ductus does not result in myocardial infarction or excessive pulmonary blood flow. As a result, affected infants tolerate closure of the pulmonary end of the ductus better and usually present later than infants in whom all of systemic perfusion is compromised by ductal closure. Infants in whom only perfusion of the lower body is compromised by ductal closure usually present after 8 hours of age with progressive acidosis. Pulmonary congestion is not prominent in such infants, unless systemic acidosis is severe enough to compromise cardiac function.

Infants in whom lower body perfusion is ductal dependent thus usually present with what appears to be a metabolic problem or sepsis rather than congestive heart failure. Typical findings include Kussmaul type of hyperpnea, mottling, but unimpaired gas exchange. Decreased lung compliance and pulmonary edema are not present in most such infants until late in their courses, when progressive metabolic acidosis impairs cardiac function. Metabolic acidosis and azotemia progressively worsen from lack of perfusion of the kidneys and lower body, and eventually shock ensues from acidosis-induced cardiac compromise. Pulmonary congestion, however, is not a prominent feature of the symptoms of infants in whom only lower body perfusion is dependent on ductal patency; instead, listlessness, pallor, cool lower extremities, and poor feeding are usually the presenting symptoms.

Systematic physical examination of the newborn provides much useful information about the criticality of illness and the preliminary distinction between lung disease and heart or systemic disease. The general physical examination of the infant often provides more important information than the cardiovascular or pulmonary examinations. Serial physical examinations are critically important in symptomatic newborns to determine (1) how symptomatic infants tolerate any required procedures or diagnostic tests; (2) whether attempted therapeutic interventions are in fact effective; and (3) when treatments that do prove to be effective need adjustments.

The first question to be answered by inspection is whether the infant is too large, too small, or just right in size. Several neonatal cardiovascular problems are associated with excessive intrauterine somatic growth. Infants who are large for gestational age (typically greater than 4 kg) may be products of diabetic pregnancies, and maternal diabetes is associated with increased risk of congenital heart disease, hypertrophic cardiomyopathy, and hypoglycemia among offspring. When maternal hyperglycemia results in profound fetal hyperinsulinemia, severe cardiac dysfunction can occur postnatally from either hypertrophic cardiomyopathy or hypoglycemia. Infants who have Beckwith-Wiedemann syndrome are also typically large for gestational age, and the associated postnatal hypoglycemia can also result in profound cardiac dysfunction. For unexplained reasons, infants with TGV are also apt to be large for gestational age.

Similarly, infants who are too small are also at increased risk of difficulties during postnatal adaptation. Infants who are small because they are premature obviously are at high risk of RDS and persistent ductal patency. Infants who are small because of intrauterine growth retardation have increased risk of polycythemia, a disorder that can result in severe cardiopulmonary compromise, particularly when central hematocrit exceeds 70%. Infants with a variety of chromosomal abnormalities that have high incidences of congenital heart disease are also often small for gestational age; trisomies 13 and 18 are the most common such abnormalities.

The second question to be answered by inspection is whether the newborn infant who may have heart disease is acutely ill or not. Newborn infants who are acutely ill look the part. Early during evolution of acute illness, sick newborns look worried and appear to be frightened. Later in the course of acute illness, sick newborns appear to retreat from interaction with the outside world and focus intently on the illness they are battling. In the final stages of acute illness, newborns become progressively less responsive; moribund newborns are unresponsive.

The third question to be answered from general inspection of the symptomatic newborn infant is whether multiple congenital anomalies are present. Infants who have more than two externally visible anomalies are highly likely to exhibit associated internal anomalies, even if the three or more external anomalies identified are relatively minor. For example, a newborn with findings as simple as a sacral dimple, extra digit, and single umbilical artery is also likely to have renal or cardiac anomalies. Certain anomalies commonly occur in association with specific chromosomal abnormalities that are accompanied by cardiac malformations; for example, cleft lip and palate are frequently present in infants with trisomy 13, and scalp defects are often present in infants with trisomy 18.

The fourth question to be answered from general inspection of the symptomatic newborn infant is whether the infant has an obvious syndrome that could account for symptoms. Such syndromes might have a chromosomal basis and characteristic cardiac defects (e.g., Turner syndrome/coarctation), an unknown basis and typical cardiac defects (e.g., VACTERL syndrome/VSD), or an unknown basis and no cardiac defects (e.g., Potter syndrome/pulmonary hypoplasia).

Observing how much work is required for each breath is also useful. In cyanotic congenital heart diseases with *decreased pulmonary blood flow*, such as pulmonary atresia, TOF, and some forms of tricuspid atresia, tachypnea is present, but work of breathing is normal because lung compliance is normal. Such infants have what appears to be effortless tachypnea. If the proper diagnosis is not recognized, however, systemic acidosis from hypoxemia eventually supervenes, and dyspnea occurs.

In cyanotic congenital heart diseases with *increased pulmonary blood flow* (such as total anomalous pulmonary venous drainage [TAPVD], truncus arteriosus, and other forms of tricuspid atresia), pulmonary congestion results in decreased lung compliance and increased work of breathing. The diminution in compliance is inversely related to pulmonary arterial pressure, not magnitude of shunt. Thus, infants with increased pulmonary blood flow have not only tachypnea but also dyspnea and increased work of breathing.

In addition, infants with *left-to-right shunts*, such as VSD, atrioventricular septal defect (AVSD), PDA, and arteriovenous malformation (AVM) also have reduced lung compliance. As in cyanotic heart diseases with increased pulmonary blood flow, the diminution in lung compliance observed in infants with uncomplicated left-to-right shunts is inversely related to pulmonary arterial pressure, not size of the shunt. Pulmonary hypertension (stiff lung vessels) can certainly cause stiff airways on a mechanical basis because tense pulmonary arterial vessels resist the motion of chest inflation. Elevations in pulmonary arterial pressure, however, also cause reduced lung compliance by exacerbating pulmonary edema, a known inhibitor of the surfactant system. Infants with large shunts typically manifest dyspnea and increased work of breathing. In the premature infant, left-to-right shunt from PDA is a common cause of dyspnea and increased work of breathing.

Similarly, in congenital heart diseases characterized by *pulmonary venous congestion* (such as aortic and mitral atresia), pulmonary venous hypertension decreases lung compliance and causes increased work of breathing. Increased work of breathing is identified by flaring of the alae nasae, intercostal retractions, subcostal retractions, and, in the premature infant, sternal retractions. Infradiaphragmatic TAPVD is an important cause of pulmonary venous congestion in symptomatic newborn infants. In addition, left ventricular dysfunction from any cause also causes pulmonary venous hypertension by elevating left atrial pressure. The net result of pulmonary venous hypertension is reduced pulmonary compliance from consequent pulmonary arterial hypertension and from pulmonary edema. In the term infant, the most common myopathic causes of left ventricular dysfunction include asphyxia, congenital myocarditis, and hypoglycemia. Endocardial fibroelastosis is not seen frequently today.

Small holes in the skin are typical of trisomy 13; these usually are 1 to 3 mm in diameter and most commonly occur over the scalp. The *color* of the skin depends on a number of factors, including gestational age, presence or absence of meconium staining, vasomotor tone, concentration of hemoglobin, oxygen saturation, pH, level of bilirubin, and cardiac output. The epidermis and dermis are virtually translucent in extremely immature infants (less than 26 weeks), and the skin appears gelatinous. *Acrocyanosis*, which usually occurs in healthy term infants, is often said to be a function of peripheral vasomotor instability. Acrocyanosis is probably instead a vestigial remnant of the vasomotor mechanisms that drive the fetus's adaptive response to hypoxemia. Acrocyanosis is characterized by cyanosis limited to the peripheral circulation, usually the hands and feet. Occasionally acrocyanosis occurs in the entire left or right side of the body (harlequin response). The lips and tongue always remain pink in acrocyanosis, and affected infants are asymptomatic. Acrocyanosis does not cause *differential cyanosis*, which is defined as cyanosis limited to the left arm, the left arm and head, the upper body, or the lower body.

Differential cyanosis is an important physical finding that *always* indicates a major cardiovascular problem in the newborn. Right-to-left ductal shunting causes differential cyanosis. Right-to-left ductal shunting can occur only when the ductus is patent and the pulmonary arterial pressure exceeds systemic pressure. Such right-to-left ductal shunts, one of several criteria diagnostic of persistent pulmonary hypertension of the newborn syndrome (PPHNS), can result from a wide variety of disorders, including many forms of congenital heart disease. Whether the cyanosis in differential cyanosis occurs in the upper body or lower body is determined by underlying cardiac anatomy.

When the cyanosis in differential cyanosis is present in the *lower body* (both legs, both legs and right arm, or both legs and right arm and head), right-to-left ductal shunt of deoxygenated blood from the pulmonary artery to the lower extremities accounts for the visibly lower oxygen content in the lower body. Differential cyanosis with cyanosis in the lower body is far more common than differential cyanosis with cyanosis in the upper body. Meconium aspiration (with associated persistent pulmonary hypertension) is the single most common cause of differential cyanosis, but congenital heart disease must be excluded in every case.

When the cyanosis in differential cyanosis is present in the *upper body* (left arm, left arm and head, or entire upper body), either TGV or supracardiac TAPVD must be present (with or without other forms of congenital heart disease). In both disorders, the most highly oxygenated blood in the body is in the pulmonary artery rather than ascending aorta. When the highly oxygenated blood from the pulmonary artery crosses the ductus right to left, the lower body and legs have visibly higher oxygen. In infants with TGV, oxygen content in the pulmonary artery is higher than the aorta because the pulmonary artery arises from the left ventricle, and the left ventricle receives oxygenated pulmonary venous return from the left atrium.

In infants with supracardiac TAPVD, oxygen content is higher in the pulmonary artery than aorta because pulmonary venous return enters the heart from the superior vena cava. It is well understood that during fetal life and in the immediate newborn period, the superior vena caval flow streams into the right ventricle and goes out to the pulmonary artery and that the inferior vena caval flow streams across the foramen ovale into the left heart and goes out to the aorta. The net result in supracardiac TAPVD is that highly oxygenated pulmonary venous blood, mixed with systemic venous blood from the superior vena cava, goes into the right ventricle and out the pulmonary artery. Right-to-left ductal shunt in afflicted infants results in good oxygenation of the lower extremities and cyanosis of the upper extremities.

Infants who are pale may have anemia or shock. Congenital heart disease does not cause anemia, but congenital heart disease is an important cause of shock. Infants who are in shock generally are pale but have a grayish appearance, and the skin is cool to touch. In the late stages of shock when death is near, the skin takes on a splotchy appearance that resembles livido reticularis in the normal newborn except that the splotches are blue rather than red.

In normal infants, refill of the capillaries after gentle pressure of the skin with the thumb for 5 seconds takes 1 to 2 seconds both in the extremities (palms and soles) and in the central circulation (forehead and central chest). Delayed capillary refill is a sign of inadequate cardiac output. Capillary refill that takes more than 3 to 4 seconds indicates moderate impairment of cardiac output; capillary refill that takes more than 5 to 6 seconds indicates severe impairment of cardiac output. As in other parts of the physical examination, serial assessments of capillary refill can be valuable in determining whether attempted therapeutic interventions are effective and when adjustments to effective treatments are needed. Because the newborn has remarkable peripheral vasomotor control and can shut down perfusion to the extremities in times of stress (e.g., cold, infection, hypoglycemia, cardiac compromise), the best places to follow capillary refill serially in infants who are compromised are the forehead and central chest.

Auscultation of the chest provides important information. The most important observation to make in auscultation of the chest in acutely ill newborn infants is symmetry of chest inflation and symmetry of breath sounds. Asymmetric chest motion and asymmetric air movement virtually always indicate a potentially life-threatening difficulty, such as pneumothorax, intubation of a main stem bronchus instead of the trachea, or chylothorax.

Visual assessment of precordial cardiac motion should determine three things: (1) whether the heart is in the left or right chest, (2) whether the heart is enlarged (or displaced laterally), and (3) whether the heart is volume-loaded or not. In symptomatic newborns, dextrocardia virtually always means complex congenital heart disease, and cardiomegaly virtually always means that cardiac compromise is contributing to the observed symptoms. Volume-loaded hearts exhibit dynamic precordial motion that can be identified easily from across the room. The most common example of volume loading of the heart in neonatal intensive care units is observed among premature infants ventilated for RDS; dynamic precordial activity in such infants virtually always indicates substantial left-to-right ductal shunts, even in the absence of murmurs and bounding pulses. In term infants, dynamic precordial activity usually indicates significant tricuspid regurgitation, which is most commonly associated with either birth asphyxia or PPHNS.

Listening to the heart provides information useful in the differential diagnosis and management of symptomatic newborns. The first matter to establish is where the heart sounds are loudest. Even in the absence of visible or palpable precordial impulses, the presence of dextrocardia should be readily divined by comparing the intensity of the heart sounds over the left and right chests. The second matter to be determined is whether both components of the second heart sound are present. If so, the aortic valve and the pulmonary valve are both present. If not, either one could be missing, or TGV could be present. At the rapid heart rates many newborns exhibit, confirming splitting of the second sound can be a challenge at times even for experienced clinicians.

The third matter to be accomplished is to localize systolic and diastolic murmurs to one of the four cardinal areas of the heart: the mitral area (apex), tricuspid/septal area (lower left sternal border), pulmonary area (upper left sternal border), or aortic area (upper right sternal border). Placing murmurs anatomically over a structure in the heart is useful in differential diagnosis. Fourth, it is important to listen for radiation of systolic murmurs to the axillae and back. Murmurs that radiate well to both axillae mean either bilateral peripheral pulmonary stenosis (common in premature infants) or pathology in the pulmonary outflow tract. Murmurs that radiate only to the left axilla often represent mitral regurgitation but can represent isolated left peripheral pulmonary stenosis as well as pulmonary stenosis (the systolic jet in pulmonary stenosis tends to be directed into the left pulmonary artery). Murmurs that radiate well to the back suggest coarctation. Finally, in infants with heart failure, it is important to listen over the anterior fontanel and liver for a bruit because AVMs of the brain and liver are important causes of high-output congestive heart failure in newborn infants.

As with other parts of the physical examination, serial auscultation of the heart can be quite useful in assessing whether attempted therapeutic interventions are in fact effective and when treatments that do prove to be effective need adjustments. For example, appearance of a systolic or continuous murmur over the pulmonary area after initiation of PGE_1 in an infant with pulmonary atresia indicates reopening of the ductus. Similarly, diminution of a systolic murmur over the lower left sternal border (i.e., diminution of tricuspid regurgitation) after initiation of nitric oxide in an infant with PPHNS indicates reduction in pulmonary arterial pressure.

The age at which a murmur is first heard has diagnostic significance. Murmurs heard in the delivery room are always due either to stenosis (such as aortic or pulmonary stenosis) or to regurgitation (such as tricuspid or mitral regurgitation) and are never due to shunts. Shunts are not heard in the delivery room because vascular resistances in lungs and body are equal at birth, and left-to-right shunts do not occur in the absence of resistance (pressure) gradients. Thus, it is irrelevant whether only the normal communications between the systemic and pulmonary circulations present at birth (foramen ovale and ductus arteriosus) are patent, or other abnormal communications between the left and right heart (such as atrial septal defect [ASD] or VSD) are also present at birth; all such lesions are inaudible in the delivery room because pulmonary and systemic vascular resistances are equal.

Typically, murmurs from uncomplicated VSDs are not audible until the second or third day after birth, and murmurs from uncomplicated ASDs are not audible until several weeks of life.

Infants born with abdominal wall defects (omphalocele or prune belly) may also have congenital heart disease. Abdomens that are intact and distended are distended by fluid (ascites or blood), gas (pneumoperitoneum, intestinal perforation, tracheoesophageal fistula), tissue (hepatomegaly, splenomegaly, or tumor), or luminal obstruction (necrotizing enterocolitis, Hirschsprung disease, duodenal atresia). Abdomens that are intact but appear to be empty usually are empty because the abdominal contents are in the chest (diaphragmatic hernia).

Palpation of the abdomen also yields much useful

information. The presence of crepitus indicates dissection of subcutaneous air leak down from the chest. In the normal newborn infant, the edge of the liver is usually palpable 1 cm below the right costal margin in the right upper quadrant. Liver distention or displacement is present if the liver edge is more than 2 cm below the right costal margin. In situs inversus totalis and in some forms of heterotaxia, the liver is on the left side, rather than on the right side. In situs ambiguus, the liver can be felt on both sides of the abdomen. If the edge of the liver is pulsatile, tricuspid regurgitation is present (Courvoisier sign). If the liver has a bruit over it, hepatic arteriovenous malformation is present.

Bilateral diminution or absence of lower extremity arterial pulses in the presence of a strong right or left upper extremity pulse is virtually pathognomonic of coarctation or interrupted aortic arch. Pulses in all four extremities must be carefully palpated and compared. If the right subclavian artery arises aberrantly from the descending aorta distal to the site of coarctation or interruption, only the pulse in the left arm may be hypertensive. Further, umbilical arterial catheterization not infrequently causes reduced femoral arterial and distal pedal pulsations on the ipsilateral side. What can initially appear to be diminished arterial pressures in the lower extremities is far more frequently unilateral femoral arterial vasospasm from umbilical arterial catheterization.

Measurements of arterial blood gases provide important insight into both cardiopulmonary function and cardiopulmonary reserve in symptomatic newborns. The most important determination provided by an arterial blood gas measurement is pH. Arterial pH is an excellent barometer of the adequacy of both cardiac and pulmonary function. If arterial pH is in the normal range, the symptomatic newborn remains compensated and is not in danger of immediate collapse. If acidosis is present, the symptomatic newborn is unstable and at high risk for rapid deterioration.

The second most important determination provided by an arterial blood gas measurement is arterial P_{CO_2}. The arterial P_{CO_2} level provides insight as to the cause of acidosis: Normal or low levels of P_{CO_2} in the presence of acidosis indicate metabolic acidosis; elevated levels of P_{CO_2} in the presence of acidosis indicate respiratory failure. The most common postnatal cause of metabolic acidosis in the neonatal intensive care unit is septic shock, but hypoplastic left heart syndrome (HLHS) and inborn errors of metabolism are also important causes.

During fetal life, P_{O_2} measurements in the high 20s were normal, and the fetus adapted to hypoxia by having fetal hemoglobin, polycythemia, and elevated levels of 2,3-diphosphoglycerate. Those adaptations do not disappear at birth. For these reasons, a P_{O_2} measurement in the 40s is not a medical emergency in the newborn as long as pH and P_{CO_2} are normal. In fact, at normal pH, newborns are 80% saturated at a P_{O_2} of 40 mm Hg. In cyanotic heart disease, depending on the lesion, a saturation of 70% may be perfectly acceptable.

Every sick newborn, term or premature, has the capacity and propensity for right-to-left ductal shunting. The possibility of right-to-left ductal shunting of unoxygenated pulmonary arterial blood into the descending aorta causing falsely low umbilical arterial P_{O_2} measurements should be considered on every umbilical arterial blood gas.

Right-to-left ductal shunting, one of the diagnostic criteria for PPHNS, occurs when the ductus is patent and the pulmonary arterial pressure exceeds systemic pressure. Such right-to-left ductal shunts can cause large differences between arterial P_{O_2} measurements obtained from the upper body and lower body. A difference in P_{O_2} of 10 mm Hg or more between the right arm and umbilical arterial catheter is diagnostic of PPHNS. Sometimes P_{O_2} differences of better than 200 mm Hg between the right arm and descending aorta are observed in afflicted infants.

In right-to-left ductal shunting, the P_{O_2} is higher in the right arm than in the umbilical artery. These positive gradients in P_{O_2} between the right arm and umbilical artery are caused by right-to-left ductal shunting of unoxygenated pulmonary arterial blood into the descending aorta. Such positive PO_2 gradients between the right arm and umbilical artery have many causes, including most commonly various forms of lung disease (e.g., meconium aspiration, pneumonia, RDS). Several forms of congenital heart disease also cause right-to-left ductal shunting and positive PO_2 gradients between the right arm and umbilical artery (e.g., interrupted aortic arch, critical coarctation, aortic stenosis, endocardial fibroelastosis, infradiaphragmatic TAPVD, AVSD, arteriovenous malformation).

In two forms of congenital heart disease, the most highly oxygenated blood is in the pulmonary artery rather than the ascending aorta: TGV and supracardiac TAPVD. When right-to-left ductal shunting occurs in infants with TGV and supracardiac TAPVD, highly oxygenated blood is shunted from the pulmonary artery into the descending aorta. The net result is higher PO_2 measurements in the descending aorta than in the right arm or negative PO_2 gradients between the right arm and umbilical artery. Negative PO_2 gradients, admittedly rare, are nevertheless diagnostic of what is termed *transposition physiology* and always mean either TGV or supracardiac TAPVD.

The chest radiograph is the single most useful general screening test in making the preliminary distinction between lung disease and heart or systemic disease in symptomatic newborns. The chest radiograph is also useful in the preliminary assessment of how sick the infant is or is likely to become. As in other components of the evaluation of symptomatic newborns, serial chest radiographs can be useful in confirming initial diagnoses, in assessing whether attempted therapeutic interventions are effective, and in making adjustments to treatments that are effective.

The number of ribs should be counted on each infant; the presence of only 11 ribs suggests underlying trisomy 21. Trisomy 21 is associated with acyanotic (typically VSDs and AVSDs) but sometimes cyanotic (typically TOF) congenital heart disease. Infants with trisomy 21 also sometimes exhibit slow postnatal relaxation of pulmonary vascular tone (e.g., PPHNS), particularly when they also have

AVSDs. Such infants can be quite blue for several days after birth (without pulmonary stenosis or right ventricular outflow obstruction) just from right-to-left intracardiac shunting secondary to pulmonary hypertension. Usually only supplemental oxygen is indicated; after several days, pulmonary vascular resistance eventually falls, and these infants begin to develop large left-to-right intracardiac shunts. In contrast, the presence of 13 ribs suggests underlying trisomy 13, a chromosomal disorder typically associated with severe and complex congenital heart disease.

The presence of hemivertebrae is suggestive of VACTERL syndrome, a syndrome usually accompanied by congenital heart disease. Congenital scoliosis is frequently associated with other congenital anomalies, including congenital heart disease.

Distinguishing the course of an umbilical arterial catheter (down from the central abdomen into the pelvis, then up along the left side of the vertebral column) from an umbilical venous catheter (up from the central abdomen along the right side of the vertebral column) is important. Early diagnosis of infradiaphragmatic TAPVD can be missed when what is thought to be umbilical arterial blood is drawn out of what is really an umbilical venous catheter. Highly oxygenated blood (pulmonary venous return) courses through the umbilical vein in infradiaphragmatic TAPVD.

It is also important to notice when catheters in the umbilical vein have really passed across the foramen ovale into the left atrium because emboli of air or clot released into the left atrium are especially hazardous. In fact, umbilical venous catheters are most safely positioned at the junction of the inferior vena cava and right atrium. This position minimizes risks of perforation and of inadvertent migration across the foramen ovale into the left atrium. On the anteroposterior radiograph, the key to recognizing left atrial position of an umbilical venous catheter is a slight leftward tilt of the tip of the catheter toward the midline. On the lateral radiograph, left atrial placement of an umbilical venous catheter is obvious from the posterior course of the catheter across the foramen ovale into the left atrium. Left atrial placement of an umbilical venous catheter is sometimes done on purpose when no other access to arterial blood is available but should never be permitted to happen by accident.

The course of umbilical arterial catheters inserted high enough to cross the diaphragm can lead to recognition of a right-sided aortic arch. Normally, high umbilical catheters always stay to the left of the vertebral column. If an umbilical catheter crosses the vertebral column above the diaphragm and ascends on the right, right-sided aortic arch is present. Right-sided aortic arch is strongly associated with TOF and truncus arteriosus.

When air is present and one can therefore see the position of the abdominal contents, the first question to be addressed is the location of the liver and stomach. Problems with heterotaxia are virtually always accompanied by complex congenital heart disease. Complete situs inversus, with the heart in the right chest, the stomach on the right, and the liver on the left, is almost always benign from a cardiac point of view. Discordance between thoracic and abdominal situs, however, is always associated with major cardiovascular malformations.

The second question to be addressed in evaluating the abdominal findings on a chest radiograph is the size of the liver. The liver in newborn infants is readily distensible, and it expands and contracts quickly with changes in blood volume and right atrial pressure. Thus, the size of the liver on serial radiographs can be useful in following adequacy of volume replacement, of diuresis, and of treatment for pulmonary hypertension.

The third question to be addressed in evaluating the abdominal findings on a chest radiograph is whether or not free air is present. Recognition of the *football sign* from free air making the hepatic ligament visible can be the only clue to perforation of the gut or peritoneal dissection of extrapulmonary air.

The fourth question to be addressed in evaluating the abdominal findings on a chest radiograph is whether ascites is present. Ascites is most commonly seen in term newborns as part of hydrops fetalis, a disorder with many causes, including fetal arrhythmias. In premature newborns, ascites is more often seen as a manifestation of hyperalimentation-induced hepatic dysfunction or necrotizing enterocolitis.

The status of the lungs is the single most important piece of information available on the chest radiograph. In evaluating the lungs, it is important to assess (1) lung inflation, (2) lung density and homogeneity, and (3) lung vascularity. In addition, the presence of pleural fluid can be an important diagnostic key. The most common disorder associated with pleural effusion in newborns is meconium aspiration, but group B streptococcal pneumonia and congenital heart disease are also associated with pleural fluid. Pleural effusion is so uncommon in infants with RDS that its presence should suggest an alternative diagnosis, such as pneumonia or infradiaphragmatic TAPVD.

One useful technique in assessing lung inflation is to count the number of posterior ribs visible on the right side of the chest above the diaphragm. In general, when fewer than eight posterior ribs are visible above the diaphragm, the lungs are hypoinflated; when more than 10 posterior ribs are visible above the diaphragm, the lungs are hyperinflated. Comparing the magnitude of inflation in serial chest films is critical to serial assessments of heart size because changes in lung inflation can mask or exaggerate apparent changes in heart size.

Hypoinflation can be an important clue to the correct underlying diagnosis (e.g., RDS, pulmonary hypoplasia) in symptomatic infants. Hypoinflation also makes interpretation of lung density, lung vascularity, and heart size far more difficult. In mechanically ventilated infants, hypoinflation can also reflect low lung compliance *(stiff lungs)* as well as inadequate inspiratory or end-expiratory pressure. Similarly, hyperinflation can be a clue to the correct underlying diagnosis (e.g., chronic lung disease, meconium aspiration) in symptomatic infants or reflect excessive inspiratory or end-expiratory pressure during mechanical ventilation.

The second assessment to make in radiographic evaluation of the lungs in symptomatic newborns is whether the parenchymal lung fields are normal or opacified and, if opacified, whether the opacifications are homogeneous or asymmetric. Vigorous positive-pressure ventilation can cause what would otherwise be a diffusely atelectatic lung to appear to be normally inflated and to have normal-appearing parenchyma. In any case, the presence of normal inflation and normal parenchymal lung fields in spontaneously ventilating, symptomatic infants rules out structural problems of the lung (e.g., diaphragmatic hernia, pulmonary hypoplasia, pneumothorax, congenital lobar emphysema) and parenchymal diseases of the lung (e.g., RDS, congenital group B streptococcal pneumonia, meconium aspiration) as possible causes. In such infants, the likelihood of a systemic illness or congenital heart disease accounting for symptoms is high.

When parenchymal opacities are present on the chest radiograph, an important question is whether those opacities are *homogeneous* or *asymmetric*. Homogeneous densities usually represent RDS or congenital pneumonia, but adult respiratory distress syndrome does occur in newborn infants. Cardiogenic pulmonary edema can also be seen as a result of cardiac dysfunction from asphyxia as well as of structural congenital heart diseases that cause left atrial hypertension. Asymmetric densities, if bilateral, are most commonly seen in meconium aspiration in term infants and in chronic lung disease in premature infants. Meconium aspiration is the most common cause of PPHNS, but every infant with PPHNS, including those with meconium aspiration, requires careful cardiovascular evaluation to rule out the many known cardiac causes of pulmonary hypertension. Similarly, every premature infant with chronic lung disease requires careful cardiovascular evaluation to ferret out the possible contribution of silent PDA to the lung dysfunction. Unilateral parenchymal densities can represent localized pneumonias, aspiration, atelectasis, and congenital anomalies.

The third assessment to make in radiographic evaluation of the lungs in symptomatic newborns is whether the pulmonary vascularity is normal, decreased, or increased. Certainly in some cases sepa rating vascular changes from parenchymal changes can be difficult. Nevertheless, attempting to distinguish whether pulmonary vascularity is normal, decreased, or increased and following changes in pulmonary vascularity serially on subsequent chest radiographs can be useful in differential diagnosis and management. The distinction between pulmonary venous engorgement from left atrial hypertension (or pulmonary venous obstruction) and pulmonary arterial engorgement from left-to-right shunt is more difficult in sick newborn infants than in older children and adults, at least in part because chest radiographs are taken supine in newborn infants. One useful marker for pulmonary venous congestion is the presence of pleural fluid.

One important radiographic appearance to recognize is the picture of *congestive heart failure with a small heart*, a pattern typical of infradiaphragmatic TAPVD. A similar pattern can be observed in some infants with retained amniotic fluid, however. In infants with various forms of hypoplasia of the right heart and inadequate pulmonary blood flow, reduction in pulmonary oligemia in response to infusion of PGE_1 (and reopening of the ductus) is usually readily evident on serial chest radiographs. Similarly, increased pulmonary vascularity is usually readily evident at least on the side of the shunt on postoperative chest radiographs after surgical placement of modified Blalock-Taussig shunts.

Systematic review of the chest radiograph should enable the clinician to determine (1) whether the heart *position* is normal or whether dextrocardia or mesocardia is present; (2) whether the heart *size* is normal or abnormal; and (3) whether the heart *contour* is normal or abnormal. In addition, the chest radiograph should enable the clinician to determine whether the pulmonary artery is normal or not. These assessments provide useful insights into differential diagnosis, but the value of the radiographic appearance of the heart is far greater when it is considered in conjunction with the status of the pulmonary vascularity and the entire clinical picture of the patient.

On the chest radiograph of the normal heart, the right border is formed by the right atrium, and most of the left heart border is formed by the left ventricle. The most characteristic feature of normal cardiac contour is the *bump* at the upper left margin of the heart derived from the normal size and position of the pulmonary artery.

Right atrial enlargement is readily evident on chest radiograph from extension of the right heart border into the right chest because the right atrium makes up the right heart border. The rest of the contour of the heart is unchanged by right atrial enlargement. Right atrial enlargement is characteristic of critical pulmonary stenosis, Ebstein anomaly, and in utero closure of the ductus secondary to maternal ingestion of over-the-counter inhibitors of cyclooxygenase (such as aspirin, ibuprofen). The right atrium also enlarges in ASD but not in the newborn period.

When the pulmonary artery is transposed, absent, or diminutive, the cardiac silhouette appears abnormal because the bump created by the normal pulmonary artery is not present. If the pulmonary artery is absent (pulmonary atresia) or hypoplastic (TOF, most forms of tricuspid atresia), absence of the normal shadow of the pulmonary artery usually makes the heart appear to be boot-shaped (*coeur en sabot*). If the pulmonary artery is transposed (TGV), the abnormal position of the pulmonary artery creates an *egg-on-side* appearance to the cardiac silhouette.

Left atrial enlargement is more difficult to detect on a chest radiograph than right atrial enlargement because the left atrium lies behind the heart in the anteroposterior projection. Left atrial enlargement can be recognized from (1) a double density behind the heart just to the right of the vertebral column and (2) splaying of the main stem bronchi from the usual angulation of 45 degrees to near 90 degrees. The latter finding occurs because left atrial enlargement can elevate the left main stem bronchus. When shunt vascularity is evident, the presence of left atrial enlargement means that the atrial septum is intact and that the shunt must be at the ventricular or ductal level.

The three most important laboratory tests in diagnosis of neonatal cardiac disorders are electrocardiog raphy, echocardiography, and cardiac catheterization. The hyperoxia test is a well-known maneuver designed to distinguish infants with congenital heart disease from those with lung disease, but it lacks both specificity and sensitivity and is therefore more misleading than useful. Electrocardiography is mainly useful in sorting out disorders of cardiac rate and rhythm. Echocardiography is by far the most valuable diagnostic tool in evaluating newborns with possible cardiac disease because it can provide the fine details of cardiovascular structure and function noninvasively. Cardiac catheterization, once the gold standard of neonatal cardiovascular diagnosis, is largely a therapeutic procedure today.

In the hyperoxia test, an infant with suspected or possible congenital heart disease is placed on 100% oxygen (or in other iterations, 100% oxygen plus constant positive airway pressure). If arterial Po_2 does not rise above some magical level (100 mm Hg in some hands, 50 mm Hg in others), the infant is supposed to have cyanotic congenital heart disease. If the Po_2 rises above 200 mm Hg, congenital heart disease is supposed to be ruled out. The problem with this test is that it does not work. All that a Po_2 less than 50 mm Hg on 100% oxygen really means is that the infant has either a large intracardiac or a large intrapulmonary right-to-left shunt—if the arterial sample in question really reflects the oxygen content being ejected from the systemic ventricle (a false assumption in many cases). For example, many infants with severe RDS have a Po_2 less than 50 mm Hg on 100% oxygen before the administration of surfactant or institution of positive airway pressure. A persistent Po_2 in the 30s in the absence of respiratory distress and in the absence of radiographic abnormalities in the lungs does suggest cyanotic heart disease, however.

Similarly, all that a Po_2 greater than 200 mm Hg really means is that highly oxygenated blood is reaching the artery from which the sample was drawn; it does not mean that highly oxygenated blood is being ejected from the systemic ventricle. For example, arterial Po_2 measurements greater than 200 mm Hg can be found in the descending aorta (umbilical arterial catheter) in TGV when the ductus is patent and pulmonary vascular resistance exceeds systemic resistance. Arterial PO_2 measurements on 100% oxygen greater than 200 mm Hg that are derived from blood ejected from the systemic ventricle can be seen in many forms of life-threatening congenital heart disease, including HLHS, infradiaphragmatic TAPVD, interrupted aortic arch, critical aortic stenosis, and critical coarctation.

The 12-lead electrocardiogram is not particularly helpful in evaluation of symptomatic newborn infants except in two circumstances. First, the 12-lead electrocardiogram is essential in diagnosing disorders of cardiac rate and rhythm. Rhythm strips from bedside monitors are not useful in identifying disorders of rhythm and should not be relied on. Typical disorders of rate and rhythm seen in newborns include supraventricular tachycardia (SVT), also known as *paroxysmal atrial tachycardia*, and complete heart block. Complete heart block is usually well tolerated if the resting ventricular rate is greater than 55 beats/min and the heart is structurally normal. Complete congenital heart block is now typically diagnosed prenatally, although occasional infants with complete congenital heart block are still delivered by emergency cesarean section for fetal bradycardia presumed to be secondary to fetal distress.

SVT is now frequently first diagnosed prenatally, particularly when the SVT is persistent enough to cause hydrops fetalis. In most newborns with SVT, good control can be achieved with digoxin alone; less commonly the combination of digoxin and propranolol is required. Recording a 12-lead electrocardiogram is indicated after abolition of SVT to look for underlying Wolff-Parkinson-White syndrome. Infants with SVT who have underlying Wolff-Parkinson-White syndrome are more likely to have recurrences and are more likely to have SVT that is difficult to suppress pharmacologically. A single normal 12-lead electrocardiogram does not exclude Wolff-Parkinson-White syndrome because the bypass tract can come and go from the surface electrocardiogram.

Multifocal atrial tachycardia has the poorest

prognosis of neonatal tachyarrhythmias but is rare. Neonatal atrial flutter can be difficult to recognize, but injections of adenosine (to abolish presumed SVT) usually induce brief periods of higher degrees of block that permit recognition of flutter.

Second, determination of axis with the 12-lead electrocardiogram is also useful. In the most common form of congenital heart disease associated with trisomy 21, left axis deviation is almost always present. Absence of left axis deviation virtually excludes the diagnosis of AVSD in infants with trisomy 21. In the absence of readily available cardiologic consultation, a screening 12-lead electrocardiogram in infants with trisomy 21 to exclude left axis deviation can provide reassurance to the pediatrician or neonatologist (and parents) that the most commonly encountered form of congenital heart disease is not present. Shunt murmurs in infants with trisomy 21 and AVSD are frequently not present for several days after birth, given the often dilatory postnatal relaxation of pulmonary vascular resistance commonly observed in infants with trisomy 21. In cyanotic infants, mild left axis deviation suggests pulmonary atresia, and extreme left axis deviation suggests tricuspid atresia.

Although echocardiography is the single most useful diagnostic test in evaluating symptomatic infants for congenital heart disease, several disorders can be missed (i.e., neonatal echocardiography lacks sensitivity, or causes false-negative diagnoses) when echocardiography is performed too soon after birth and not repeated later. The most important (and most difficult to diagnose) example is coarctation. As long as the aortic end of the ductus is patent, many infants who have coarctation are not diagnosable by either echocardiography or cardiac catheterization. Normally the aortic end of the ductus does not close until after 10 days of age, although the pulmonary end usually shuts by the end of the first day of life in term infants. It is only closure of the aortic end of the ductus that precipitates significant obstruction in many infants with coarctation. Coarctation cannot be excluded until the aortic end of the ductus closes.

A second example of a malformation that can be

missed when echocardiograms are performed shortly after birth is a small or moderate VSD. Such defects are usually identified by color flow Doppler–detected left-to-right shunts, rather than by direct visualization of ventricular septal dropout. Yet left-to-right shunts in VSDs cannot occur until pulmonary vascular resistance falls below systemic resistance, a development that occurs slowly in some infants.

A third example of a malformation that can be missed when echocardiograms are performed too infrequently is failure to demonstrate ductal patency in premature infants who have chronic lung disease. Silent PDA in infants with chronic lung disease is the most common diagnosis missed by neonatal echocardiography. In infants with chronic lung disease, pulmonary vascular resistance is usually not only high, but also highly variable. Infants with chronic lung disease who have not had the ductus ligated almost always have intermittent left-to-right ductal shunts that wax and wane over periods of minutes in response to changes in pulmonary vascular resistance. Thus, absence of left-to-right ductal shunting at a single point in time by echocardiography in infants with chronic lung disease provides little reassurance that ductal patency is not contributing to pulmonary compromise.

Two disorders that are commonly overdiagnosed by neonatal echocardiography when the study is performed too soon after birth are PDA and ASD. In the case of PDA, the ductus is obviously normally patent at birth. In term infants, the pulmonary end of the ductus often does not fully constrict until 24 hours after birth. In premature infants, the ductus is not likely to shut for quite some time.

Similarly the foramen ovale is normally patent at birth and typically remains patent in up to 90% of infants for the first year of life. Distinguishing left-to-right atrial shunt across a patent foramen ovale from left-to-right shunt across a small or even moderate ASD is usually impossible in the first days and often first months after birth. Sometimes the final assessment of what is a patent foramen ovale versus ASD cannot be made until the end of the first year of life.

With the advent and refinement of echocardiographic and Doppler ultrasound techniques over the past two decades, the role of cardiac catheterization and angiocardiography in the diagnosis of neonatal congenital heart disease has diminished. In many cases, cardiac catheterization may be entirely unnecessary or may be tailored to provide limited anatomic information that complements the echocardiographic diagnosis. In practice, the utilization of cardiac catheterization for the diagnosis of congenital heart disease in the newborn varies widely from center to center, depending on the quality of echocardiographic support, the type of surgery planned, and the preferences of the attending cardiologist and surgeon. The overriding principle determining the indications for cardiac catheterization in an individual patient should be whether or not all important anatomic and physiologic questions have been answered sufficiently to guide proper treatment. The decision about diagnostic catheterization should not be influenced by whether the patient has a congenital heart anomaly that is typically diagnosed only by echocardiography.

The technique of neonatal cardiac catheterization varies widely from center to center, depending on the preferences of the operator. These preferences affect the chosen route of vascular access, the selection of catheters and other equipment, and many other technical aspects. For most diagnostic right heart studies, the authors prefer a percutaneous approach to a femoral vein for ease of catheter manipulations and exchanges, although the authors have occasionally used the umbilical vein. (The authors prefer the umbilical vein approach for bedside Rashkind atrioseptostomy.) For retrograde left heart studies, the umbilical artery is frequently available and ideal, obviating risk of femoral arterial injury. With improvements in catheter and introducer sheath design, a 3, or at most 4, French system is sufficient for diagnostic studies and is minimally traumatic when used after percutaneous entry into a femoral artery. In selected circumstances, unusual access sites may be used, such as the right radial artery when the aortic arch is interrupted, the right subclavian artery is not aberrant, and a left ventricular angiogram does not opacify the ascending segment. Isolation and cannulation of vessels by a cutdown technique is an option but is rarely necessary.

Of all the diagnostic information obtained at cardiac catheterization in newborns, angiographic demonstration of the anatomy is of primary importance and may be tailored to supplement well-documented echocardiographic anatomy.

The common acyanotic forms of congenital heart disease with left-to-right shunts *dependent* on low pulmonary vascular resistance rarely require diagnostic angiographic assessment in the neonatal period. Critical obstructions (i.e., pulmonary and aortic stenosis) are studied in the setting of a therapeutic intervention and are discussed later. Coarctation of the aorta may be challenging to diagnose or exclude, particularly in patients with major intracardiac defects and a large ductus arteriosus. A retrograde juxtaductal or transverse aortogram or an antegrade balloon occlusion descending thoracic aortogram demonstrates the intraluminal filling defect and extent of proximal aortic hypoplasia. Occasionally angiography is necessary to distinguish between coarctation and interruption of the aortic arch. Rarely in interrupted aortic arch, contrast material injected into the left ventricle does not sufficiently opacify the aortic arch, and hand injection of contrast material via a right radial artery intravenous catheter is diagnostic (if the right subclavian artery does not arise aberrantly from the descending aorta). In transposition of the great arteries, coronary artery anomalies are common and may be demonstrated by aortography. The *laid-back* view, obtained by an antegrade aortic root injection filmed with extreme caudal angulation of the x-ray beam, provides a look down the barrel of the ascending aorta and is especially valuable for visualizing the coronary origins and course.

TOF occurs in its classic form with right ventricular outflow obstruction and in a more complex form with complete pulmonary atresia. Newborns with pulmonary atresia usually have more severe and variable associated vascular abnormalities, such as extreme hypoplasia, nonconfluence, or abnormal arborization of the native pulmonary arteries and major aortopulmonary collateral arteries, and benefit from angiographic assessment. When the ductus arteriosus is widely patent, a juxtaductal aortogram allows visualization of the pulmonary arterial anatomy. When an infant presents after ductal closure, pulmonary venous wedge angiography by hand injection of contrast material fills the native pulmonary arteries retrograde via the pulmonary capillary bed. Selective contrast injections into aortopulmonary collateral vessels often fill the native pulmonary arteries and aid in identifying arborization abnormalities. Although some operators prefer selective coronary arteriography to detect coronary anomalies even in newborns, aortography or left ventriculography is generally sufficient to diagnose or exclude anomalous origin of the anterior descending coronary from the right coronary artery (the most prevalent variation associated with TOF).

Pulmonary atresia with an intact ventricular septum presents an entirely different set of diagnostic considerations that guide angiographic assessment. Right ventriculography allows quantitation of the degree of hypoplasia of the chamber and tricuspid valve annulus, determination of whether the chamber is tripartite or not, and proximity of the outflow tract to the pulmonary trunk (the position of which may be identified by simultaneous placement of a retrograde catheter via the ductus). Right ventriculography also identifies sinusoidal connections to the coronary arteries and may fill the ascending aorta. Aortic root angiography should opacify both coronary artery beds, or the coronary circulation may be dependent on suprasystemic right ventricular perfusion pressure.

Total anomalous pulmonary venous drainage is usually associated with pulmonary venous obstruction when it requires angiographic assessment in the newborn. A pulmonary arteriogram generally allows visualization of the anomalous site of drainage except when pulmonary blood flow is critically reduced because of the venous obstruction. Alternatively, the venous catheter may be passed to the common pulmonary venous chamber for selective angiography, although this may be most difficult when it is most necessary (i.e., the obstruction is severe). Occasionally, selective bilateral branch pulmonary arteriography improves angiographic identification of mixed sites of drainage (supradiaphragmatic and infradiaphragmatic in the same patient).

Truncus arteriosus may be associated with truncal valve dysfunction, branch pulmonary artery stenosis, interrupted aortic arch, or coronary artery anomalies. A large-volume, rapidly injected, truncal root angiogram, usually with the antegrade catheter, can demonstrate most, if not all, of these features in a single injection.

Tricuspid atresia may occur with transposed or normally related great arteries, a large or small VSD, and varying degrees of pulmonary stenosis and pulmonary arterial hypoplasia. A large-volume, rapidly injected, left ventriculogram, with the venous catheter, can demonstrate most, if not all, of these features in a single injection. In newborns with ductus-derived pulmonary blood flow, a juxtaductal aortogram visualizes the pulmonary artery anatomy.

Several other complex cyanotic congenital heart malformations may require angiographic assessment. In double inlet left ventricle with transposed great arteries, ventriculography may aid in the evaluation of the bulboventricular foramen and its egress to the aorta. In the heterotaxia syndromes (asplenia/polysplenia), anomalous systemic and pulmonary venous drainage and pulmonary atresia with associated pulmonary arterial hypoplasia are common, and angiography is particularly valuable in their assessment.

COMMON PRESENTATIONS AND SPECIFIC CARDIAC PROBLEMS

The range of developmental abnormalities and problems with pregnancy, labor, and delivery that can result in post-natal symptoms is quite broad. Nevertheless, the great majority of infants with serious or life-threatening problems present in one of eight different ways: respiratory distress, cyanosis, shock, murmur, multiple congenital anomalies, prematurity, or asphyxia. Familiarity with the common cardiovascular causes of these eight presentations can provide earlier insight into the correct diagnosis and management for better than 9 out of 10 infants with potentially serious cardiovascular problems.

Complete Transposition of the Great Arteries

In transposition of the great arteries, the position of the great arteries is reversed; that is, the aorta arises anteriorly from the right ventricle and the pulmonary artery posteriorly from the left ventricle. The pulmonary and systemic circulations are therefore arranged in parallel rather than in series, with the systemic venous blood passing through the right heart chambers then back out to the body, and pulmonary venous blood traversing the left heart and returning to the lungs. Survival after birth depends on mixing between the circuits.

Transposition of the great arteries in the newborn is often an isolated defect, but other associated malformations involving defects of the atrial or ventricular septum, stenosis or atresia of the pulmonic valve, and anomalies of the atrioventricular valves are not uncommon and may alter the physiology considerably. Interestingly, extracardiac anomalies are unusual in newborns with transposition of the great arteries. Transposition of the great arteries occurs in slightly more than 1 per 4500 live births. There is a strong sex predilection in transposition of the great arteries, with males outnumbering females by almost 2:1.

The pulmonary and systemic circulations are arranged in parallel rather than in series, with the aorta arising from the right ventricle and the pulmonary artery from the left. In utero, there is little disruption in fetal hemodynamics because blood returning from the systemic and pulmonary veins passes unimpeded into the atrium and ventricles in the normal fashion. Blood from the right ventricle is pumped into the ascending aorta then to the systemic arteries and placenta. Blood from the left ventricle passes into the pulmonary artery, then, because of the high pulmonary resistance, most is diverted into the ductus arteriosus and descending aorta. The only variation from the normal fetal circulation is that the slightly less saturated blood from the superior vena cava is preferentially shunted to the head vessels rather than through the ductus arteriosus, and the more saturated blood from the inferior vena cava is shunted to the lungs rather than to the cerebral circulation. Despite these differences, in utero development appears normal, and thus far no major extrauterine abnormalities have been identified.

After birth, newborns completely depend on mixing between pulmonary and systemic circulations for survival. For a while the fetal pathways, the ductus arteriosus and foramen ovale, suffice. By a few hours of age, the pulmonary resistance is significantly lower than the systemic, so shunting of hypoxemic blood from the aorta to the pulmonary artery is facilitated. Because the pulmonary circuit cannot be overloaded, obligatory shunting of pulmonary venous return from left atrium to right atrium occurs. This bidirectional shunting from aorta to pulmonary artery and left atrium to right atrium improves mixing and prevents severe cyanosis. As the ductus arteriosus closes, however, the obligatory shunting is eliminated, and the only site of mixing is the foramen ovale. Although some bidirectional shunting may occur allowing deoxygenated blood to get to the lungs and oxygenated blood to the systemic circulation, this is usually inadequate, and severe systemic hypoxemia (PO_2, 15 to 40 mm Hg; O_2 saturation, 30 to 60) results.

The physical examination is usually unrewarding except for generalized cyanosis. Although peripheral pulses may be somewhat bounding and the right ventricular impulse slightly hyperactive, the heart sounds are usually normal, with physiologic splitting of the second sound present about half the time. Prominent heart murmurs are uncommon, although there may be a short grade 2/6 systolic murmur along the left sternal border. A loud murmur should alert one to the possibility of associated heart disease (e.g., a VSD). Signs of congestive failure are usually absent, although tachypnea may be present, probably as a compensatory mechanism for the hypoxemia.

Because there is little disturbance in the intrauterine blood flow, the electrocardiogram is usually normal showing right axis deviation and right ventricular hypertrophy that is within the normal limits for age. The chest radiography is also usually normal for a newborn, although the relative anteroposterior position of the great vessels and the usual (although unexplained) absence of a thymic shadow give the narrow appearance of the superior mediastinum frequently described as an *egg-on-side* appearance. The pulmonary blood flow is rarely increased in the first few days of life, although it may be increased in infants who present later.

Transposition of the great arteries should be strongly suspected in any cyanotic newborn showing normal-to-increased pulmonary blood flow on the radiograph and right ventricular hypertrophy on the electrocardiogram. A severely hypoxemic infant breathing comfortably with a normal physical examination, chest radiograph, and electrocardiogram almost invariably has transposition. All other types of cyanotic congenital heart disease are associated with diminished or congested pulmonary vascular markings on the radiograph and a single second heart sound. Persistent fetal circulation can usually be distinguished by echocardiography.

Untreated, transposition of the great arteries in infants is associated with a dismal prognosis; 30% die in the 1st week, and 50% die in the first months of life. The management involves three phases: rapid correction of metabolic derangements, palliation, and later correction. If the infant is acidotic with a pH of less than 7.25 when first seen, sodium bicarbonate should be given to correct the base deficit. In those who are severely acidotic or in whom further palliation must be delayed, PGE_1 is used to open the ductus arteriosus and improve mixing and oxygenation.

If infants present with acidosis secondary to hypoxemia, a true emergency exists. Correction of the acidosis and improvement in intracardiac mixing with PGE_1 to reopen the ductus arteriosus and balloon atrial septostomy to improve interatrial mixing are mandatory.

Surgical correction historically has involved rerouting the blood at the atrial level (Senning or Mustard procedures). More recently, most centers have performed an arterial switch including coronary relocation as a primary operation in the perinatal period. Surgical mortality has been reduced to about 5% to 10% in most centers, with excellent medium-term survival (up to 10 to 15 years).

Tetralogy of Fallot

In 1888, Fallot described a series of cyanotic patients with a VSD, pulmonary stenosis, right ventricular hypertrophy, and an aorta that appeared to be over the ventricular septum. For many years, it has been appreciated that the last two manifestations are secondary to the first two lesions.

The VSD location is predictably high in the ventricular septum; additional defects are present in 15% of the patients. The degree of pulmonic obstruction at the infundibulum (subvalvular) or secondarily at the pulmonary valve or peripheral pulmonary arteries is variable, ranging from mild stenosis to complete atresia, and accounts for the variability of presentation. Associated anomalies include ASDs, right aortic arch (25%), and anomalies of the coronary arteries (5%). TOF occurs slightly less frequently than transpositions (1 of every 5000 live births) and accounts for 9% of infants presenting in the 1st week of life.

In utero there does not seem to be any major hemodynamic disturbance, and consequently, newborns with TOF are well developed at birth. During fetal life, the aorta carries an increased percentage of combined ventricular output with the exact proportion a function of the degree of pulmonic stenosis. The ductus arteriosus is smaller than normal because its flow is diminished, and it may be quite tortuous. Because there is no volume or pressure overload within the heart, the ventricles and atrioventricular valves usually develop normally.

After birth, the degree of shunting depends on

the severity of the pulmonary stenosis and the relative pulmonary and systemic arteriolar resistance. In the newborn with severe pulmonary stenosis, the resistance to blood passing out the right ventricular outflow tract is high, and desaturated venous blood preferentially passes through the VSD into the aorta, resulting in arterial hypoxemia and cyanosis. If the pulmonary stenosis is mild, there may be little resistance to blood passing out the pulmonary artery; infants with this condition may behave similar to those with a VSD, with increasing left-to-right shunt and heart failure as the pulmonary arteriolar resistance drops over the first weeks of life. The usual hallmarks of TOF, arterial hypoxemia and cyanosis, may be completely absent in this group at first. Occasionally, mild-to-moderate pulmonary stenosis may occur in a balanced situation in which pulmonary and systemic resistances are equal and little shunt in either direction occurs; often these infants shunt right to left with crying.

The presentation of infants with tetralogy is a function of the degree of pulmonary stenosis. Those with severe obstruction usually present in the first days with extreme cyanosis as the ductus arteriosus closes. Those with lesser degrees of pulmonary stenosis may be only mildly cyanotic and present with a systolic ejection murmur along the left sternal border in the delivery room or in the nursery. The pulmonary component of the second heart sound is diminished or inaudible. Signs of congestive heart failure are absent except in a small group with an absent pulmonary valve who present with a to-and-fro murmur at the left upper sternal border owing to pulmonary stenosis and regurgitation. Tetralogy *spells*, which are attacks of paroxysmal dyspnea associated with irritability, extreme cyanosis, and loss of the systolic murmur, are an emergency because cerebral hypoxemia may lead to convulsions, coma, and death. Spells are unusual in the first months of life.

Because the right ventricle receives normal flow in utero, the electrocardiogram of the newborn with TOF is normal, showing right axis deviation and right ventricular hypertrophy. The heart size on the chest radiograph is usually normal because neither the atria nor the ventricles are exposed to a volume overload. In those who are hypoxemic, the pulmonary blood flow is decreased because venous blood is being diverted away from the lungs to the systemic circuit. The main pulmonary artery segment is often diminished, giving the classic *coeur-en-sabot* appearance. A right aortic arch is present in one fourth of the cases.

The cyanotic infant with decreased pulmonary blood flow and a normal heart size on the chest radiograph, right axis deviation and right ventricular hypertrophy on the electrocardiogram, and a systolic ejection murmur on examination usually has TOF. Infants with a systolic murmur without cyanosis may be confused with patients with isolated valvular pulmonary stenosis or even those with a VSD. More complicated lesions with a physiology similar to that of TOF, ventricular defect, and pulmonary stenosis must be differentiated by echocardiography or angiocardiography. Examples are double-outlet ventricle with pulmonary stenosis, single ventricle with pulmonary stenosis, and transposition.

Historically, the approach to TOF has been either early palliation with an aortopulmonary shunt or corrective surgery. Most centers now reserve palliative surgery for those younger than 1 year, but an increasing number of surgeons are doing corrective operations at the time of presentation. Surgery involves closing the VSD, usually through a right ventriculotomy; resecting infundibular muscle; and if the infundibular muscle, pulmonary valve, and main pulmonary artery are hypoplastic, using a pericardial patch to open the narrowed area. Failure to close the VSD is unusual, although some degree of residual right ventricular outflow tract obstruction is common. When the patch crosses the pulmonary annulus, the children are left with pulmonary regurgitation. Recently, long-term (30-year) follow-up studies have become available, with an actuarial survival of more than 86% at 30 years for those repaired during childhood.

Tetralogy of Fallot with Pulmonary Atresia

TOF with pulmonary atresia is the severest form of TOF, with the deviated parietal band of the infundibulum completely occluding the right ventricular outflow tract. Because there is no antegrade flow through the pulmonic valve, development of the pulmonary arteries depends on flow from the ductus arteriosus and embryologic intersegmental or bronchial arteries. If the flow into the pulmonary arteries is proximal, the mediastinal portion of the right and left pulmonary arteries may be of good size. If, however, the collaterals insert well within the hilum of the lungs, the mediastinal portions may be hypoplastic or even atretic. Even when central pulmonary arteries are present, there may be incomplete arborization of the pulmonary arteries with some or most of the lung parenchyma supplied via the collateral systemic arteries rather than the mediastinal pulmonary arteries.

A cyanotic infant showing decreased pulmonary blood flow on the radiograph, right ventricular hypertrophy on the electrocardiogram, and no murmur or a continuous murmur usually has TOE with pulmonary atresia. Newborns with transposition and an intact ventricular septum have no murmurs and may be just as cyanotic but have normal or increased pulmonary blood flow visible on chest radiographs. Infants with total anomalous pulmonary venous return usually show a pulmonary venous congestion pattern on the chest radiographs. More complicated lesions simulating TOF with pulmonary atresia must be distinguished by two-dimensional echocardiogram or angiography.

Those infants with large collaterals and congestive heart failure can usually be distinguished from infants with a VSD, PDA, or aortopulmonary window on the basis of their arterial hypoxemia as well as from those with truncus arteriosus and transposition with a VSD on the basis of the continuous murmurs.

Since there is no forward pulmonary blood flow, these infants frequently become very sick when the ductus arteriosus closes. For those who present with severe hypoxemia and acidosis, PGE_1 is usually sufficient to give temporary improvement. Reparative surgery is more problematic than in infants with a pulmonary stenosis because of the common accompaniment of hypoplasia or even discontinuity of pulmonary arteries.

Some centers use a palliative systemic-to-pulmonary artery shunt in the perinatal period with later repair. Other centers have been doing primary repair in those with an adequate pulmonary tree by closing the VSD and using an external conduit (usually aortic homograft) between the right ventricle and pulmonary artery. Surgery is necessary later in childhood because of the fixed size of the conduit, which becomes relatively smaller with somatic growth. For children with hypoplastic or discontinuous pulmonary arteries, a staged procedure is frequently necessary involving palliative surgical operations (unifocalization) and catheterization laboratory intervention to dilate or stent the hypoplastic pulmonary arteries.

Pulmonary Atresia with an Intact Ventricular Septum

In pulmonary atresia with an intact ventricular septum (approximately 1 in 14,000 births), the pulmonary valve is an imperforate membrane. In more than 80% of the newborn patients, the right ventricle is moderately or severely hypoplastic, often having a volume of only 1 or 2 mL at birth. The tricuspid valve annulus is also hypoplastic, corresponding to the size of the right ventricle, and the valve may be stenotic owing to fusion of the chordae. The right atrium is invariably enlarged and hypertrophied and may be enormous in infants with severe tricuspid regurgitation. The high pressure within the right ventricular cavity causes dilation of the normal myocardial sinusoids, and connections are often present between the sinusoids and coronary arteries, with flow going from right ventricle to ascending aorta. Obstructions in the coronary arteries are not uncommon in this group with sinusoids, and myocardial perfusion may be via the right ventricle, the aorta, or both. In contrast to patients with TOF associated with pulmonary atresia, the infants with pulmonary atresia and an intact ventricular septum almost invariably have normal pulmonary arteries.

Prenatally, egress of blood from the right ventricle is prevented by the pulmonary atresia. All the venous blood returning to the right atrium must pass through the foramen ovale to the left atrium, left ventricle, and ascending aorta; these chambers are dilated compared with those in the normal fetus. Conversely, because flow to the right ventricle is minimal, this chamber is usually hypoplastic. The pulmonary blood flow in utero is derived entirely from the aorta via a small, usually tortuous, ductus arteriosus. This physiologic arrangement does not disrupt the normal growth and development during fetal life. After birth, there is a continuation of the fetal pattern; the pulmonary blood flow continues to be totally dependent on the small ductus arteriosus. As this closes in the first hours or days of life, the minimal pulmonary blood flow diminishes further, and severe hypoxemia and acidosis follow.

Infants with pulmonary atresia are mildly cyanotic soon after birth but are often intensely cyanotic by 24 hours of age as the ductus arteriosus constricts. On physical examination, the second heart sound is single. A continuous murmur, from left-to-fight shunting through the ductus arteriosus, or a systolic regurgitant murmur along the left sternal border, secondary to tricuspid regurgitation, may be heard; however, in about 20% of infants, no murmur is audible. The liver is enlarged if tricuspid regurgitation is severe and the foramen ovale is restrictive.

On chest radiographs, the cardiothoracic ratio is increased because of dilation of the right atrium and left ventricle, and the pulmonary vascular markings are invariably reduced. The aortic arch is to the left of the trachea in almost all infants. The electrocardiogram is characteristic and extremely helpful in the differential diagnosis. Because of the right ventricular hypoplasia and low volume of blood in the right ventricle and large left ventricle in utero, there is a left ventricular predominance in the precordial leads, with a QRS axis of +30 to +120 degrees. Right atrial hypertrophy is also often seen.

A cyanotic newborn with pulmonary atresia and an intact ventricular septum can usually be distinguished from an infant with transposition of the great arteries with an intact ventricular septum because the latter child has a split second heart sound, increased pulmonary flow on the radiograph, right ventricular hypertrophy on the electrocardiogram, and a characteristic echocardiogram. Infants with tricuspid atresia and a hypoplastic right ventricle show decreased pulmonary flow on the radiograph and left ventricular predominance on electrocardiogram, but they almost invariably have a QRS axis of -30 to -90 degrees on the electrocardiogram, whereas infants with pulmonary atresia have a QRS axis of $+30$ to $+120$ degrees. Infants with pulmonary stenosis and a hypoplastic right ventricle may be difficult to distinguish from those with pulmonary atresia before angiography but usually have a pulmonary ejection murmur rather than a regurgitant murmur and a valve that can be seen on two-dimensional echocardiography.

The initial treatment must be directed at correcting the metabolic acidosis with oxygen and bicarbonate. The value of PGE_1 to dilate the ductus arteriosus, increase pulmonary blood flow, and improve oxygenation has been well demonstrated. PGE_1 is useful in allowing time for stabilization of the infants before initiation of surgery.

The surgical therapy of pulmonary atresia with an intact ventricular septum depends on the degree of hypoplasia of the right ventricle and tricuspid valve. When near normal in size, a pulmonary valvulotomy or right ventricular outflow tract patch may suffice. If the right ventricle and tricuspid valve are intermediate in size, a right ventricular outflow tract patch and palliative aortopulmonary shunt are frequently performed in the perinatal period. If the right ventricle and tricuspid valve grow, the palliative shunt can be closed either in the interventional catheterization laboratory or surgically. If there is no significant growth, a Fontan operation is required, directing systemic venous blood to the pulmonary artery, bypassing the right ventricle. For children with extreme hypoplasia of the right ventricle and tricuspid valve, frequently with sinusoidal connections and right-to-left shunting between the right ventricle and the coronary arteries, the long-term approach should be directed toward the Fontan, although a palliative aortopulmonary shunt must be done in the perinatal period since the Fontan will not work with the elevated pulmonary vascular resistance of the perinatal period.

Pulmonary Stenosis with an Intact Ventricular Septum

In this lesion (1 in 14,000 live births), the pulmonary valve has a narrowed orifice that is usually due to fusion of the three pulmonary commissures. The size of the right ventricular cavity can be normal but is usually somewhat hypoplastic in those infants who present with cyanosis in the 1st month of life. The size of the chamber is rarely, if ever, as small as that seen in infants with pulmonary atresia and an intact ventricular septum, and abnormalities of the tricuspid valve and right ventricular sinusoidal–coronary artery fistulas are less common. The main and peripheral pulmonary arteries are usually normal.

In utero the obstruction at the pulmonary valve results in hypertrophy as well as a loss of compliance of the right ventricle. This leads to diversion of an increased proportion of venous return through the foramen ovale to the left side of the heart and ascending aorta. If the stenosis appears early in gestation and is severe, significant hypoplasia of the right ventricle with corresponding enlargement of the left ventricle occurs, resembling that seen in pulmonary atresia and an intact ventricular septum. If the stenosis is milder and occurs later in gestation, the right ventricle can be normal or near normal in size.

After birth, the degree of right-to-left shunting at the atrial level and thus arterial hypoxemia depends on the degree of pulmonary stenosis and right ventricular hypoplasia. If the stenosis is severe, right-to-left shunting at the atrial level may be massive and adequate pulmonary blood flow dependent on left-to-right shunting through the ductus arteriosus. If the stenosis is milder, with most of the pulmonary blood flow through the pulmonary valve, there may be little effect from ductal closure. As the pulmonary arteriolar resistance (in series with the pulmonary valve resistance) decreases over the first few weeks of life, the right-to-left shunt at the atrial level and, thus, the systemic hypoxemia may decrease.

In mild pulmonary stenosis, a loud systolic ejection murmur at the left upper sternal border may be the only finding. In moderate or severe stenosis, the murmur is less prominent, but cyanosis is present, increasing as the ductus arteriosus constricts. There is a prominent *a* wave in the jugular venous pulse reflecting reduced right ventricular compliance, and the liver is often enlarged and may even be pulsatile. The pulmonary component of the second heart sound is delayed and diminished and may be inaudible.

On chest radiograph, there is mild cardiomegaly owing to an enlarged right atrium and diminished pulmonary blood flow. Poststenotic dilation in the main pulmonary artery in the newborn is unusual. The electrocardiogram is normal if the pulmonary stenosis is mild or moderate. With severe pulmonary stenosis and a diminutive right ventricle, the electrocardiogram usually demonstrates right atrial enlargement and left ventricular predominance with a QRS axis of +30 to +120 degrees, similar to that seen in pulmonary atresia with an intact ventricular septum.

With severe obstruction and right ventricular hypoplasia, pulmonary stenosis can be confused with pulmonary atresia with an intact ventricular septum. Usually an ejection rather than regurgitant murmur at the left upper sternal border allows one to differentiate these conditions, but occasionally echocardiography, angiography, or even surgical inspection is necessary to make the diagnosis with certainty. Newborns with tricuspid atresia usually have a superior axis (-90 to -30 degrees) on the electrocardiogram, and those with transposition rarely have a loud murmur and have normal or increased flow on the chest radiograph. If the right ventricle is not diminutive, the electrocardiogram has right ventricular predominance, and it may be difficult to differentiate pulmonary stenosis with an intact ventricular septum from pulmonary stenosis with a VSD (TOF). Echocardiography usually detects the latter because of the overriding aorta and absence of echoes in the area of the ventricular septum. The murmur of mild valvular pulmonary stenosis can be confused with the murmur of a VSD, ASD, or peripheral pulmonary stenosis.

The treatment of the cyanotic newborn with critical pulmonary stenosis is surgical intervention or balloon dilation. For the severely hypoxemic neonate, oxygen and PGE_1 are the initial therapy, with bicarbonate added if metabolic acidosis is present. While the gold standard used to be surgical valvotomy, balloon valvuloplasty has replaced surgical therapy as a first approach at most centers. The procedure can be done at low risk and a very high likelihood of long-term palliation.

Tricuspid Atresia

In tricuspid atresia (1 in 20,000 live births), there is a failure of development of the right atrioventricular valve; therefore an intra-atrial communication, usually a patent foramen ovale, is necessary for survival. There is usually a VSD connecting a large left ventricular cavity with a hypoplastic chamber that represents the infundibulum or outflow portion of the right ventricle. The great arteries may be either normally related (Type I) or transposed (Type II), and there may be pulmonary atresia (a), pulmonary stenosis (b), or no pulmonary stenosis (c). About 70% of infants with tricuspid atresia have Type I, with three fourths of these having pulmonary stenosis (b). In contrast, of the 30% who have Type II (transposition), more than three fourths have no pulmonary stenosis (c). The presentation of newborns with tricuspid atresia depends on the anatomy. Those with severe pulmonary stenosis or atresia present with cyanosis in the first few days of life. Infants with a large VSD and no pulmonary stenosis present with congestive heart failure, usually late in the 1st or during the 2nd month as the pulmonary vascular resistance falls.

The presence of tricuspid atresia in utero must be compatible with a relatively normal intrauterine circulation because growth and development proceed normally. Because the tricuspid valve is atretic, all systemic venous return is diverted across the foramen ovale into the left atrium and left ventricle. If the great arteries are normally related and the ventricular septum is intact or if the pulmonary valve is atretic, all the left ventricular output passes through the aorta, and pulmonary blood flow is via the ductus arteriosus. If the VSD is large, some of the left ventricular output passes through the VSD into the hypoplastic right ventricle, exiting the pulmonary artery if the vessels are normally related and exiting the aorta if transposition is present. Either way, there is antegrade flow through the pulmonary artery and ductus arteriosus.

After birth, there is little change in the circulation, but the normal postnatal alterations impose significant handicaps. The newborns with pulmonary atresia or severe pulmonary stenosis continue to depend on the ductus arteriosus for pulmonary blood flow. When the ductus begins to close, severe hypoxemia, acidosis, and eventually death follow.

Infants with pulmonary stenosis or atresia (a, b) are usually cyanotic soon after birth, with the cyanosis increasing as the ductus arteriosus closes. Those with pulmonary stenosis usually have a loud systolic ejection murmur along the left sternal border; those with pulmonary atresia may have no murmur at all or a continuous murmur from the ductus arteriosus. Infants with type c (no pulmonary stenosis) may have minimal cyanosis with an ejection murmur and heart failure as the major manifestations of heart disease. The heart size and the pulmonary blood flow visible on the radiographs are determined by the degree of pulmonary stenosis. Infants with pulmonary atresia or stenosis have a small heart with decreased pulmonary blood flow; those without pulmonary stenosis have a large heart with increased pulmonary flow. A right aortic arch is occasionally present.

The electrocardiogram is usually helpful. Because of the right ventricular hypoplasia and increased left ventricular flow in utero, left ventricular predominance with diminished right ventricular forces is almost universal. The QRS axis is almost always superior (0 to -90 degrees) in Type I, probably in large part owing to early origin of the left bundle of the conducting system and the resultant abnormal depolarization sequence. Right atrial hypertrophy is frequently present.

In the cyanotic infant, tricuspid atresia can be differentiated from transposition, TOF, and Ebstein disease of the tricuspid valve by the demonstration of left ventricular predominance on the electrocardiogram and from pulmonary atresia or stenosis with a diminutive right ventricle on the basis of the superior QRS axis. In the minimally cyanotic infant, tricuspid atresia can be differentiated from the atrioventricular canal type of VSD by electrocardiography or echocardiography and from the more complicated types of acyanotic heart disease by the presence of arterial hypoxemia, which is especially evident while the infant is crying.

In the severely hypoxic infant, the primary treatment is oxygen, bicarbonate, and PGE_1, followed by a systemic-to-pulmonary artery shunt. For those with a large enough VSD sufficient to provide adequate pulmonary blood flow, no palliation may be necessary in the perinatal period. For those with a large, nonrestrictive VSD and no pulmonary stenosis, the increased pulmonary blood flow may lead to congestive heart failure and require a palliative banding procedure. The Fontan operation (right atrium–to–pulmonary artery connection) provides palliation for children with tricuspid atresia. This cannot be done in the perinatal period because of increased pulmonary vascular resistance and is usually performed somewhere between 6 months and 3 years of age. It has provided good long-term palliation with a complication rate (arrhythmias, stroke, protein-losing enteropathy, or atrial arrhythmias) of about 1% per year.

Ebstein Anomaly of the Tricuspid Valve

In 1866, Ebstein described the heart of a 19-year-old man with cyanosis and palpitations who died of heart failure with an anomaly of the tricuspid valve. The lesion (1 in 80,000 live births), now known as Ebstein anomaly of the tricuspid valve, is due to redundancy and dysplasia of the tricuspid valve with adherence of a variable portion of the septal and, often, posterior leaflets to the right ventricular wall so that the free portion of the leaflets is displaced downward, away from the normal atrioventricular ring. Thus, the atrium and ventricle are divided in three segments: a normal right atrium, a portion of the atrium above the displaced valve that is partly ventricular myocardium, and the true right ventricle. The tricuspid valve is usually regurgitant and, at least in the newborn, stenotic. The right atrium is often large, in part owing to the muscularized segment but primarily because of the tricuspid stenosis and regurgitation; the right ventricle is correspondingly small. An ASD (or patent foramen ovale) is almost always present in the newborn, and pulmonary stenosis and atresia are not uncommon. Other associated lesions such as VSDs, coarctation, and transposition are rarely seen.

In utero the incompetent or stenotic tricuspid valve diverts systemic venous return through the foramen ovale into the left side of the heart, resulting in increased left atrial and ventricular flow. The tricuspid regurgitation into the right atrium leads to severe right atrial dilation and hypertrophy before birth and may cause in utero heart failure with edema or anasarca.

After birth, the degree of hypoxemia is a function of the right-to-left shunting at the atrial level. This depends on the degree of difficulty with which blood passes through the right ventricle and pulmonary artery into the lungs. With high pulmonary vascular resistance of the newborn increasing right ventricular afterload, the tricuspid regurgitation may be exacerbated and the right-to-left shunting at the atrial level massive. These severely hypoxic infants may depend on the ductus arteriosus for most of their pulmonary blood flow, and when the ductus closes, the hypoxemia may be severe, and acidosis may develop. If the foramen ovale is restrictive, preventing decompensation of the right atrium, right-sided heart failure with hepatomegaly may be prominent.

If the tricuspid stenosis and regurgitation are less severe, right-to-left shunting and, therefore, cyanosis may be less prominent. In either case, as the pulmonary vascular resistance drops over the first few days and weeks of life, reducing right ventricular afterload and tricuspid regurgitation, dramatic improvements in arterial saturation and congestive heart failure may be seen.

The infants with Ebstein anomaly who present during the neonatal period are almost invariably cyanotic. Right-sided congestive heart failure with hepatomegaly owing to severe tricuspid regurgitation is frequently present. On auscultation, there may be a quadruple rhythm composed of a loud first sound, single second sound, and loud third and fourth sounds. A pansystolic murmur of tricuspid regurgitation is often audible.

On chest radiographs, the cardiac silhouette is usually enlarged because of massive dilation of the right atrium. The largest hearts in infants with congenital disease are seen in this condition. Often it is difficult for one to see enough lung field to note the diminished pulmonary flow.

The P waves on the electrocardiogram are often tall and peaked, suggesting right atrial hypertrophy. Right ventricular conduction abnormalities prolonging the QRS duration are common, although they are not seen as frequently in the newborn as in the older child. Wolff-Parkinson-White syndrome with a short PR interval and a delta wave may be seen in as many as 20% of children, and atrial tachycardias and flutter are not uncommon.

On chest radiographs, the hearts of children with Ebstein disease are large. In the minimally distressed infant with cyanosis, a murmur along the left sternal border, right ventricular hypertrophy on the electrocardiogram, and massive cardiomegaly, the diagnosis is almost certain.

Patients with pulmonary atresia with an intact ventricular septum or tricuspid atresia may have cyanosis and cardiac enlargement, but they usually have left rather than right ventricular hypertrophy on the electrocardiogram, and the tricuspid valve is hypoplastic or atretic on echocardiogram rather than large and redundant as in Ebstein disease. Infants with transposition of the great arteries or TOF may be just as cyanotic, but the former have increased pulmonary vascularity, and the latter rarely show cardiac enlargement on chest radiographs.

The treatment of Ebstein anomaly in the newborn period is based on two premises: (1) many infants improve markedly over the first weeks of life as the pulmonary resistance drops, and (2) surgical approaches to treating these critically ill newborns have been problematic. PGE_1 may be helpful in improving oxygenation in a severely cyanotic infant by maintaining patency of the ductus arteriosus until the pulmonary resistance falls. In older children, tricuspid annuloplasty or valve replacement may be successful in those with significant congestive heart failure or hypoxemia. Pharmacologic therapy or ablation is useful for those with atrial arrhythmias. In those with minimal symptoms, a conservative, nonsurgical approach is probably preferable. Attempts to close the tricuspid valve transforming Ebstein disease to a single ventricle physiology and then performing a Fontan operation (right atrium–to–pulmonary artery anastomosis) has been tried with mixed results.

Truncus Arteriosus

Truncus arteriosus (about 1 in 33,000 live births) has been defined as the cardiac defect in which a single great artery arises from the base of the heart supplying the coronary, pulmonary, and systemic arteries. Embryologically, truncus probably results from atresia (rather than hypoplasia as is seen in TOF) of the subpulmonary infundibulum, partial or complete absence of the pulmonary valve, and an aortopulmonary septal defect. The truncal valve usually resembles a normal aortic valve and overrides a large VSD.

In utero the main consequence of truncus arteriosus is complete mixing of the systemic and pulmonary venous return above the truncal valve. The truncus is usually large, and the ductus arteriosus arising from the pulmonary arteries may be smaller than normal. Because blood flow through the heart is normal, the atrium and ventricles develop normally.

After birth, the flow to the pulmonary arteries and systemic arteries is a function of the relative resistances in the two circuits. Initially the pulmonary resistance is high, and pulmonary flow equals or slightly exceeds systemic flow. Over the first hours or days of life, however, the pulmonary arteriolar resistance decreases, and pulmonary blood flow increases. As the pulmonary venous return increases, the left ventricle must eject an increasing volume load, which eventually leads to congestive failure. Because there is common mixing of systemic and pulmonary venous blood above the truncal valve, the degree of hypoxemia decreases as the pulmonary flow increases so that these infants are only mildly cyanotic until left heart failure and pulmonary edema interfere with oxygen exchange, and pulmonary venous desaturation ensues. In some infants, the pulmonary arteries are hypoplastic or stenotic at their origin; in these patients, the pulmonary blood flow is restricted, and cyanosis rather than congestive failure may be the presenting symptom.

Children with truncus arteriosus usually present in the 1st month (and often in the 1st week) with predominantly left-sided heart failure. Tachypnea, poor feeding, increased perspiration, and intermittent cyanosis are usually prominent, and hepatomegaly is occasionally present. On physical examination, the cardiac impulse is hyperactive, and the pulses are usually bounding secondary to the diastolic runoff from the aorta. On auscultation, the second heart sound is single, although the phonocardiogram can often detect multiple components, presumably from the abnormal truncal valve cusps. Commonly a systolic ejection click is audible. Although a continuous murmur is often thought to be characteristic of truncus, it is actually unusual because pulmonary hypertension is the rule. Systolic ejection murmurs of moderate intensity (grade 2 or 3/6) as a result of relative truncal stenosis are common, and a mid-diastolic flow rumble across the mitral valve is often present.

The heart is enlarged on the chest radiograph because of dilation of the left atrium and ventricle. The pulmonary vascular markings are increased, and pulmonary venous congestion is frequently seen. A right aortic arch is present in about one fourth of cases. The QRS axis is usually normal, with biventricular hypertrophy present in about 60% of infants, left ventricular hypertrophy in 20%, and pure right ventricular hypertrophy in the remainder.

A newborn with mild cyanosis, congestive heart failure, and bounding pulses probably has truncus arteriosus. Infants with a VSD, PDA, aortopulmonary window, arteriovenous fistula, or coarctation of the aorta are not cyanotic, and infants with TOF and pulmonary atresia and large collaterals who may have cyanosis and heart failure have loud continuous murmurs. In infants with tricuspid atresia and a large VSD, the electrocardiogram shows a superior axis and left ventricular hypertrophy, and infants with transposition and a large VSD do not usually have bounding pulses.

For the newborn with congestive heart failure, digoxin and diuretics may be tried but rarely suffice. Surgical repair, closing the VSD so that left ventricular blood is diverted exclusively through the truncal valve, dividing the pulmonary artery, removing it from the site of the aorta, and connecting the right ventricle to the distal pulmonary artery using a conduit (usually aortic homograft) is the procedure of choice by age 3 months to prevent pulmonary vascular disease. This approach continues to carry a significant risk but has been done in many centers with survival in the 80% to 90% range. Inevitably, surgery to replace the conduit as the children grow is necessary.

Total Anomalous Pulmonary Venous Connection

In this anomaly (1 in 17,000 live births), the pulmonary veins have no connection with the left atrium and drain either directly or, more commonly, indirectly into the right atrium via one of the normal embryonic channels. The embryologic defect seems to be a failure of development of the common pulmonary vein normally connecting the developing pulmonary venous plexus with the posterior aspect of the left atrium. As a consequence, one or more of the normal anastomotic channels between the pulmonary venous plexus of the lung buds and the cardinal or umbilicovitelline vein persists, allowing drainage of the pulmonary blood flow into the systemic venous atrium. If the connection to the left common cardinal system persists, postnatal drainage is to the left innominate vein (35% of cases) or to the coronary sinus (19%). Other pathways that may persist include the right common cardinal system (drainage to right superior vena cava or azygos, 11% of cases) and the umbilicovitelline system (ductus venosus or portal system, 21%). Alternatively, the pulmonary veins may drain directly into the right atrium (4%). The presence of an interatrial communication, either a patent foramen ovale or a true ASD, is necessary to sustain life after birth.

The postnatal presentation depends on the degree of obstruction to pulmonary venous drainage. If obstruction is severe (almost invariable with drainage into the umbilicovitelline system and frequent with drainage into the right superior vena cava or innominate vein), the children present within the 1st week of life. If obstruction is mild or absent, presentation is usually during the second half of the 1st year or later.

In utero there is little hemodynamic disruption from total anomalous pulmonary venous connection because before birth the pulmonary blood flow represents only 5% to 10% of combined ventricular output, an amount that can be handled by the anomalous systemic venous connection. The drainage of pulmonary venous blood to the right side of the heart rather than the left causes no apparent sequelae; the newborns are normal in size and development.

After birth, the fetal pathways persist. The pulmonary venous return continues to drain to the right atrium via one of the systemic venous channels, where it mixes with the normal systemic venous return. A portion of the totally mixed pulmonary and systemic venous return passes into the left atrium, left ventricle, and aorta, and the rest passes into the right ventricle and pulmonary artery. As the pulmonary arteriolar resistance drops, the pulmonary blood flow increases, and if there is obstruction to the increased pulmonary venous flow, pulmonary edema follows.

The pulmonary venous obstruction increases the pulmonary vascular resistance above systemic, diverting blood from the pulmonary artery into the descending aorta as long as the ductus arteriosus remains open. When the ductus begins to close, the increased pulmonary resistance elevates right ventricular and right atrial pressure and leads to increasing right-to-left shunting at the atrial level. The increased pulmonary resistance secondary to the obstruction reduces pulmonary flow, and the pulmonary edema reduces the oxygen content of the blood that is not obstructed, resulting in arterial hypoxemia and, eventually, acidosis and death.

In infants with severe pulmonary venous obstruction, the predominant finding is cyanosis. The heart is not hyperactive, and other than experiencing tachypnea, the infant is usually comfortable, at least initially. The second heart sound is single or narrowly split and accentuated. Often no murmurs are audible.

In newborns with lesser degrees of pulmonary venous obstruction, cyanosis may be less impressive, and the signs and symptoms of heart failure—tachypnea, dyspnea, and feeding difficulties—may predominate. In these infants, the right ventricular impulse is hyperdynamic, and the second heart sound is widely split, with the pulmonary component increased. A systolic ejection murmur at the left upper sternal border and a mid-diastolic murmur at the left lower sternal border secondary to increased blood flow across the pulmonary and tricuspid valves may be audible.

In infants with severe obstruction, the heart is normal in size on the chest radiograph, and pulmonary venous congestion is obvious. Those with milder obstruction have right ventricular dilation and increased pulmonary blood flow. Occasionally the dilated accessory venous channels to the left or right superior vena cava can be seen on the anteroposterior projection.

The electrocardiogram almost invariably shows right axis deviation and right ventricular hypertrophy. In the 1st week, this may be difficult to distinguish from normal, but in those who present in the 2nd week, the right ventricular hypertrophy becomes more obvious and may be associated with right atrial hypertrophy. Angiocardiography, either in the common pulmonary vein entered from the systemic venous connection or in the pulmonary artery with usual long filming, outlines the site or sites of pulmonary venous drainage except when the obstruction is almost complete.

In the infant with severe cyanosis that is unresponsive to oxygen and a small heart and pulmonary venous congestion visible on the radiographs, the diagnosis is usually clear. It is occasionally difficult to distinguish infants with total anomalous pulmonary venous return from those with persistent fetal circulation with or without primary lung disease because (1) both groups of patients demonstrate tachypnea, dyspnea, and cyanosis on physical examination as well as haziness of the lung fields on radiographs, and (2) both may transiently improve with 100% oxygen because a perfusion imbalance may occur in either condition. In preterm infants, lung disease is more common, but in the term infant, the index of suspicion must be high for total anomalous pulmonary venous return. Echocardiography or even catheterization may occasionally be necessary to distinguish the two with certainty. HLHS may also be associated with pulmonary edema on radiographs, but there is usually extreme cardiac enlargement with increased pulmonary blood flow visible on the films and severe circulatory collapse.

The treatment of total anomalous pulmonary venous connection (TAPVC) with obstruction is surgical. The horizontal common pulmonary vein posterior to the heart is connected to the back wall of the left atrium and the anomalous systemic venous channel is ligated. Initially, surgical mortality was high, although repair can now be accomplished in more than 85% of children. Long-term results have usually been quite good, with a small incidence of residual stenosis at the anastomotic site present in some.

Asplenia

Asplenia is one of the heterotaxia syndromes (1 in 12,000 live births) that are characterized by positional abnormalities of the abdominal viscera (midline liver, stomach on the right, malrotation of the gut); splenic abnormalities (absence of spleen or multiple tiny splenules); and complex, usually cyanotic, congenital heart disease. For convenience, heterotaxia syndromes have been classified as asplenia and polysplenia, although the disease associated with asplenia may be present with a normal spleen, and polysplenia heart disease may exist with no spleen, many splenules, or a normal spleen.

In asplenia, there is *bilateral right-sidedness*. The liver tends to be midline, with right and left lobes equal in size. Both lungs are trilobed with epiarterial bronchi (bronchus over the pulmonary artery) similar to the bronchus seen in the normal right lung. There is often no rotation or reverse rotation of the midgut loop, with abnormal mesenteric attachments. Often the entire small bowel is on one side of the abdomen and the large intestine on the other. Cardiac malformations usually include bilateral superior vena cava, inferior vena cava either to the right or left of the spine, common atrium, complete atrioventricular canal, single ventricle, and total anomalous pulmonary venous return. Transposition of the great arteries is common, and severe pulmonary stenosis or atresia is almost invariably present. A helpful pathognomonic feature of asplenia, demonstrable by echocardiography, catheter passage, or angiocardiography, is the finding of the abdominal aorta and inferior vena cava on the same side of the spine.

The infants are usually normal at birth, a finding that suggests relatively normal intrauterine development. This is not surprising because virtual common mixing of systemic venous and pulmonary venous blood normally occurs before birth, and the pulmonary stenosis or atresia and TAPVD are less important in utero because pulmonary blood flow is minimal.

After birth, the presentation is usually similar to that of newborns with a large VSD and severe pulmonary stenosis or atresia—profound cyanosis, especially as the ductus arteriosus closes.

Cyanosis is usually the presenting symptom. If the infant has pulmonary stenosis rather than atresia, a systolic murmur is audible along the left sternal border. The second heart sound is single. The asplenia syndrome may be diagnosed by the plain chest radiograph. The liver is midline and symmetric, and the stomach is found in the midline or on the right or left side of the abdomen. If the chest film is of good quality, the bilateral epiarterial bronchi are visible. The heart may be in the right chest (dextrocardia), midline (mesocardia), or in the left chest (levocardia) and is usually normal in size with reduced pulmonary vascularity. The electrocardiogram is variable. There is often a superior QRS axis (0 to -120 degrees) with a counterclockwise loop in the frontal plane typical of an endocardial cushion defect. The configuration of the QRS complex depends on the position of the heart in the chest and the presence or absence of a ventricular septum. The P-wave axis is usually inferior and anterior with a normal PR interval.

Infants with asplenia must be differentiated from those with large VSD and pulmonary stenosis or atresia (TOF). The characteristic picture of abdominal heterotaxia with bilateral epiarterial bronchi on chest radiographs should alert one to the probability of the asplenia syndrome. Finding the inferior vena cava and abdominal aorta on the same side of the spine seems to be pathognomonic. The finding of Howell-Jolly and Heinz bodies in red cell smears is presumptive evidence of asplenia, and the absence of spleen on ultrasound or radionuclide scan is confirmatory.

It is often more difficult to differentiate between asplenia and polysplenia. In general, the heart disease is more complex with asplenia; the lungs are trilobed, the bronchi are epiarterial, the P-wave axis is normal, and the inferior vena cava is present on the same side as the abdominal aorta. In the polysplenia syndrome, the lungs are bilobed, the bronchi hyparterial (bronchus beneath the pulmonary artery), the inferior vena cava absent, and the P-wave axis superior. Severe pulmonary stenosis is frequent in infants with asplenia and less common in polysplenia.

Temporary infusion of PGE_1 helps those who depend on the ductus arteriosus for pulmonary blood flow. Occasionally, the increased pulmonary blood flow may unmask latent pulmonary venous obstruction from total anomalous pulmonary venous connection that is frequently present. Palliation in the form of a systemic-to-pulmonary artery shunt has been successful in most. The Fontan operation directly connecting the systemic venous return to the pulmonary artery, leaving the single ventricle to pump pulmonary venous blood to the body, has been attempted with increasing success. The surgical mortality should be less than 15%, with the long-term complications rate (arrhythmias, strokes, protein-losing enteropathy, and congestive heart failure) approximately 1% per year.

Because children without spleens have a high risk of sepsis and, at least in the authors' experience, a higher rate of mortality from sepsis than from heart disease, the authors believe that pneumococcal vaccine and prophylactic antibiotics should be administered to all asplenic patients who survive beyond the neonatal period.

Coarctation of the Aorta

The sine qua non of this anomaly (1 in 7000 live births) is the presence of a constriction in the aorta distal to the left subclavian artery, usually at the site of insertion of the ductus arteriosus. There may be, in addition, tubular hypoplasia of the aortic arch and intracardiac anomalies. Because there is normally little flow across the aortic isthmus in utero, the tubular hypoplasia of the arch does not affect fetal growth and development. In the presence of a posterior shelf, there is also no significant hemodynamic difficulty because the flow is small and the large ductus arteriosus allows ample room for it to bypass the narrowing.

After birth, the constriction in the aorta increases left ventricular afterload. In the presence of a VSD, this increased systemic resistance leads to a large left-to-right shunt. As the pulmonary vascular resistance falls, the left-to-right shunt increases, resulting in a volume as well as a pressure overload of the left ventricle. In addition to congestive heart failure, there is failure of the blood to pass from ascending to descending aorta if the coarctation is severe. The results are tissue hypoxia, lactic acidosis, and eventual death after the ductus arteriosus closes.

Those infants with a juxtaductal coarctation but no associated anomalies have a slightly different hemodynamic picture. In these newborns, closure of the ductus arteriosus leads to an acute increase in afterload to the left ventricle because blood must be pumped through the narrowed segment. Because no obstruction was present in utero, no collateral vessels have developed. Owing in part to a reduced number of sympathetic receptors, the neonatal myocardium is not able to respond to increased work as well as the left ventricle of an older child or adult can. Consequently, congestive heart failure, with elevation of left ventricular end-diastolic, left atrial, and pulmonary venous pressures follows. Occasionally the acute left atrial dilation causes the septum secundum to become incompetent, resulting in an atrial left-to-right shunt. If the coarctation is not too severe, congestive failure may be mild, and there may be time for compensatory mechanisms (e.g., left ventricular hypertrophy or collateral vessels that bypass the obstruction) to develop.

The newborn with coarctation of the aorta presents with the usual signs and symptoms of congestive heart failure: dyspnea, tachypnea, tachycardia, hepatomegaly, poor feeding, and increased perspiration. A careful examination of the peripheral pulses demonstrates that pulses and blood pressure (by Doppler or flush method) in the legs are diminished compared with those in the arms. Blood pressure in both arms must be measured because it may be diminished in the left arm if the coarctation involves the origin of the left subclavian artery, and it may be decreased in the right arm in the rare situation in which the right subclavian artery arises anomalously below the coarctation as the last vessel of the aortic arch rather than as the first branch of the innominate. Occasionally the pulses in the legs *wax and wane* as the ductus arteriosus opens and closes. In the newborn with an isolated juxtaductal coarctation, there may be no murmur or, occasionally, a short systolic ejection murmur in the axilla or back. In newborns with tubular hypoplasia and a VSD, there is usually a harsh pansystolic murmur at the left lower sternal border, but its absence does not rule out a ventricular defect.

In the absence of complex intracardiac anomalies, there is right axis deviation and right ventricular hypertrophy on the electrocardiogram reflecting normal intrauterine blood flow. On the chest radiograph, the heart is enlarged with the pulmonary vasculature congested, and if a left-to-right shunt is present from a stretched foramen ovale, the heart is actively engorged. Poststenotic dilation in the descending aorta and rib notching, usually present in older children with coarctation, are not seen in newborns.

The diagnosis of coarctation of the aorta is obvious if there is a marked discrepancy in blood pressure between the arms and legs. As already mentioned, however, in some newborns the pulses wax and wane, presumably as the ductus arteriosus closes. Therefore, one must check the pulses and blood pressure more than once if there is any possibility of coarctation.

Coarctation of the aorta must be differentiated from other causes of congestive heart failure in the 1st or 2nd week of life. HLHS usually causes a symmetric decrease in pulses with equal blood pressures in the arms and legs and severe right ventricular hypertrophy on the electrocardiogram. Aortic stenosis also causes a symmetric decrease in pulses but is usually associated with left ventricular hypertrophy and ST-T changes on the electrocardiogram. Echocardiography or catheterization may be necessary to differentiate these lesions if no difference in pulses or blood pressure is apparent.

The medical treatment of a newborn with congestive heart failure from coarctation of the aorta includes digitalis and diuretics and, if acidosis or low output is present, PGE_1, to dilate the ductus arteriosus. Those with a juxtaductal coarctation without associated heart disease are usually repaired surgically by excision of the narrowed segment and end-to-end anastomosis. Some centers with an active, aggressive, interventional catheterization laboratory have performed balloon dilation in the perinatal period. This may have to be repeated in the first year of life because of recurrence, but it has become the procedure of choice in some centers.

For those with complex intracardiac anomalies (usually with tubular hypoplasia of the aortic arch), palliative or corrective operations for the underlying heart disease are frequently necessary in addition to surgical or balloon therapy of coarctation of the aorta.

Interrupted Aortic Arch

Infants with an interrupted aortic arch (1 in 50,000 live births) have a discontinuity between the ascending and descending aorta. Almost any cardiac anomaly can be associated with interrupted aortic arch, but a PDA and a VSD are almost invariably present, and aortic stenosis, double outlet right ventricle, truncus arteriosus, and single ventricle are not uncommon. The embryologic defect in interrupted aortic arch is not known. More than two thirds of the newborns with interrupted aortic arch have been found to have DiGeorge syndrome, now known to be due to a deletion in chromosome 22 (22q11).

In the normal fetus, the left ventricle supplies the ascending aorta and the right ventricle supplies the descending aorta through the ductus arteriosus, with only 10% of combined ventricular output passing through the arch of the aorta from ascending to descending aorta. In the fetus with an interrupted aortic arch, no blood passes through the aortic isthmus, but this results in no major observable hemodynamic abnormalities. After birth, however, the descending aorta continues to depend on the ductus arteriosus to provide systemic output. When the ductus begins to close, flow to the descending aorta diminishes, and tissue hypoxia, acidosis, and death follow. Rarely the ductus arteriosus remains open. In these infants, congestive heart failure occurs as the pulmonary vascular resistance falls over the first weeks of life and pulmonary blood flow increases.

The clinical presentations of the various types of interruption are similar. As the pulmonary vascular resistance falls, the newborns develop the signs and symptoms of congestive heart failure: respiratory distress, tachypnea, tachycardia, hepatomegaly, poor feeding, and increased perspiration. As the ductus arteriosus closes, the pulses and perfusion in the lower body diminish and mottling appears. Although differential cyanosis should be observable, because the upper body receives fully saturated blood from the left ventricle and the lower body receives desaturated venous blood from the pulmonary artery, it is rarely clinically apparent because a large left-to-right shunt through a VSD tends to increase the pulmonary artery oxygen saturation, and pulmonary venous desaturation from pulmonary edema lowers the aortic saturation, making the differences minimal and not clinically visible, even to the experienced observer. The presence of strong pulses in the left carotid but not in the left subclavian artery or in the right carotid but not left carotid artery can often localize the site of the interruption. Heart murmurs are rarely impressive in these infants, but a systolic murmur can sometimes be heard along the left sternal border, presumably from the VSD. The second sound is usually loud and single.

Because intrauterine flows are normal, the electrocardiogram is rarely helpful at birth; there is usually right axis deviation and right ventricular hypertrophy that is normal for age. No specific anomalies are present on the chest radiograph other than generalized cardiac enlargement and increased pulmonary vascular markings often associated with pulmonary venous congestion.

The diagnosis of an interrupted aortic arch is difficult but should be suspected in any newborn with early congestive heart failure. The finding of differential blood pressures between the arms and legs suggests either coarctation of the aorta or interruption: differences in the pulse between the right and left carotid arteries make the latter condition more probable. Other acyanotic heart diseases in the newborn in which congestive heart failure occurs (e.g., aortic stenosis and hypoplastic left heart syndrome) can usually be excluded by the differential pulses in interrupted aortic arch or by the electrocardiographic finding of left ventricular hypertrophy and strain in aortic stenosis and the echocardiographic demonstration of a small ascending aorta in HLHS.

The initial treatment of newborns with interrupted aortic arch should be aimed to reopen the ductus with PGE_1 and treat the congestive heart failure and acidosis. After stabilization, the interrupted aortic arch can usually be repaired by direct anastomosis between the proximal and distal ends of the aortic arch. Since virtually all infants have a VSD, the operation is usually done under cardiopulmonary bypass with closure of the VSD at the same time. Perinatal survival is now above 75%, with long-term prognosis usually quite good, although balloon dilation of the anastomotic site is frequently required later in childhood.

Aortic Stenosis

Although left ventricular outflow obstruction in childhood may occur below or above the valve, for all practical purposes only valvular aortic stenosis (1 in 16,000 live births) causes severe symptoms in the neonatal period. The valve is usually unicommissural and unicuspid, and the tissue is thickened, nodular, and severely deformed. The myocardium is always hypertrophied, but the left ventricular cavity varies in size. It may be dilated, normal, or hypoplastic; when small, the defect gradually becomes a part of HLHS. In many infants, the left ventricular endocardium is thickened and covered with a gray layer of fibrous and elastic tissue that may involve the papillary muscles, resulting in mitral regurgitation. This *endocardial fibroelastosis* is probably secondary to myocardial hypoxia from the thick myocardium, which, in the presence of high intracavitary pressures, cannot be adequately perfused in the endocardial layers. Associated lesions, such as coarctation of the aorta, VSD, and ASD, are occasionally seen.

In utero the presence of left ventricular outflow obstruction imposes a pressure load on the left ventricle. If the stenosis occurs early in gestation and is severe, the afterload reduces flow through the ventricle, and left ventricular hypoplasia and HLHS may result. If the stenosis is less severe, the left ventricular size is normal, but the myocardium is hypertrophied, and fibroelastosis from inadequate endocardial perfusion may be present.

After birth, the left ventricular output normally must increase by about 50% with the switch from a parallel to an in-series circulation. In the presence of severe aortic obstruction, the marginally compensated left ventricle may be unable to handle increased volume load. If the foramen ovale is closed, the left atrial pressure rapidly increases, leading to pulmonary edema. Occasionally, left atrial dilation makes the septum primum incompetent, allowing the left atrium to decompress through the foramen ovale. This left-to-right shunt at the atrial level may exacerbate the congestive heart failure.

The infant with critical aortic stenosis is usually normal at birth. A systolic murmur is invariably audible along the left sternal border with radiation to the right upper sternal border but may be only grade 2 or 3/6. The symptoms of congestive heart failure—respiratory distress, poor feeding, and tachypnea—may be delayed by hours to weeks; however, once symptoms occur, they may progress rapidly, leading to a low output state with cool, mottled extremities; diminished pulses; and a murmur that is barely audible. The murmur is rarely associated with a thrill, even when output is adequate, but a systolic ejection click at the apex may be present. In stark contrast with its radiographically visible enlargement, the heart is rarely hyperactive on palpation.

The most frequent electrocardiographic pattern is left ventricular hypertrophy with inverted T waves over the left precordium, suggesting left ventricular ischemia. Occasionally, right ventricular hypertrophy may be seen, but in our experience, this is associated with at least some hypoplasia of the left ventricle. Even in those with right ventricular predominance, inverted T waves over the left precordium are common.

In infants with congestive heart failure, the heart is invariably enlarged on chest radiographs and may be massive. The pulmonary vessels are indistinct owing to pulmonary venous congestion and may also be actively engorged if there is a large left-to-right shunt at the atrial level from a stretched foramen ovale. Using a long-axis view of the left ventricular outflow tract, two-dimensional echocardiography shows severe immobility of the aortic valve with little or no systolic opening, left ventricular hypertrophy, left atrial dilation, and poststenotic dilation in the ascending aorta. Evaluation of the ascending aorta with Doppler technique shows increased velocity of blood flow, allowing estimation of the gradient.

At cardiac catheterization, the left ventricle can usually be approached through the foramen ovale, but occasionally a retrograde study across the aortic valve or even a transatrial septal puncture may be necessary. There is usually a pressure gradient of greater than 40 mm Hg between the left ventricle and ascending aorta, with the left ventricular systolic pressure exceeding 120 mm Hg, but occasionally in infants with severe congestive heart failure, the left ventricle cannot generate such a high pressure, and the gradient may be less. The left ventricular end-diastolic pressure is invariably elevated and has been observed to be as high as 35 mm Hg. If the foramen ovale is incompetent, a left-to-right shunt at the atrial level may be present, with the pulmonary flow–to–systemic flow ratio occasionally exceeding 3:1. A left ventricular angiocardiogram in the left anterior oblique projection outlines the domed, thickened aortic valve.

Aortic stenosis must be differentiated from other causes of heart failure in the 1st month of life. With aortic atresia and HLHS, there is congestive failure but no left ventricular hypertrophy on the electrocardiogram. In coarctation of the aorta with or without a VSD, the pulses are weak or absent in the legs but are usually palpable in the arms and carotids, and left ventricular strain on the electrocardiogram is usually not present. The murmur of aortic stenosis is loudest at the right or left upper sternal borders, whereas in infants with coarctation the murmur is louder at the lower left sternal border or into the axilla. Finally, aortic stenosis is associated with an ejection click that is rarely present in the newborn with coarctation of the aorta. With acyanotic lesions causing congestive heart failure, such as VSDs and PDA, there is usually a hyperactive precordium associated with the large left-to-right shunts. In tricuspid atresia, truncus arteriosus, and single ventricle, there is usually cyanosis with crying.

These infants are usually very sick when first seen, and the usual medical management with digoxin, diuretics, and correction of the acidosis must be accomplished without delay. Aortic valvotomy under inflow occlusion or a cardiopulmonary bypass has been the procedure of choice. More recently, many interventional catheterization laboratories have attempted balloon dilation of the aortic valve with success that approaches that of the surgical procedure. The long-term prognosis is fair, with repeat dilation of the valve commonly necessary later in childhood. Valve replacement either with a prosthetic valve or, more recently, a pulmonary autograft has been necessary in some infants surviving initial palliation and is likely to be necessary for most patients later in childhood or as an adult.

Hypoplastic Left Heart Syndrome: Aortic or Mitral Atresia or Severe Stenosis with a Hypoplastic Left Ventricle

On gross pathologic examination, the hearts of children with HLHS (1 in 6000 live births) are all similar, with severe hypoplasia of the left ventricle and ascending aorta and a dilated right ventricle and pulmonary artery. The aortic valve may be atretic with a complete absence of any recognizable valve tissue or may be fused and domed with an eccentric pinhole orifice. The mitral valve is atretic in one fourth of the cases and hypoplastic in the rest. The left ventricle may be slitlike if both mitral and aortic valves are atretic but is somewhat more developed when there is some flow through the mitral valve. The ascending aorta is hypoplastic between the coronaries and the innominate artery, and a coarctation of the aorta may be present. VSDs are uncommon.

In a fetus with a hypoplastic left heart, the right ventricle must support the entire circulation. Almost all the systemic venous return that enters the right atrium passes into the right ventricle and is ejected into the pulmonary artery. A small portion of blood may pass through the foramen ovale, but with mitral or aortic atresia this is minimal. Because the pulmonary resistance is high, virtually all the blood entering the pulmonary artery is diverted through the ductus arteriosus into the aorta rather than passing into the lungs. Most blood flow is retrograde into the aortic arch and ascending aorta. Flow to the subclavian, carotid, and coronary arteries is therefore also retrograde. The ascending aorta is small because the coronary arteries are the only continuation after the takeoff of the innominate artery.

After birth, the pulmonary vascular resistance falls, and the systemic resistance increases so that an increasing proportion of blood from the single pulmonary trunk goes to the lungs rather than through the ductus arteriosus. The increased pulmonary blood flow leads to an increase in pulmonary venous return that cannot freely exit from the left atrium because of hypoplasia of the left atrium and foramen ovale. Pulmonary venous hypertension and pulmonary edema result. As the ductus arteriosus begins to close at 12 to 48 hours of age, the perfusion to the systemic circulation is reduced, resulting in systemic and coronary ischemia. Newborns with this disease are the sickest patients seen by the pediatric cardiologist, with the median age of death 4.5 days in untreated infants.

The infants are usually normal at birth, but tachypnea and dyspnea soon develop as the pulmonary blood flow increases. Cyanosis is rarely prominent, despite the total mixing of the systemic and pulmonary circulations, because the pulmonary blood flow is so increased. Congestive heart failure with tachypnea, hepatomegaly, and poor feeding is usually present by 24 to 48 hours of age. Finally, as the ductus arteriosus begins to close, the signs of low output—mottling, grayness of the skin, and markedly diminished pulses—follow. One third are in vascular collapse by the time they reach the physician, with blood pressures of 40 mm Hg or less, and they are hypothermic, hypoglycemic, and ashen in color. Auscultation is rarely helpful because prominent murmurs are unusual, and the second heart sound is single.

The electrocardiogram reflects the intrauterine circulation, showing right axis deviation and right ventricular predominance that may be normal for age. Occasionally, diminished left-sided forces owing to left ventricular hypoplasia can be appreciated. Right atrial hypertrophy is seen in about two thirds of the infants. Coronary ischemia frequently results in ST-T wave changes. A marked sinus tachycardia is usually present. The heart is markedly enlarged on chest radiographs, with both increased pulmonary blood flow and pulmonary venous congestion prominent. Angiography demonstrates severe hypoplasia of the ascending aorta.

Infants with HLHS must be differentiated from those with other causes of respiratory distress in the 1st month of life. In the early stages, the tachypnea may suggest lung disease, but the appearance of congestive heart failure with tachycardia, hepatomegaly, and cardiac enlargement on radiographs should allow the two to be differentiated. Nonstructural heart diseases, myocarditis, transient myocardial ischemia, and intrauterine supraventricular tachycardia must be ruled out as must other causes of vascular collapse, such as sepsis.

After the onset of congestive heart failure, HLHS must be differentiated from the two other common structural causes of failure early in the 1st week of life: aortic stenosis and the coarctation syndrome. There is usually left ventricular hypertrophy on the electrocardiogram in the former, and a difference in pulses and blood pressure between the upper and lower extremities is normally present in the latter.

Since the hypoplastic left heart syndrome has been uniformly fatal, treatment was initially terminated at the time of definitive diagnosis and comfort care given. More recently, centers have tried a more aggressive approach, either with staged surgical repair or cardiac transplantation. If either of the latter procedures are considered, congestive heart failure should be treated with digoxin, and diuretics and PGE_1, should be given to dilate the ductus arteriosus to improve systemic perfusion. Bicarbonate should be given to treat the metabolic acidosis.

The staged surgical procedure involves turning the defect into a single ventricle that can later be repaired by a modified Fontan procedure. The first stage in the perinatal period involves dividing the pulmonary artery connecting the proximal portion to the aorta so that the right ventricle becomes the systemic pump. Pulmonary blood flow is provided via an aortopulmonary shunt. An atrial septal defect is created to decompress the hypertensive left atrium. A second stage involves dividing the aortopulmonary shunt and directly connecting the systemic venous return to the pulmonary artery (Fontan).

Other centers have gone directly to neonatal cardiac transplantation. Since the availability of hearts is limited in the perinatal period, approximately 25% of children have died on the transplant list.

The most recent data would suggest an initial mortality of 25% to 35% with either the staged surgical approach or transplantation, including those who die on the transplant waiting list. Survival to the age of 8 years is about 65% and is almost identical with either staged surgical repair or transplantation. Further data will be necessary to decide which of these two surgical approaches is preferable.

Ventricular Septal Defects

VSDs (1 in 3000 live births) may be isolated, part of a more complex cardiac anomaly such as TOF, or associated with other congenital cardiac defects such as coarctation of the aorta. In this section, only the isolated defect is considered; the more complicated types are discussed elsewhere in this chapter. Ventricular defects have been classified according to their location in the ventricular septum. The most common site is the membranous portion of the septum that lies between the crista supraventricularis and the papillary muscle of the conus when the heart is viewed from the right ventricular side. Less common sites are the area above the crista (subpulmonary), the muscular portion of the septum below the tricuspid valve (atrioventricular septal defect), and the anterior trabecular portion of the ventricular septum near the apex of the right ventricle. The size of VSDs varies: They can be as small as a pinhole or large enough to make the ventricular septum almost completely absent. In about 10% of infants, multiple defects are present.

Because the right and left sides of the heart are arranged in parallel before birth, the presence of a large communication at the ventricular level in addition to the normal ductus connection at the great vessel level does not significantly alter the fetal circulation. After birth, the hemodynamics depend on the size of the defect and the pulmonary and systemic vascular resistances. If the defect is large (greater than $1 \text{ cm}^2/\text{m}^2$ body size or equal to at least half the size of the aortic valve), it offers no resistance to flow. The systolic pressures in both ventricles and both great vessels are approximately equal, and the degree of intracardiac shunting is determined by the systemic and pulmonary vascular resistances. For the first few hours of life, the resistances are about equal, and little shunting (left-to-right or right-to-left) occurs. Over the following hours, days, and weeks, the pulmonary vascular resistance gradually falls, increasing the proportion of blood ejected by the left ventricle that goes through the VSD into the pulmonary artery. When the pulmonary blood flow is about three times greater than the systemic flow, the left ventricle can no longer accommodate the volume load, and signs and symptoms of congestive heart failure develop. In full-term infants with an isolated ventricular defect, this usually occurs late in the 1st or during the 2nd month of life, but failure is occasionally seen earlier, sometimes in the 1st week, presumably owing to a more rapid fall in the pulmonary vascular resistance. The left-to-right shunting at the ventricular level results in increased flow in the pulmonary artery, pulmonary veins, left atrium, and left ventricle, with the latter chamber ejecting blood directly into the pulmonary artery. The right atrium and right ventricle are not volume overloaded, but in the presence of a large defect the right ventricle must generate pressures equal to those of the left ventricle, so there is usually right ventricular hypertrophy without significant dilation.

If the ventricular defect is small, it does offer resistance to flow, and the pressures in the two ventricles may differ. These infants are a heterogeneous group, with the hemodynamics depending on the size of the hole rather than the pulmonary vascular resistance. If the defect is small, the right ventricular and pulmonary artery pressures may be normal and the pulmonary blood flow less than twice the systemic flow. These infants are rarely symptomatic, and a murmur is usually the sole indication of heart disease. If the defect is larger, the right heart pressures may be close to systemic pressures, with flow ratios exceeding 3:1. These infants may have congestive heart failure.

Newborns with a small VSD have a grade 2 or 3/6 high-pitched, pansystolic murmur along the left sternal border and are asymptomatic. Even if the defect is large, the elevated pulmonary resistance prevents significant shunting in the first few days and weeks of life, so heart failure is unusual. Later, as the left-to-right shunt increases, signs and symptoms of congestive failure—tachypnea, tiring with feeding, poor weight gain, diaphoresis, and hepatomegaly—develop.

On physical examination, the cardiac impulse is usually hyperactive, and the apex is displaced laterally. A systolic thrill and grade 4/6 pansystolic murmur can be appreciated along the left sternal border. If the left-to-right shunt is large, a mid-diastolic rumble is audible at the apex from the increased flow across a structurally normal mitral valve. If the pulmonary artery pressure is increased, the pulmonary component of the second heart sound is single or narrowly split and accentuated.

Although the electrocardiogram is usually an accurate tool for assessing the hemodynamics in older children with a VSD, it is less valuable in the newborn because the normal pattern of right ventricular predominance masks the typical changes. A normal progression from right to left ventricular predominance over the 1st month is usual for a small VSD, and an increase in both right and left ventricular forces over the 1st month of life is typical of a large ventricular defect with pulmonary hypertension.

The chest film is a better tool than the electrocardiogram in the evaluation of a newborn with a ventricular defect. If the heart is normal in size and the pulmonary vascular markings are normal, the left-to-right shunt is small. With large shunts, the cardiac silhouette is enlarged, and the pulmonary vascular markings are increased and, if there is an elevated pulmonary venous pressure, indistinct. The two-dimensional echocardiogram can usually allow visualization of defects that are larger than 2 mm and rule out associated cardiac anomalies. Doppler assessment of the flow through the defect gives an estimate of the interventricular gradient and may be helpful to estimate the size. Color Doppler can frequently pick up small defects that cannot be imaged otherwise. VSDs also can be visualized with angiography.

An infant who has congestive heart failure and a systolic murmur in the first 2 weeks of life is not likely to have an isolated ventricular defect. If cyanosis is absent, coarctation (with or without a ventricular defect), critical aortic stenosis, or HLHS is more likely. They can usually be differentiated by the absence of femoral pulses in coarctation, the presence of left ventricular hypertrophy with strain on the electrocardiogram in aortic stenosis, and the appearance of a shocklike picture in HLHS. If cyanosis is present, truncus arteriosus, tricuspid atresia, or TOF must be considered. In the asymptomatic newborn with a murmur, mild aortic stenosis, valvular or peripheral pulmonary stenosis, and TOF can be confused, especially if the lesions are mild.

One must treat newborns with a VSD with the knowledge that many, if not most, small defects close spontaneously and that up to 20% of large defects also get much smaller or close. Newborns with a small or moderate size VSD often require no treatment. For those with mild heart failure, digoxin and diuretics and the usual anticongestive measures often suffice. Occasionally a child with a large defect responds poorly to anticongestive measures with continued severe heart failure and poor weight gain despite maximal medical management. For these infants, reparative surgery is necessary.

Surgery can be done at a very low risk (less than 5%) with a very high probability of a surgical cure. For those with multiple muscular defects, pulmonary artery banding is sometimes performed in the hope that some or most of the defects will close spontaneously, making later surgical repair easier.

Atrioventricular Septal Defects (AVSD)

The atrioventricular canal portion of the heart is formed from the endocardial cushions, a mass of embryonic mesenchymal tissue that forms the structures in the middle portion of the heart: the lower portion of the atrial septum, the upper portion of the ventricular septum, and the septal portions of the mitral and tricuspid valves. Any one or all of the components may be abnormal in an endocardial cushion defect, the modern term for which is AVSD. The spectrum of abnormalities in AVSD range from an isolated cleft in the mitral or tricuspid valve to a complete atrioventricular canal with a huge deficiency of the atrial and ventricular septum and a common atrioventricular valve. A variety of classifications have been proposed, but the tremendous spectrum of variations makes sharp distinctions difficult, and a description of the anomalies is preferable: atrial septal defect of the ostium primum type, ventricular septal defect of the atrioventricular canal type, clefts of the mitral or tricuspid valve, single atrioventricular valve, and complete atrioventricular septal defect. Atrioventricular septal defects are the most common type of heart disease present in Down syndrome. Up to 45% of infants with atrioventricular septal defects have trisomy 21. Other cardiac anomalies are often present in association with AVSDs. Heterotaxia syndromes, single ventricle, double outlet right ventricle, transposition, and pulmonary stenosis are the most common.

The hemodynamics of AVSDs are complex. Shunting in these infants may be dependent or obligatory. Dependent shunting through either an ASD or VSD is a function of the pulmonary and systemic vascular resistance. In the newborn period, when the pulmonary vascular resistance is high, little left-to-right shunt may be present. As the pulmonary resistance drops over the first days and weeks of life, the pulmonary blood flow increases, eventually leading to congestive heart failure as the left ventricle becomes overloaded. Obligatory shunting occurs from a high pressure chamber to a low pressure chamber, usually from ventricle to atrium, and is independent of resistance. In AVSDs, obligatory shunting is usually from left ventricle through the mitral portion of the atrioventricular valve into the left atrium and across the atrial defect into the right atrium or, less frequently, directly into the right atrium. This left-to-right shunt caused by atrioventricular valve regurgitation is independent of the status of the pulmonary vasculature and may occur even with the high pulmonary vascular resistance seen in the newborn period.

The degree of intracardiac shunting at any given time is the result of a complex interplay between the pulmonary and systemic resistances affecting the dependent shunting and the obligatory shunting. In the first weeks of life, however, when the pulmonary vascular resistance tends to be high, the newborns who present with congestive failure tend to have obligatory shunts owing to atrioventricular valve regurgitation.

When there is only an ostium primum atrial defect present, infants with AVSD rarely, if ever, are seen in the neonatal period. Infants with AVSD who have an isolated ventricular defect present similarly to the previously described newborns with membranous or muscular ventricular defects. The age at presentation of infants with a complete AVSD is related to the presence of atrioventricular valve regurgitation; if it is severe, the infants may present in the first 1 or 2 weeks of life with the usual manifestations of heart failure, tachycardia, tachypnea, feeding difficulties, and sweating. If the atrioventricular valves are competent, infants present later in the 1st month or even in the 2nd month of life. The precordium is usually hyperactive on palpation, with the maximal impulse displaced laterally and inferiorly. A thrill at the lower left sternal border may be present. If there is significant atrial shunting, the first heart sound is accentuated. In the usual case with pulmonary hypertension, the pulmonary component of the second heart sound is loud. Heart murmurs may be quite variable, but usually there is a loud pansystolic murmur at the lower left sternal border and a flow rumble across the mitral valve best heard at the apex. In the presence of mitral regurgitation, a pansystolic murmur at the apex is audible, but it may be hard to distinguish from the murmur of the VSD.

The electrocardiographic features in infants with AVSDs are characteristic. Because of posterior displacement of the atrioventricular node, His bundle, and distal left bundle as well as hypoplasia of the anterior portion of the left fascicle and an early origin of the left bundle, there is a characteristic superior QRS axis (0 to -150 degrees) on electrocardiogram. These children also have a prolonged PR interval, biatrial hypertrophy, and biventricular hypertrophy.

The heart is almost invariably enlarged on the chest radiograph, and the pulmonary blood flow is increased and often congested. The size of the cardiac silhouette is often out of proportion with the increased pulmonary blood flow, presumably owing to the atrioventricular valve regurgitation.

AVSDs should be considered in all infants who show congestive heart failure, a left-to-right shunt, and a superior axis on the electrocardiogram. Infants with tricuspid atresia without significant pulmonary stenosis may also demonstrate a large heart with increased pulmonary blood flow on the radiograph and a superior axis on the electrocardiogram, but they are desaturated and almost invariably have pure left ventricular hypertrophy on the electrocardiogram, as opposed to the right or biventricular hypertrophy seen in infants with atrioventricular canal defects. Echocardiography can resolve any remaining questions. When congestive failure is present, the usual medical management consisting of digoxin, diuretics, and high-calorie formula should be started. In some infants, this suffices for many months, but frequently surgery is required because of persistent congestive heart failure and failure to thrive.

Surgical repair involves dividing the common atrioventricular valve and closing the ASD and VSD using either one patch or two, attaching the mitral portion of the atrioventricular valve on the left side of the patch and the tricuspid portion on the right side of the patch. Hospital mortality following correction of a complete atrioventricular canal in infancy ranges from 3% to 10%. The development of significant atrioventricular valve regurgitation or subaortic stenosis is occasionally encountered, but a 10-year survival is now expected to be in the 85% to 90% range.

Arteriovenous Fistulas

Arteriovenous fistulas (1 in 100,000 live births) are a rare cause of congestive heart failure in the newborn. There are two types of fistulous connections: a direct communication between an artery and vein bypassing the capillary bed and, less commonly in the newborn, an angioma with multiple arterial and venous supply. Although arteriovenous fistulas causing heart failure have been described in the subclavian, internal mammary, and vertebral arteries and hemangiomas may be found in the skin, pelvis, and coronary arteries, most of the newborns with heart failure have either a cerebral arteriovenous fistula or a hemangioma of the liver.

Arteriovenous fistulas are present in utero but do not seem to cause significant hemodynamic embarrassment. At birth, infants are well developed without evidence of heart failure, but profound heart failure may develop within a few hours. This dramatic change is a result of the shift from the parallel to the in-series circulation after birth. In utero, the systemic venous return including the arteriovenous fistula is divided into two streams. Part of the venous return goes through the right heart chambers into the pulmonary artery, and the rest goes through the foramen ovale to the left-sided heart chambers. After birth, the entire systemic return, including return from the fistula, must pass through the right heart as well as the pulmonary arteries and then to the left heart and aorta. In addition, the removal of the low-resistance placenta circuit after birth increases the systemic resistance and forces more blood through the arteriovenous fistula. These changes occurring with the transitional circulation suddenly impart a large volume overload to the right and left sides of the heart. The neonatal heart is unable to tolerate the increased systemic venous return, and heart failure and circulatory collapse result.

Congestive heart failure with tachypnea, dyspnea, and feeding difficulties is usually present within the first few days of life. Cyanosis is occasionally seen secondary to pulmonary venous desaturation and to right-to-left shunting at the atrial or ductal levels. The peripheral pulses are generally diminished but may be increased in the arteries feeding the fistula. Infants with a cerebral arteriovenous fistula may have dilated veins in the neck. Cardiac enlargement with a hyperdynamic cardiac impulse is present on palpation, and a soft systolic ejection murmur over the semilunar valves or a diastolic flow murmur across the atrioventricular valves may be audible on auscultation. Occasionally a continuous bruit may be heard over the fistula.

Right axis deviation, right ventricular hypertrophy, and ST-T wave changes are usually present on the electrocardiogram. On the chest radiograph, there is generalized cardiac enlargement with increased pulmonary blood flow and pulmonary venous congestion. In infants with a cerebral arteriovenous fistula, the superior mediastinum is often widened because of dilation of the ascending aorta, carotid arteries, jugular vein, and superior vena cava.

The presence of vascular collapse and congestive heart failure in the 1st week of life suggests myocarditis or a left-sided obstructive lesion, such as HLHS, coarctation of the aorta, or aortic stenosis. If there is a bruit over the head with normal or brisk pulses in the head vessels and dilated veins in the neck, a fistula is likely. Occasionally the clinical diagnosis remains unclear, and echocardiography or catheterization is necessary.

For the newborn with circulatory collapse, the usual treatment of congestive heart failure is correction of acidosis and administration of digoxin and diuretics followed by diagnostic study. For newborns with a cerebral or hepatic arteriovenous fistula, coiling of the feeding vessels has occasionally been successful. For those with smaller fistulas, successful therapy has been possible; for the majority of infants with large arteriovenous fistulas with multiple feeding vessels, the prognosis is guarded. Interferon has been tried with limited success.

TRANSIENT MYOCARDIAL ISCHEMIA

A number of newborns suffer a form of myocardial ischemia that frequently is transient but that may be associated with significant cardiovascular symptoms and even death. In some of these infants, the signs of respiratory distress and congestive heart failure or shock are predominant; in others, myocardial dysfunction and tricuspid regurgitation are the presenting symptoms.

The infants are usually born at term by a delivery complicated by hypoxic stress that occurs before or during birth. Fetal scalp pH measurement is in the range of 6.9 to 7.1. The Apgar score is usually less than 3 at 1 minute. Respiratory distress and cyanosis are frequently present soon after birth, with affected infants developing the signs and symptoms of congestive heart failure (tachypnea, tachycardia, hepatomegaly, and a gallop rhythm) within a few hours. Some develop hypotension and cardiovascular collapse and shock. About half the newborns have systolic heart murmurs. In most, the murmur is at the left lower sternal border and suggests tricuspid regurgitation, but in a few the murmur is loudest at the apex and sounds like mitral regurgitation.

The chest radiograph invariably shows cardiomegaly. There is usually a diffuse haziness with pulmonary venous congestion in those with predominantly left-sided heart failure. In those with right-sided heart failure, pulmonary congestion may be absent and pulmonary blood flow may be diminished by right-to-left atrial shunting. The electrocardiogram shows right ventricular predominance that is normal for age and right atrial hypertrophy in the majority. Diffuse ST-T changes are usually present, with the most common pattern being ST depression in the midprecordium and persistent T-wave inversion over the left precordium.

Transient myocardial ischemia should be suspected in all newborns who experience birth asphyxia and who have respiratory distress, cyanosis, or signs of congestive failure soon after birth. Echocardiography is helpful in distinguishing infants who have tricuspid regurgitation associated with transient ischemia from those who have tricuspid regurgitation caused by Ebstein disease of the tricuspid valve or critical pulmonary stenosis or pulmonary atresia with an intact ventricular septum.

The treatment is symptomatic. Digitalis and diuretics should be given for congestive heart failure and metabolic abnormalities of hypoglycemia, and acidosis should be corrected promptly. Those with severe respiratory distress may need intubation and assisted ventilation. Those with cardiovascular collapse may benefit from ionotropic support with dopamine or dolbutamine. Afterload reduction with nitroprusside should be reserved for those most severely affected. For those who are first seen with severe acidosis and cardiogenic shock, the prognosis remains grim, with death likely occurring from heart failure, low cardiac output, or failure of a necessary organ system.

Myocarditis

Myocarditis (1 in 80,000 live births) occurs in all age groups, but there is higher frequency in the 1st month than in any other period of life. It is a well-recognized entity with a clinical pattern sufficiently distinctive for one to make an antemortem diagnosis. Although often a fulminant disease, it is not invariably fatal, and early recognition and prompt treatment may alter the outcome. Any infective agent can cause myocarditis, although the enteroviruses, particularly coxsackie B and echo viruses, are the most common.

On gross examination, the heart is enlarged and dilated. The cardiac muscle feels flabby and is often pale or nutmeg-like in color. Microscopic examination reveals a multicellular infiltration of the myocardium. Lymphocytes, large mononuclear cells, eosinophils, and polymorphonuclear leukocytes are present in varying numbers with either patchy or diffuse distribution. Necrosis and fragmentation of muscle fibers may be present. Although rare in patients with primary myocarditis, involvement of the endocardium and pericardium may occur. When the coxsackievirus is the causative agent, involvement of other organs, particularly the central nervous system, is common. Involvement of multiple organs is even more common with rubella and herpesviruses.

Most serious coxsackievirus infections occur in the first 10 days of life. The clinical course of young infants with myocarditis is variable. The initial symptoms may be mild and include lethargy, failure to feed, vomiting, or diarrhea. Jaundice may be present, and evidence of a mild upper respiratory tract infection is sometimes noted. In the milder forms of the disease, clinical manifestations may be limited to slight tachypnea, tachycardia, and poor heart sounds. Frequently there are no premonitory symptoms. The infant becomes seriously ill suddenly. Respirations increase, become labored, and are often accompanied by a grunt. The infant appears restless and anxious. The skin is pale, mottled, and mildly cyanotic. The temperature may be slightly or greatly elevated or subnormal. The pulse rate is usually rapid, between 150 and 200, and weak. Occasionally bradycardia is present. The percussion note over the chest may be normal or hyperresonant. Dullness is uncommon. The breath sounds are usually harsh, and rales may be heard at the bases. Although there is always some degree of cardiac enlargement, it is often difficult to detect clinically. The heart sounds are mushy, particularly the first sound, and a gallop rhythm may be present. The liver is almost invariably enlarged. Edema is an uncommon finding, and venous engorgement is almost never detected. There may be signs referable to central nervous system involvement, including lethargy, seizures, or coma with occasional focal signs suggesting meningoencephalitis.

Chest radiographs show generalized cardiac enlargement as well as haziness of the lung fields. At times, it is not possible to make the distinction between congestion and pneumonia. Electrocardiograms often show abnormalities. Low-voltage QRS complexes and low, isoelectric, or inverted T waves are the most frequent findings. There may also be significant disturbances in conduction, such as heart block, extrasystoles, and ventricular or atrial tachycardia. The electrocardiographic abnormalities are frequently transient. Elevations of aspartate transaminase, lactic dehydrogenase, and cardiac creatine phosphokinase are variably present with levels dependent on the extent of tissue damage.

The diagnosis of myocarditis should be suspected in any newborn with congestive heart failure in whom structural heart disease has been excluded by two-dimensional echocardiogram. The suspicion should be heightened if there is a known respiratory infection in the mother or proven viral illness in other nursery infants. The acute form of myocarditis is commonly mistaken for overwhelming sepsis or a severe lower respiratory tract infection. This is especially true for the latter because cyanosis and respiratory distress may initially suggest pneumonia. Myocarditis should be suspected if there are tachycardia, poor heart sounds with or without gallop rhythm, a degree of dyspnea disproportionate with the pulmonary findings, and radiographic evidence of cardiac enlargement. Myocarditis must also be differentiated from other cardiac conditions that may occur in the neonatal period, such as congenital heart disease with congestive failure precipitated by infection, the acute form of endocardial fibroelastosis, and paroxysmal tachycardia. Coarctation of the aorta, a not uncommon cause of heart failure in the newborn, must always be excluded by careful evaluation of the pulses and blood pressures in the arms and legs.

Endocardial fibroelastosis is usually associated with left ventricular hypertrophy indicated in electrocardiographic tracings by high-voltage R waves in precordial leads taken over the left side of the heart. The left ventricular pattern may not be as striking in the first few days or weeks of life. In myocarditis, low-voltage complexes are characteristic and are the result of severe disturbances in myocardial function. Occasionally, infants with endocardial fibroelastosis in severe heart failure may have low voltage temporarily.

Congestive heart failure is frequently present with paroxysmal tachycardia, but in this condition the heart rate is usually much more rapid than in myocarditis. Almost invariably the rate is greater than 220 beats/min if the tachycardia itself is severe enough to cause heart failure. Mild forms of myocarditis are particularly difficult to recognize. Signs of heart failure may not be prominent or may be absent entirely. The clinical manifestations may include pallor, slight increase in the respiratory rate, tachycardia, and poor heart sounds. Such findings in an infant who has signs of infection and who appears to have a disproportionate degree of cardiac embarrassment should suggest the possibility of myocarditis. Although electrocardiographic studies may aid in the diagnosis, there is no specific pattern, and a normal tracing does not rule out the disorder.

Young infants with myocarditis may become critically ill with such rapidity that treatment should be instituted as soon as the diagnosis is suspected. Oxygen therapy and digitalis should be started at once with the usual anticongestive measures. Afterload reduction with nitroprusside may be helpful for those who are not hypotensive. A clinical trial is underway to test the efficacy of intravenous gamma globulin, but data are not yet available to know if this is effective. For those most severely involved, cardiac transplantation may be the most reasonable option, although the availability of neonatal hearts on short notice remains highly problematic.

Endocardial Fibroelastosis

Endocardial fibroelastosis (approximately 1 in 70,000 live births) may occur as an isolated or primary condition or in association with a variety of congenital and acquired cardiac lesions. In the latter groups, the clinical entity is that of the underlying cardiac disease, and the fibroelastosis is a secondary finding on postmortem examination. The description that follows is limited mainly to infants with the primary or isolated form of endocardial fibroelastosis.

Gross enlargement of the heart is a constant finding. The weight is increased, and there are hypertrophy and dilation of one or more chambers. This is especially true of the left ventricle, which is the most frequent site of endocardial thickening. Involvement of the left atrium is fairly common, but less than half have an additional lesion of the right ventricle and right atrium. Fibroelastosis confined to the right side of the heart is rare. On gross examination, the endocardium is diffusely thickened and smooth and has a porcelain-white appearance. About half the cases show involvement of one or more valves, the mitral more commonly than the others. In contrast to the usual pattern of congenital abnormalities, there is a striking absence of other malformations. Microscopic examination shows an increase in the fibrous and elastic tissue within the endocardium with some extension into the myocardium. When the valves are involved, the picture is similar to that of the endocardium. There is no evidence of inflammation in the heart. Pneumonia and signs of congestive heart failure are commonly associated autopsy findings.

On auscultation, the heart sounds may be normal or muffled, and a third heart sound is frequently present. Heart murmurs may be present in more than 50% of patients, usually a grade I to grade II pansystolic murmur at the apex from mitral regurgitation secondary to papillary muscle dysfunction.

Diastolic murmurs are uncommon. Chest radiographs invariably show cardiac enlargement that is usually significant, with increased pulmonary vascularity secondary to pulmonary venous congestion. Left atrial enlargement is common. The electrocardiogram almost invariably reveals left ventricular hypertrophy with tall R waves over the left precordium, frequently associated with prominent Q waves and T-wave inversion. Supraventricular or nodal tachycardia, complete heart block, or other arrhythmias may occasionally be seen.

Endocardial fibroelastosis should be suspected in the newborn if abnormalities of cardiac rhythm (e.g., heart block, atrial tachycardia) are present. In the most acute form, diagnosis is difficult. These infants often resemble patients with sepsis or pneumonia. The presence of tachycardia, cardiomegaly, and hepatomegaly should lead to the suspicion of heart failure owing to primary heart disease. Differentiation from primary myocarditis may be particularly difficult. The findings in both conditions are remarkably similar. One distinguishing feature is the strikingly low voltage noted on the electrocardiogram in severe myocarditis, but low voltage may occasionally occur in endocardial fibroelastosis. The left ventricular pattern commonly found in endocardial fibroelastosis may be slight or absent in the patient less than 1 week old with an acute case. The diagnosis should be suspected in any young infant with an enlarged heart, particularly when there is little or no cyanosis and no audible heart murmurs. Absence of the latter signs should exclude most other forms of congenital heart disease. The presence of palpable femoral pulsations eliminates coarctation of the aorta. Infants with anomalous origin of the left coronary artery may have a similar clinical and radiographic picture. The electrocardiogram in this condition is often distinctive, however, and shows a pattern of coronary insufficiency with inverted T waves in leads I and II plus a prominent Q wave in lead I. Glycogen storage disease of the heart is a rare cause of cardiac enlargement in infancy. Here the enlargement is usually globular, without specific chamber enlargement. The electrocardiographic pattern is more bizarre in glycogen storage disease, and a short PR interval is often present. A specific diagnosis can be made by analysis of the glycogen content of skeletal muscle.

Treatment is symptomatic. Transplantation may be necessary for those most seriously affected.

Cardiomyopathy of the Infant of the Diabetic Mother

Many large-for-gestational-age infants born to diabetic mothers have an asymmetric hypertrophic cardiomyopathy involving primarily the ventricular septum. Fetal hyperinsulinemia contributes directly to septal hypertrophy. Microscopic examination has demonstrated hypertrophy of the fibers with areas of cellular disarray. The exact mechanism of the cardiac hypertrophy and the reason that the hypertrophy primarily affects the ventricular septum remain a matter of conjecture.

Affected infants, who are usually puffy and plethoric, may present with the signs and symptoms of congestive heart failure: tachypnea, tachycardia, and hepatomegaly. They usually have respiratory distress and frequently cyanosis from birth. Systolic ejection murmurs are common and, at least according to one study, seem to be correlated with the degree of obstruction to left ventricular ejection by the septal hypertrophy. Cardiac enlargement on the chest radiograph is almost universal, and pulmonary venous congestion is seen in most symptomatic patients. These abnormalities, however, do not correlate with the echocardiographic findings of wall or septal thickness. On echocardiographic evaluation of symptomatic infants, the right ventricular anterior wall, the ventricular septum, and the left ventricular posterior wall are thickened, but the septal wall is disproportionately hypertrophied so that the septal wall–to–left ventricular posterior wall ratio is increased above normal in about one half of infants. In one study the internal dimensions of the right and left ventricle were normal, as was the percentage of dimensional change, a measure of cardiac function. In five of the 24 infants, there was evidence of left ventricular outflow tract obstruction owing to apposition of the anterior leaflet of the mitral valve to the hypertrophied interventricular septum during systole. The echocardiogram is diagnostic and should be performed on all infants of diabetic mothers with signs or symptoms of respiratory distress or congestive heart failure. Other forms of heart disease must be excluded because the incidence of congenital heart disease in infants of diabetic mothers is five times that of the normal population.

The treatment is symptomatic. Hypoglycemia, hypocalcemia, and hypomagnesemia and polycythemia should be corrected, and maintenance fluid should be provided intravenously if oral intake is not possible. Occasional increasing respiratory distress requires intubation and assisted ventilation. Unless severely depressed myocardial contractility can be demonstrated on echocardiogram, digitalis and other ionotropic agents are contraindicated since they may lead to increasing left ventricular outflow tract obstruction.

The prognosis in this group of newborns is excellent. Of 11 symptomatic infants reported by Way and colleagues, all were asymptomatic by 1 month of age, with the radiograph in all and the electrocardiogram in 10 returning to normal. Echocardiograms showed regression of septal thickness in all the patients, and repeat cardiac catheterizations in two of the 11 have shown normal hemodynamics with elimination of gradients of 30 and 74 mm Hg between the left ventricle and the aorta. The findings of Gutgesell and coworkers are similar.

Glycogen Storage Disease of the Heart

Glycogen storage disease is a rare condition that may produce symptoms from birth. There are at least 22 types of which only three affect the heart. The most common is Pompe disease, usually classified as Type IIa. It is transmitted through a single recessive autosomal gene. The defect is due to the congenital absence of alpha-1,4-glycosidase (lysosomal acid maltose) from intracellular lysosomes.

This results in the accumulation of normal glycogen in lysosomal sacs of virtually all tissues, where it cannot be degraded by glycolytic enzymes.

The heart is always enlarged, often to enormous proportions. The walls of both ventricles are thick, but the atria are normal. Microscopic examination shows infiltration of the muscle fibers with large vacuoles of glycogen. Varying amounts of glycogen deposition are also found in the skeletal muscles, liver, kidneys, and central nervous system. Frequently the infant appears normal at birth but goes on to have a history of poor feeding, lassitude, a feeble cry, protruding tongue, and failure to gain weight. Hypotonia may be striking, and the tongue may appear thick. Cardiac enlargement is the rule. A systolic heart murmur may be noted, but it is often soft and variable. The liver is not usually enlarged.

The usual parameters for glycogen metabolism are normal, including glucose tolerance and response to epinephrine and glucagon. These infants do not suffer from hypoglycemia. Radiologic examination shows gross generalized cardiomegaly, although the heart need not be enlarged at birth. The electrocardiogram may show abnormalities at birth or after a period of some weeks: The presence of a short PR interval, huge precordial voltages, and evidence of left ventricular hypertrophy is universal. T-wave inversion, ST-T elevation, and deep Q waves are frequently seen. On echocardiogram, thickening of the left ventricular free wall disproportionate to the thickness of the interventricular septum is seen. Cardiac catheterization and angiography are rarely indicated.

The diagnosis is rarely made in the neonatal period unless there is a family history of the disease. The early symptoms are ill defined and, with the exception of intermittent episodes of dyspnea, do not suggest a cardiac abnormality. The patient is more likely to be several weeks or months old before the cardiac enlargement is detected. The diagnosis should be suspected in any infant with an enlarged heart in the absence of structural heart disease, especially if the enlargement is great. Muscle weakness is an important additional clue. Macroglossia is often present and may be confused with cretinism or Down syndrome.

Tumors of the Heart

Cardiac tumors are rare but when present the manifestations of heart disease may appear infrequently in the neonatal period. Several types of tumors have been described—rhabdomyomas are the most common and are frequently associated with tuberous sclerosis. Most commonly the tumors are multiple, but occasionally only one is found. They are situated in the walls of the right or left ventricle or occasionally in the interventricular septum and, on occasion, project into the lumen and obstruct one of the valves or the outflow tract of the right or left ventricle. Histologically they consist of numerous nodular areas with vacuoles that contain glycogen. On electron microscopy the glycogen is seen in the cytoplasm and in the mitochondria. Fibromas, solitary tumors in the septal or parietal wall of the left ventricle, are usually not encapsulated with tissue mixing with the myocardial cells in the wall. They have been described in the neonatal period and occasionally cause problems by compressing the anterior descending coronary artery, interfering with the conduction system, or obstructing right or left ventricular outflow. Other tumors, including teratoma, lipoma, hemangioma, hamartoma, and sarcoma, are considerably less common, especially in the perinatal period.

The clinical picture is extremely variable. Many infants, especially those with multiple intramural rhabdomyomas, are asymptomatic and are identified on two-dimensional echocardiogram performed because minor obstructions lead to turbulence and murmurs. Occasionally, newborns present with arrhythmias, including atrial flutter or fibrillation or ventricular tachycardia, or complete heart block because of interference with the conduction system. Heart murmurs are usually not present unless the tumor projects into the cardiac cavity and obstructs blood flow. Changes in the cardiac examination depend on the location and severity of the intracavitary obstruction to flow. The electrocardiographic findings are variable, with right, left, and combined ventricular hypertrophy being reported, although occasionally the electrocardiogram is normal. Often there is evidence of abnormal repolarization with inverted T waves. On chest radiographic studies, the heart is usually normal in the absence of significant hemodynamic disruption, although in children with large fibromas the tumor may distort the cardiac contour. Two-dimensional echocardiogram is now the best tool to evaluate the size, location, number, and hemodynamic severity of the tumor or tumors.

Most rhabdomyomas and fibromas need no therapy. The natural history has not been determined conclusively because these tumors are so uncommon. Most of the intramural lesions do not progress and enlarge, however, and some may become relatively smaller with time.

Cardiac Dysrhythmias

Cardiac dysrhythmias are not uncommon in the newborn, accompanying the significant changes in circulatory hemodynamics and gas exchange that occur with the switch from the in utero to extrauterine circulations. In a review of more than 3000 apparently normal newborns, Southall and colleagues found dysrhythmias in about 1% on a routine 10-second electrocardiogram before discharge. The vast majority of these dysrhythmias were of little significance, but life-threatening arrhythmias may occur on rare occasions.

Sinus Arrhythmia, Sinus Tachycardia, and Sinus Bradycardia

Sinus arrhythmia is a phasic variation of the sinus node discharge that may occur either in cycle with respiration or independent of it. It is quite common and, as far as can be determined, is of no clinical significance. On electrocardiogram, the PP interval is irregular and the P wave, PQ interval, and QRS complexes are normal.

Sinus tachycardia can be defined as a heart rate

that exceeds the upper range of normal, usually 175 to 190 beats/min in a full-term infant and 195 beats/min in a premature infant. The PP interval is short, but the P wave, PQ interval, and QRS complexes are normal. It is usually a manifestation of increased adrenergic activity that may be the result of crying, feeding, or blood letting, but it may also be secondary to congestive heart failure, shock, anemia, or fever. No treatment is necessary if the significant secondary causes of the tachycardia can be ruled out.

Sinus bradycardia is a heart rate that falls below what is generally accepted as normal (i.e., below 90 to 100 beats/min), with a normal P wave preceding each QRS. Occasionally the sinus mechanism is so depressed that the junctional tissue depolarizes first, resulting in a junctional escape rhythm. Sinus bradycardia has been associated with defecation, hiccupping, yawning, and nasopharyngeal stimulation, probably as a result of parasympathetic stimulation, and is frequently seen with prolonged apnea. Also, it may be seen with severe systemic disease, particularly that associated with acidosis, hypoxemia, or increased intracranial pressure. Occasionally, otherwise normal infants have a sinus bradycardia of 80 to 90 beats/min in the absence of other findings, probably because of immaturity of the autonomic nervous system and increased vagal tone. In deep sleep, healthy newborn infants can occasionally exhibit heart rates as low as 60 beats per minute. If systemic and primary cardiac disease can be excluded, no treatment is necessary.

Ectopic Beats: Supraventricular and Ventricular

Although during routine predischarge screening in one series the incidence of ectopic beats was less than 1%, continuous monitoring of healthy newborns shows that the incidence of ectopic beats is much greater, as high as 13%. Supraventricular ectopic beats are usually preceded by a P wave with an abnormal contour, have a normal-appearing QRS, and are followed by an incomplete compensatory pause before the next P wave. Ventricular ectopic beats usually have a wide abnormal QRS, a tall T wave in the opposite direction from the QRS, and a full compensatory pause. These arrhythmias may be seen with metabolic abnormalities, hypoxia, or digoxin toxicity or after cardiac surgery, but they are also frequently seen in otherwise normal newborns. Treatment includes correction of the predisposing factors when possible; in otherwise normal infants, no treatment is necessary unless couplets or atrial or ventricular tachycardia is present because the prognosis is excellent, with ectopy usually disappearing within the 1st month of life.

Paroxysmal Supraventricular Tachycardia

Paroxysmal SVT is one of the most common serious arrhythmias occurring in the fetus and newborn. Although precise incidence data are not available, the generally accepted frequency is approximately 1 in every 25,000 children. Although usually relatively benign in the older child, the arrhythmias may be life-threatening in the fetus or newborn, who generally has a higher ventricular rate and is less able to rely on other mechanisms for support of a failing circulation. On electrocardiogram there is a rapid regular rhythm, usually 230 to 320 beats/min, that originates in the atria or junctional region with normal, abnormal, or inapparent P waves; a normal or slightly widened QRS; and ST segments that are normal or slightly depressed. Several mechanisms play a part in the genesis of SVTs, but a rapid ectopic pacemaker or a circus type of re-entry secondary to different refractory periods of adjacent conducting bundles is the most common. Wolff-Parkinson-White syndrome, in which there is a direct muscular connection between the atrium and ventricle that allows re-entry, is recognizable on the electrocardiogram by a short PQ interval and slow initial ventricular depolarization (delta wave) and is present in about 50% of the cases.

SVT may occur in the fetus. It may not cause symptoms before birth, but occasionally the rapid rate may lead to in utero congestive failure with fetal edema or hydrops and fetal death. Rarely the fetal SVT is intermittent, and the authors have observed infants with hydrops born with normal electrocardiograms who subsequently demonstrate recurrent SVT.

The newborn with SVT presents with signs and symptoms of low cardiac output and congestive heart failure; fussiness, refusal to feed, vomiting, tachypnea, and hepatomegaly are common. At first, the infants have some duskiness or cyanosis of the skin, but later their skin turns ashen gray, and their extremities become cool owing to extreme peripheral vasoconstriction. Cardiac examination usually reveals no problem other than tachycardia. Underlying heart disease may be difficult to detect, even if present, because of the rapid heart rate. At first, the chest radiograph may be normal, but, by the time symptoms occur, there is usually cardiac enlargement, often with pulmonary venous congestion. The echocardiogram is helpful in ruling out associated heart disease.

SVT is diagnosed electrocardiographically. Occasionally, normal newborns with increased adrenergic activity may have heart rates exceeding 200 beats/min, but these infants do not have congestive failure, and the rate slows down when they are quiet. Sometimes, however, it may be difficult to distinguish newborns with a tachycardia associated with severe congestive failure caused by myocarditis or congenital heart disease from those with SVT. Rates of 220 beats/min or more in the newborn are rarely, if ever, of sinus origin and thus require treatment. Rates of 220 beats/min or less in the newborn usually represent sinus rhythm. The presence of heart failure with a rate of 200 to 220 beats/min suggests underlying heart disease because this rate alone is rarely rapid enough to cause significant congestive heart failure in the newborn. Another helpful electrocardiographic sign is that SVT is almost always regular, with variation in heart rate of more than 1 to 2 beats/min being an unusual occurrence. Therefore, any variation in rate with crying or feeding is likely to signify a sinus mechanism. Rarely a therapeutic trial of adenosine may be necessary to sort out the underlying mechanism.

SVT in a newborn represents an emergency, and treatment should not be delayed. Vagal stimulation, including gagging, carotid sinus massage, or ice compresses to the head, is rarely effective. Adenosine is approved for intravenous use for paroxysmal SVTs in adults and children. It has now become the first-line treatment for paroxysmal atrial tachycardia. Adenosine is given as an intravenous bolus starting at 0.05 mg/kg and increased by 0.05 mg/kg until tachycardia resolves (usually within seconds). Adenosine is a remarkably safe and effective agent for treating both term and preterm infants with SVT. It acts by inducing complete atrioventricular block transiently. By this mechanism, the re-entry circuit is interrupted. Half-life of adenosine in the blood after injection is only seconds. Adenosine is ineffective in treatment of other tachycardias; therefore a response is diagnostic as well as therapeutic. Older treatments include digoxin with half the total intravenous digitalizing dose of 0.02 mg/kg in term infants (0.015 mg/kg in premature infants) given immediately and the rest in divided doses over the next 12 to 18 hours. Other regimens that have been used include over-drive atrial pacing DC cardioversion (0.25 to 1 joule/kg) synchronized to the peak of the QRS complex to avoid the vulnerable period of the T wave, propranolol (0.01 to 0.1 mg/kg intravenously), phenylephrine (0.005 to 0.02 mg/kg intravenously), or edrophonium (0.2 mg/kg intravenously). Calcium channel blockers should be avoided in neonates, because they can cause cardiovascular collapse.

Atrial Flutter

Atrial flutter is a relatively rare dysrhythmia in the neonatal period. The atrial rate ranges between 360 and 480 beats/ min, with the ventricular response one half or, less commonly, one third of that. The atrial activity is best seen as a saw-toothed pattern of the P waves in leads II and V_{4R} to V_2. Newborns with atrial flutter may have congestive heart failure from the tachycardia, but more commonly the 2:1 or 3:1 block reduces the ventricular rate so that the dysrhythmia is well tolerated.

The treatment involves digitalization and, if this

fails to revert the rhythm to sinus, cardioversion. The prognosis is not as favorable as with atrial tachycardia because recurrences are more common, but most infants without associated structural heart disease usually do well. Ongoing treatment with digoxin is usually successful in preventing recurrences. If this approach is not successful, propranolol or quinidine can be added.

Ventricular Tachycardia

Ventricular tachycardia (three or more premature complexes in a row) in the newborn is uncommon. When it does occur, it is usually in association with structural heart disease and is triggered by cardiac catheterization, surgery, anesthesia, metabolic abnormalities, or digitalis toxicity. The QRS complexes are wide and tall, and the T waves are directed opposite to the QRS complex. The rate is usually less than 200 beats/min, but higher rates have been reported. The initial treatment should be lidocaine (1 mg/kg intravenously) or cardioversion. Other drugs that may occasionally be useful include phenytoin (diphenylhydantoin), procainamide, quinidine, and propranolol. In the idiopathic variety, echocardiography and angiocardiography should be performed to rule out the possibility that a resectable tumor is the source of the tachycardia. Treatment must be individualized, with the long-term prognosis depending primarily on the underlying cardiac problem.

Atrioventricular Block

First-Degree and Second-Degree Heart Block. First-degree heart block is a prolongation of the PR interval beyond the normal limits, 0.164 second on the first day of life, and 0.14 second for the rest of the neonatal period. It is of no hemodynamic significance by itself and requires no treatment. In second-degree heart block, there is an intermittent failure of impulse transmission from atria to ventricles. It may be exhibited as a progressive prolongation of the PR interval in successive cycles followed by an unconducted atrial impulse (Wenckebach or Mobitz Type I) or failure of atrial impulse transmission with dropped ventricular beats and no progressive prolongation of the PR interval (Mobitz Type II). Both Type I and Type II may be manifestations of infection or digitalis toxicity. Neither type needs treatment, but both should be watched carefully because either may lead to third-degree, or complete heart block.

Third-Degree Heart Block. In complete heart block, there is complete failure of the atrial impulse to lead to a ventricular response; the atria and ventricles beat independently, with the latter having a slower rate. On the surface electrocardiogram, there is no fixed relationship between the P waves and the QRS complex. Complete heart block is a relatively common problem in the newborn, occurring in 1 of every 15,000 to 20,000 live births. Histologically there may be an absence of a connection between the atrial conduction tissue and the atrioventricular node, absence or degeneration of the connection between the atrioventricular node tissue and the distal conducting tissue, or a lesion beyond the atrioventricular node that interrupts the bundle of His.

CHAPTER 8

Nervous System

CENTRAL NERVOUS SYSTEM MALFORMATIONS

NEURAL TUBE DEFECTS

Neural tube defects, encompassing craniorachischisis totalis, anencephaly, myeloschisis, encephaloceles, and meningomyeloceles (and Arnold-Chiari malformation), were, until recently, one of the most frequent congenital malformations encountered in newborns, occurring in about 3 per 1000 births on the East Coast of the United States, in about 1 per 1000 births on the West Coast of the United States, and at a higher rate in various regions of the United Kingdom. In 1970, the occurrence rate for England and Wales was 4.5 per 1000 births; in 1991, this rate had dropped to 0.18 per 1000 births. For the most part, the lower occurrence rates reflect two major interventions: in utero diagnosis with termination of affected pregnancies and maternal periconceptional folate therapy (which is estimated to prevent 60% of neural tube defects).

Anencephaly and Encephaloceles

The defects referred to as *neural tube defects* are those that result from abnormalities of neural tube closure or from splitting of the neural tube (schisis). Anencephaly is a lethal malformation in which the calvaria is absent and the intracranial contents are replaced by vascularized, disorganized glial tissue (area cerebrovasculosa). The hypothalamus and cerebellum are usually malformed, the anterior lobe of the pituitary is present, and the internal carotid arteries are hypoplastic, which may be secondary to abnormal brain formation.

Because the anencephalic infant has a period of exencephaly, in which the brain tissue extrudes through the unformed calvaria and then is degraded by exposure to the amniotic fluid, some investigators have hypothesized that the primary defect is the abnormal skull formation. There are some cases in which remnants of calvarial bones are present, with normal brain under the protective bones (Roessmann, 1995).

Anencephaly can be diagnosed by fetal ultrasound examination and by measuring alpha-fetoprotein (AFP) in maternal serum. AFP is the major serum protein in the early embryo and is fetus specific. It normally passes from the fetal serum into fetal urine and then into amniotic fluid; in the amniotic fluid, it is swallowed by the fetus and catabolized in the fetal gastrointestinal tract. In anencephaly, open spina bifida, and open encephalocele, there is leakage of fetal serum directly into the amniotic fluid, and amniotic fluid ATP levels as well as maternal serum levels are elevated. When a neural tube defect is closed (i.e., covered by intact skin), however, the AFP level is not elevated; this occurs in about 5% of neural tube defects.

Both anencephaly and cranium bifidum with occipital encephaloceles affect girls more than boys. Examination of the infant with occipital and parietal encephaloceles can be aided by transillumination, skull radiographs, ultrasound examination, computed tomography (CT) scans, and magnetic resonance imaging (MRI). Decisions about which modality to use depend on the individual cases and whether other cerebral anomalies or hydrocephalus is suspected. Frontonasal encephaloceles pulse or bulge with brief bilateral jugular vein compression, indicating communication with the subarachnoid space. Nasal gliomas, dermoids, and teratomas can all occur in the same region. Intranasal encephalocele should be suspected when an intranasal mass is found in a child with a broad nasal bridge and widely spaced eyes. Some of these children may also present with recurrent meningitis. Basal encephaloceles are not usually diagnosed until childhood and can be located in the nasopharynx, sphenoid sinus, or posterior orbit. Treatment of encephaloceles, when possible, is surgical removal, early in life.

Meningocele, Meningomyelocele, and Lipomeningomyelocele

When there is herniation of the meninges or the meninges and spinal cord through the spinal defect, the lesion is referred to as *spina bifida cystica;* 80% of these lesions are meningomyeloceles, and 20% are meningoceles. The lesion most often occurs in the lumbar or lumbosacral region (69% of cases), and 95% of children with lumbar or lumbosacral meningomyelocele have the brain abnormalities referred to as the Arnold-Chiari II malformation. The incidence of meningomyelocele in the United States is about 0.2 to 0.4 per 1000 live births.

When the lesion is a meningocele, it is usually skin covered, and neurologic function is usually normal (sometimes there are other abnormalities of spinal cord or brain). Meningomyeloceles are usually not skin covered unless a lipoma overlies the defect, forming a lipomeningomyelocele.

Arnold-Chiari Malformation

Almost all patients with meningomyelocele have the Arnold-Chiari malformation. Hydrocephalus in patients with meningomyeloceles can be correlated with the site of the lesion. Increased intracranial pressure is present in about 15% of newborns with meningomyelocele; in some infants, there are no signs of increased pressure because of decompression owing to cerebrospinal fluid leakage through the meningomyelocele. In these infants, hydrocephalus and increased pressure can become evident after surgical closure of the meningomyelocele. Most infants with hydrocephalus develop abnormal increases in head size within a month after birth.

As in anencephaly, fetal diagnosis of open meningomyelocele is made by quantitating maternal serum AFP and by ultrasound or MRI of the fetus in cases in which the protein is elevated. Another marker, amniotic fluid acetylcholinesterase, is also used to diagnose neural tube defects in utero, along with amniotic AFP levels, increasing the sensitivity of the screening when the maternal serum AFP level is questionable or high. The best time for determination in maternal serum is 16 to 18 weeks of gestation and in amniotic fluid 14 to 16 weeks of gestation. Ultrasound or MRI is done routinely in many centers now, certainly in any questionable case or in any case in which there is an affected sibling. The risk of recurrence for neural tube defects in general is 2% to 5% when there has been one affected previous child; the risk increases when there has been more than one affected sibling (from 5% to 12% when there have been two).

Occult Dysraphisms

It is important to examine newborns for evidence of occult dysraphisms by looking for midline skin findings—hair, hemangiomas, pigmented spots, skin tags, aplasia cutis congenita, cutaneous dimples or tracts, or any subcutaneous mass. Problems occurring in infancy and childhood related to these lesions include delay in walking, delay in sphincter control, anatomic abnormalities of the feet or legs, and pain in the back or legs. Gait and sphincter abnormalities, foot deformities, and scoliosis occur in older patients.

Clinical management of the newborn with a neural tube defect has to be individualized. Aggressive surgical therapy is advocated for most infants; to date, this has resulted in patients with increased cognitive abilities, increased ambulation, a lower incidence of incontinence, and lower mortality.

Patients with occult dysraphisms require radiographs of the spine to diagnose the bony defect. CT, myelography, MRI, and real-time ultrasonography are used to visualize the anatomy, the tissue–cerebrospinal fluid relationships, and mobility of the cord.

Disorders of the Prosencephalon
Agenesis of the Corpus Callosum

Although agenesis of the corpus callosum is sometimes found at autopsy as an incidental finding in otherwise normal individuals, this lesion is frequently associated with other defects that lead to symptoms. When there is agenesis of the corpus callosum, the medial portion of each hemisphere has abnormal gyration with absence of the cingulate gyrus and sulcation that is perpendicular to the long axis of the hemisphere.

Migration Disorders
Neurocristopathies

Disorders thought to arise from abnormalities of neural crest formation, migration, proliferation, or differentiation include the LEOPARD syndrome (*l*entigenes, *e*lectrocardiographic abnormalities, *o*cular hypertelorism, *p*ulmonary stenosis, *a*bnormal genitalia, *r*etardation of growth, and *d*eafness); multiple lentigenes syndrome; NAME syndrome (*n*evi, *a*trial myxoma, *m*yxoid neurofibroma, and *e*phelides); LAMB syndrome (*l*entigenes, *a*trial *m*yxoma, mucocutaneous myxomas, and *b*lue nevi); and the Peutz-Jeghers-Touraine syndrome. Tumors derived from neural crest cells include those arising from Schwann cells, perineural cells, or fibrocytes; from neural sense organs; from ganglionic or neuroendocrine cells; or from melanogenic cells. Some neurocutaneous syndromes, such as neurofibromatosis, hypomelanosis of Ito, and neurocutaneous melanosis, as well as other entities, such as multiple schwannoma syndrome (without neurofibromatosis), multiple mucosal neuromas, multiple hamartomas syndrome, cutaneous meningiomas, and multiple endocrine neoplasia, are all thought to involve neural crest cells in some way. Many of the diseases previously classified as neurocutaneous syndromes are now being called *hereditary tumor syndromes of the nervous system*, with more definition of their pathogenesis becoming available through molecular genetic studies.

Hirschsprung disease is a disorder of neural crest development and occurs in 1 in 5000 births. It is characterized by absence of hindgut intramural ganglion cells, which causes intestinal obstruction in the neonatal period. A gene associated with some cases of Hirschsprung disease has been mapped to chromosome 10 and localized to the *RET* proto-oncogene. Mutations that affect the RET protein seem also to be present in patients with multiple endocrine neoplasia Type 2A.

Neuroblastoma is a neuroectodermal tumor that occurs mostly in children. It usually arises from the adrenal gland but can arise from sympathetic ganglia, the neuroendocrine system, or the ovary. It is sometimes seen in association with neurofibromatosis. Cutaneous metastases from neuroblastoma can occur as multiple skin nodules and have been seen in the newborn.

Möbius Syndrome

Möbius syndrome typically consists of bilateral facial and abducens palsies caused by absence or hypoplasia of the cranial nerve nuclei. In some cases, there is involvement of other cranial nerves. Associated features, such as mental retardation, dextrocardia, and endocrine and muscular abnormalities, have been described.

Proliferation Disorders

Micrencephaly

Micrencephaly is a condition in which smallness of the brain or of the cerebral hemispheres is the only lesion; microcephaly is used to describe a small cranial vault induced either by micrencephaly or by acquired atrophic lesions (e.g., multicystic encephalopathy, hydranencephaly, diffuse cortical atrophy).

Micrencephaly vera is the term used to describe small brains that are usually well formed (although usually not as small as radial microbrains) with simple gyral patterns. In these brains, the number of cortical neuronal columns is normal, but the cell-number in each column is reduced. Evrard and colleagues have shown the absence of residual germinal matrix in one such brain at 26 weeks' gestation. This abnormality would most likely occur between 6 and 18 weeks' gestation, when the later proliferative events are occurring. Both of these forms of micrencephaly may be caused by genetic abnormalities, teratogenic influence, or sporadically. Autosomal dominant, autosomal recessive, and X-linked recessive types have been described. Irradiation before 18 weeks' gestation is a well-known teratogenic agent that can produce micrencephaly, and use of alcohol and cocaine during this time in pregnancy can also result in micrencephaly. Maternal hyperphenylalanine has also been associated with these defects in nonphenylketonuric offspring.

Macrencephaly

Just as micrencephaly implies a small brain, macrencephaly describes a large brain that is generally well formed. It is distinguished from macrocephaly, which defines a large head from a number of causes. Syndromes associated with macroencephaly include generalized growth disturbances; others include familial macrencephaly (autosomal dominant or autosomal recessive), neurocutaneous syndromes, macrencephaly associated with known chromosomal disorders (fragile X syndrome and Klinefelter syndrome), and unilateral macrencephaly (hemimegalencephaly).

Neurocutaneous Syndromes

Neurocutaneous syndromes that can be diagnosed in the newborn in some cases include neurofibromatosis 1, Sturge-Weber disease, and tuberous sclerosis. The gene for neurofibromatosis 1, on chromosome 17, is involved in the regulation of cell proliferation through the *ras* proto-oncogene. Neurofibromas usually contain a mixed population of cells, including Schwann cells, perineurial cells, and mast cells. Forty percent of infants with neurofibromatosis have five café-au-lait lesions greater than 5 cm in size at birth, and 20% to 40% of these infants have macrocephaly eventually. Occasionally, optic nerve glioma and plexiform neuroma of the eyelid are seen in the newborn with neurofibromatosis.

Sturge-Weber disease, a sporadic disease of mesoblastic origin, is characterized by a cutaneous nevus or port-wine stain in the areas of the sensory branches of the trigeminal nerve as well as a vascular malformation that involves the leptomeninges, choroid, and cortex homolaterally. The port-wine stain is evident at birth, and cerebral atrophy can be present at birth. Glaucoma is sometimes present at birth, and all children with Sturge-Weber disease should be followed for development of glaucoma. Cerebral calcifications can sometimes be seen on neuroimaging in the newborn with Sturge-Weber disease but are usually not manifest until 6 months of age or later.

Tuberous sclerosis is characterized by abnormal proliferations of both neurons and glial cells as well as hamartomas in other organs. The genetics are complicated with two genes now identified for this disease, one on chromosome 16 and the other on chromosome 9. The typical cutaneous hypopigmented spots are frequently present in the neonatal period, and seizures may occur in the newborn with tuberous sclerosis. Infants with tuberous sclerosis at several months of age may manifest infantile spasms. Subependymal nodules and cortical tubers can sometimes be diagnosed by CT, ultrasound, or MRI in the newborn period.

Incontinentia pigmenti is a rare disorder with a predilection for females. In eight families with hereditary incontinentia pigmenti, genetic linkage analysis has shown a gene locus at Xq28. Other families have shown X/autosomal translocations with the same phenotype, however. The disease is manifest by well-described dermatologic features that pass through four stages. Lesions seen during the neonatal period in 90% of cases are macular, papular, vesicular, erythematous, and bullous; may be pustular; and are characterized by the presence of eosinophils. Half of the cases show skin lesions at birth. These early-phase lesions usually are present for several months (and may be present for several years). In the second stage, the skin lesions have been described as lichenoid or keratotic, verrucous, or pustular. This stage usually occurs at 2 to 6 weeks of age but may be present at birth if the first stage was present in utero. In the third stage, the lesions become pigmented, occurring usually between 3 and 6 months of age (but they may be delayed). The pigmentation is usually tan, brownish, or grayish and can be in streaks, whorls, flecks, or other configurations. These lesions, too, can be seen at birth, suggesting that the other lesions have been present in utero.

Cerebellar Malformations

The Dandy-Walker malformation and related disorders are primarily associated with aplasia or hypoplasia of the vermis of the cerebellum. The Dandy-Walker malformation consists of complete or partial agenesis of the vermis; cystic dilation of the fourth ventricle; and enlargement of the posterior fossa with upward displacement of the lateral sinuses, tentorium, and torcular. Dandy and Blackfan, then Taggart and Walker originally described the syndrome and ascribed its components to nonpatency of the foramina of Luschka and Magendie. Others have pointed out that atresia of the foramina does not have to be present to have the syndrome. More than 80% of those with the Dandy-Walker malformation develop signs of hydrocephalus during the first postnatal year; some have hydrocephalus at birth. Those diagnosed after 12 months of age usually have delayed developmental milestones, with or without increased head size. Neurologic signs may include cranial nerve palsies, apnea, nystagmus, and truncal ataxia. The diagnosis can be made by ultrasonography in utero or by CT or MRI scan postnatally. Treatment usually requires ventricular and posterior fossa shunting.

Aplasia and hypoplasia of the cerebellar hemispheres are usually associated with other brain malformations.

Arteriovenous Malformation of the Vein of Galen

An arteriovenous malformation (AVM) of the vein of Galen frequently causes symptoms in the newborn period. This malformation consists of a meshwork of arteries extending from the vertebrobasilar system that feeds, sometimes along with branches of the anterior and middle cerebral arteries, into the vein of Galen. Because of the large shunt of blood through the malformation, the newborn usually presents with cardiomegaly and heart failure. The preferential steal (diversion) of blood through the malformation can also cause infarction of brain tissue. Despite the poor prognosis, surgery can be helpful for some infants by slowing or arresting the otherwise progressive deterioration associated with the lesion. Other types of vascular malformations occur in the brains of infants and children, but they are not as likely to present in the newborn period as AVM of the vein of Galen.

DESTRUCTIVE LESIONS IN UTERO

Varying degrees of destruction of the brain can occur in utero related to events that cause brain necrosis and cavitation. Such lesions include a range of defects from isolated cysts to hydranencephaly. Similar lesions have been produced in experimental models by trauma, arterial vascular obstruction, infection, hyperthermia, and endotoxin. Usually it is not possible to define the exact cause of such lesions.

Aqueductal Stenosis

Although aqueductal obstruction can be the result of several types of pathology, including stenosis, forking, atresia, or septum formation, when due to gliosis, it has been classified as postinflammatory. A form of stenosis without evidence of gliosis is apparently sex linked and is also associated with other malformations, including abnormal thumbs, agenesis of the corpus callosum, and agenesis of the corticospinal tracts. Because the fetal brain before 17 to 20 weeks gestation does not show gliosis as a result of acquired damage, it is not always possible to tell if an aqueductal lesion is a true malformation or is secondary to intrauterine infection or other insult.

Hydrocephalus

The term *hydrocephalus* implies an increased amount of cerebrospinal fluid (CSF) within the ventricles, under pressure, as a result of an obstruction to the outflow of CSF or an overproduction of CSF. Obstruction to outflow can be at the foramen of Monro, in a ventricle, at the aqueduct, at the foramina of Luschka and Magendie, in one or more cisterns, or at the places of absorption in the arachnoid villi. Hydrocephalus as a result of overproduction of CSF can occur with choroid plexus papillomas, carcinomas, or hyperplasia. Choroid plexus papillomas can be seen as congenital brain tumors, and hydrocephalus associated with choroid plexus papilloma may be a combination of obstruction to outflow by the papilloma and overproduction of CSF. The term *communicating hydrocephalus* is used to define cases in which the ventricular system and cisterns communicate. In *noncommunicating hydrocephalus*, there is obstruction at some point within the ventricular system or between the cisterns.

Hydrocephalus is frequently associated with developmental anomalies of the brain, including the Dandy-Walker malformation and variants, Chiari malformations, lissencephalies and cerebro-ocular muscular syndromes, holoprosencephaly, and other defects with maldevelopment or loss of cerebral tissue. Hydrocephalus can also be a consequence of aqueductal occlusion (see earlier), tumors or cysts that obstruct various parts of the ventricular system, or postinflammatory states (postmeningitic, posthemorrhagic). Surgical treatment of hydrocephalus, most commonly by ventriculoperitoneal shunting, has increased survival of affected infants dramatically with improved cognitive outcome.

Hypoxic-Ischemic Lesions

Intrauterine hypoxic-ischemic lesions are usually manifest as complete or incomplete necrosis or hemorrhage in either or both white and gray matter. Fetal brains are particularly prone to rarefaction or cavitary lesions of white matter, especially in the periventricular regions, centrum semiovale, and subcortical white matter. The cerebellum may also be affected. The areas most likely to be infarcted are those that correspond to areas of poor vascularization between dorsal and basal penetrating arteries. Such lesions are also found frequently in premature infants who die after having sustained prenatal or postnatal hypoxia-ischemia. When lesions with necrosis, cavitation, and mineral deposits are apparent by ultrasound scanning at birth, they are due to intrauterine injury because these findings take days to weeks to develop.

Gray matter lesions are more likely to be found in term infants. They may be found as parasagittal lesions, as laminar cortical necrosis, as pontosubicular necrosis, and as necrosis of the basal ganglia. Experimental studies in primates have suggested that total asphyxial injury results in brain stem damage; partial asphyxia with acidosis results in cerebral cortical injury with edema; partial asphyxia without acidosis results in white matter injury; and a combination of partial and total asphyxia results in basal ganglia injury plus lesions of the neocortex (the more severe the total asphyxia, the more brain stem injury also occurs). Human newborns also show cerebellar lesions after significant hypoxia-ischemia.

Hydranencephaly

One of the most devastating intrauterine encephaloclastic lesions is hydranencephaly, which is loss of tissue in the territories supplied by the internal carotid arteries. The brain stem is usually intact, but the hemispheres are usually replaced by fluid-filled cavities surrounded by a leptomeningeal membrane with remnants of the damaged cortex.

Hemorrhagic Lesions

Fresh hemorrhage, especially petechial hemorrhages and subependymal germinal matrix hemorrhages, occurs in fetal brains; choroid plexus hemorrhage also occurs. Periventricular and subcortical infarctions can also be hemorrhagic.

Lesions Caused by Infections

Aqueductal stenosis has already been mentioned as a postinfectious or postinflammatory sequela; it has been documented in particular after mumps infection in utero. Rubella, cytomegalovirus, *Listeria monocytogenes,* and *Toxoplasma gondii* are agents known to affect the developing nervous system. They can cause meningitis, choroiditis, and multicystic encephalopathy with resulting microcephaly or hydrocephalus. Varicella zoster and herpes simplex type 2 viral infections can affect the fetus, although herpes simplex type 2 more commonly affects the fetus at birth. When varicella zoster infection occurs in utero, a congenital defects syndrome can occur with damage to sensory nerves and cutaneous manifestations, ophthalmic involvement, encephalitis, and damage to the spinal cord. Intrauterine infection with herpes simplex type 2 involves the skin, eyes, and central nervous system (CNS). Infection with human immunodeficiency virus (HIV) is thought to occur in utero in a minority of cases, and neuropathology in the fetus is not yet well documented.

Lesions Associated with Metabolic Disease

Metabolic disease in the mother or the fetus can result in neuropathology in the fetus. Abnormalities in infants of untreated phenylketonuric mothers and of mothers heterozygous for ornithine transcarbamylase deficiency are mentioned elsewhere. Diabetes mellitus in the mother has been associated with neural tube defects in the offspring. Infants dying of metabolic disease in the fetal or neonatal period may show secondary findings of hypoxia-ischemia; in lipid storage diseases, they may show characteristic cells containing abnormal by-products (such as cerebroside in Gaucher disease).

DRUGS AND THE DEVELOPING NERVOUS SYSTEM

Retinoic Acid

Retinoic acid is a vitamin A metabolite that plays a role in many developmental processes. Alcohol may act on the fetus through this compound because ethanol competitively antagonizes the enzyme that converts vitamin A to retinol, which then is converted to retinoic acid; retinoic acid may play a role in the genesis of neural tube defects. Important from a public health standpoint is the fact that the vitamin A analogue isotretinoin is a teratogen itself, causing craniofacial abnormalities with cleft palate, ear defects, CNS defects, and heart lesions. The ears can be small and malformed or absent with abnormal ear canals. The CNS abnormalities include aqueductal stenosis, migrational defects, micrencephaly, vermian atresia, and migration abnormalities of the brain stem and cerebellum.

Because isotretinoin is prescribed for acne in women in the early child-bearing years, the potential for this embryopathy must be kept in mind. This drug should not be prescribed casually, and careful attention to the sexual histories of the patients using this drug and to their use of contraception is extremely important before its use. The patients should be counseled about the teratogenic effects of isotretinoin.

Hydantoins

The fetal hydantoin syndrome is a constellation of findings that may occur with several of the anticonvulsant drugs when they are taken during pregnancy. The syndrome consists of growth disturbance, characteristic facies, cranial abnormalities, hypoplastic nails and distal phalanges, and neurodevelopmental delay. Similar findings may be present after intrauterine exposure to barbiturates, primidone, and carbamazepine. Usually these infants have small heads with enlarged fontanels (approximately 30% are microcephalic), ocular hypertelorism, a broad nasal bridge, and hypoplasia of the nails and distal phalanges. Other findings, such as cleft lip and palate, heart anomalies, gingival hypertrophy, wide-set nipples, bilateral inguinal hernias, simian creases, digital thumbs, and pilonidal sinuses, have been reported to lesser, varying extents.

Environmental Toxins: Mercury and Polychlorinated Biphenyls

Knowledge of the effects of exposure to toxins such as mercury and polychlorinated biphenyls (PCBs) has come from industrial accidents, in which pregnant women have ingested badly contaminated foods or water. After the mercury poisoning of the water and fish of Minamata Bay, Minamata, Japan, many fetuses were affected. Infants showed multiple neurologic defects, including spastic cerebral palsy with ataxia, mental retardation, dysarthria, and hypersalivation.

PCB poisoning has occurred in both the United States and Japan. Infants with in utero exposure have had intrauterine growth restriction, brown coloration of the skin and mucous membranes, widely open fontanels, abnormal calcifications in the skull, teeth present at birth, and neurodevelopmental delay. Long-term follow-up of PCB-exposed children has been carried out by Chen and Hsu, with assessments of intelligence, somatosensory evoked potentials, and pattern visual evoked potentials. Their findings have suggested that prenatal exposure to PCBs affects higher cortical functions.

THE NEWBORN NERVOUS SYSTEM

CLINICAL ENCEPHALOPATHIES
Postasphyxial (Hypoxic-Ischemic) Encephalopathy

Whether imposed by lack of oxygen in the blood or lack of blood reaching the brain, hypoxia is the main insult causing hypoxic-ischemic encephalopathy. Asphyxia implies hypoxia caused by respiratory insufficiency of one type or another, with the added component of some degree of carbon dioxide retention. During ischemia, metabolic by-products build up in the tissues, and during reperfusion, the reintroduction of oxygen can lead to the buildup of toxic oxygen radical species, which then lead to membrane lipid peroxidation. Metabolic changes occur immediately in the brain during hypoxia-ischemia (and asphyxia), leading to suppression of electrical activity, cortical depression, and stupor or coma. These events have been associated with changes in many cellular parameters, and the amount of recovery from such insults depends on a number of factors, not least of which are the degree of asphyxia or hypoxia-ischemia and the duration. Other factors, such as temperature, glucose availability, gestational age, and previous insults, all play roles in determining the amount of resulting brain compromise and ultimate injury.

Metabolic Encephalopathy

Metabolic encephalopathies occur when either vital substrates are withdrawn (such as glucose) or when there is accumulation of a metabolite that is toxic in concentrations that are higher than normal (ammonia, branched-chain amino acids and ketoacids, phenylalanine, glycine, valine, methionine, and others). Other acids that are well known to accumulate are those associated with disorders of *organic acid metabolism*. Such disorders have been recognized for propionate and methylmalonate metabolism, pyruvate and mitochondrial metabolism, defects of medium-chain acyl-coenzyme A (CoA) dehydrogenase, glutaric acidemia, glutathione synthetase deficiency, molybdenum cofactor deficiency, and defects of carbohydrate metabolism (galactosemia, glycogen storage disease Type I, fructose-1,6-diphosphatase deficiency, and phosphoenolpyruvate carboxykinase deficiency, among others).

Hypoglycemia is defined as a plasma glucose level less than 40 mg/dL, regardless of gestational age (despite the lack of knowledge about acceptable glucose levels in very preterm infants). Plasma levels of glucose this low, although defined as hypoglycemia, do not necessarily correlate with symptoms.

Hepatic encephalopathy is probably the most frequent clinical symptom complex associated with hyperammonemia. In the newborn, however, there are possible inborn errors of urea cycle metabolism that cause hyperammonemia and encephalopathy. Infants with such disorders are usually affected in the perinatal period with the introduction of protein into the diet through milk. Symptoms include irritability, lethargy, poor feeding, seizures, coma, and death. The enzyme deficiencies include carbamylphosphate synthetase deficiency, ornithine transcarbamylase deficiency, arginosuccinate deficiency, arginosuccinase deficiency, and arginase deficiency. Neuropathologic changes have been particularly apparent in astrocytes after hyperammonemic states. In addition, the ammonia ion can substitute for sodium and potassium, with effects on membrane electrical properties, the chloride pump, and postsynaptic inhibitory mechanisms. Almost all metabolic functions of the nervous system are affected by hyperammonemia.

Bilirubin

Bilirubin is toxic to the brain in several ways. In brain slices, bilirubin has been shown to depress oxygen consumption. Bilirubin at high concentrations uncouples oxidative phosphorylation in mitochondria in vitro, and inclusion of albumin in the incubation medium could protect the mitochondria from the effects of the bilirubin. Bilirubin has also been shown to affect water and sodium transport across the toad bladder membrane, and in cultured ascites cell lines, bilirubin inhibits potassium transport and increases sodium and water retention. Neuronal swelling is found in kernicteric brains and may result from similar physiologic effects of bilirubin. Neuronal transport and enzyme systems are affected by bilirubin. Notably, bilirubin inhibits the activation of protein kinase and decreases the phosphorylation of synapsin I in synaptic vesicles. In cultured neuroblastoma cell lines, bilirubin impairs mitochondrial action, impairs the activity of Na$^+$, K$^+$-ATPase, causes decreased thymidine uptake, and causes decreased incorporation of methionine. Physiologic studies have shown that bilirubin impairs nerve conduction; action potentials are decreased by bilirubin in hippocampal brain slices. Unconjugated bilirubin has been shown in adult brains to lower cortical electroencephalographic (EEG) amplitudes and, in some cases, to abolish the EEG tracing. Bilirubin also reduces the transport of tyrosine and the synthesis of dopamine, especially at high concentrations. These effects all provide some reasons for the encephalopathic effects of bilirubin.

The clinical condition of bilirubin encephalopathy has been well described, and its autopsy correlative findings, or kernicterus, have been known since 1903. The clinical manifestations of full-blown kernicterus are usually recognized as lethargy (developing after the first 48 postnatal hours), an incomplete Moro response, and often opisthotonic posturing after abrupt postural changes. The infant's suck is ineffective, and the cry is cerebral (high pitched). The infant may have abnormal eye movements, characterized by persistent downward gaze and rotary nystagmus, and episodes of hypothermia and hyperthermia. At the end stage of the disease, decerebrate posturing occurs. Bilirubin pigment is found at autopsy, along with swelling and vacuolization of neurons, in numerous nuclei and structures, but not usually in the cerebral cortex.

Infectious Encephalopathy

Most pediatricians are familiar with infants who are encephalopathic because of CNS infection. Viral encephalitides are, in particular, associated with neurochemical abnormalities and cellular dysfunction in the brain, characterized by direct cytolysis, impairment of synaptic transmission, alteration of metabolism of neurotransmitters, and fusion of cell membranes. A number of viral infections are characterized by intracellular inclusion bodies (herpesvirus, cytomegalovirus, measles, subacute sclerosing panencephalitis, polio, and rabies). In infants and children, encephalitides are clinically characterized by alterations of consciousness, headache, neurologic abnormalities, and fever. Viral encephalitis is recognized in newborns by alterations in consciousness, neurologic signs, hypothermia or hyperthermia, and seizures and is especially likely to be due to herpesvirus type 2. In recent years, infants with HIV have been recognized with progressive encephalopathies developing between 2 months and 5 years of age, after infection during the prenatal or perinatal period. Newborn infants, especially preterm infants, are at particular risk for bacterial or spirochetal infections of the nervous system and in some cases for fungal or for parasitic infections (such as toxoplasmosis).

ASPHYXIAL AND HYPOXIC-ISCHEMIC INJURY

Neonatal encephalopathy is recognized as mild, moderate, or severe and can be graded in various ways. The grading scheme of Sarnat and Sarnat has been in use since 1976; this scheme has been modified by Volpe and others. In general, mild encephalopathy is characterized by alternating levels of consciousness—including periods of lethargy, irritability, and hyperalertness. The infants are jittery, feed poorly, and do not have normal sleep cycles. The cranial nerve examination is normal, muscle tone may be increased, and deep tendon reflexes are frequently increased. Some autonomic signs are present, such as pupillary dilation and tachycardia. Most of the primitive reflexes are normal, with the exception of the Moro, which may be increased. Infants with mild encephalopathy do not have seizures.

The infant with moderate encephalopathy is more lethargic with poor feeding and hypotonia. Clonus is usually present, and the gag reflex is usually depressed. There may be abnormal movements, including spontaneous myoclonus or extrapyramidal dysfunction. The pupils are usually constricted, and the infant may have bradycardia. Seizures frequently occur within the first 24 hours.

The severely encephalopathic infant is comatose and flaccid with absent reflexes. The pupils often are fixed or sluggishly reactive, and the doll's eye reflex is absent. The infant may be bradycardic and frequently has apnea and hypotension.

The neurologic sequelae in infants with hypoxic-ischemic encephalopathy are related to the degree of the encephalopathy; infants with low Apgar scores, delayed respirations, meconium staining, or problems of fetal heart rate patterns, who do not show signs of encephalopathy, are not likely to show neurologic sequelae unless intrauterine brain damage is already present.

Cellular susceptibilities to injury seem to depend on maturational factors, metabolic factors (sparing of neurons with NADPH diaphorase-nitric oxide synthase, sparing of dopamine-synthesizing neurons), metabolic rate, and presence and density of glutamate receptor types. Glutamate receptors seem to be highly concentrated in the basal ganglia in the perinatal period, and the glutamate receptor subtype most clearly related to neuronal death in the striatum is the receptor subtype of greatest density in that region in the perinatal period.

Periventricular leukomalacia (white matter injury) occurs in both term and preterm infants but is particularly prevalent in the preterm infant. The incidence of cystic periventricular leukomalacia in one study was 3.2% of infants weighing less than 1500 g at birth. The two most common sites of occurrence of this lesion are at the level of the occipital radiation at the trigone of the lateral ventricles and at the level of the cerebral white matter around the foramen of Monro, two regions that are particularly prominent border zones between penetrating branches of major arteries in the preterm brain. The end result is frequently multiple cysts or a large cavitary lesion; there may be hemorrhage into the area of necrosis (25% at autopsy). Although cavitation may be apparent in 1 to 3 weeks, it is also possible for gliosis to occur over a period of time, with subsequent loss of cavities.

The constriction of the white matter may lead to secondary enlargement of the ventricles. Cavitation occurs as a consequence of necrosis in the immature brain more frequently than in the mature brain probably because of the high water content, low myelin component, and relatively limited glial response in the immature brain.

Periventricular leukomalacia may be a sequela in premature infants who are subject to episodes of ischemia. A correlation has been shown between the occurrence of hypocarbic alkalosis in the first 24 postnatal hours in very-low-birth-weight infants and subsequent development of periventricular leukomalacia. Episodes of apnea and bradycardia have also been shown to reduce cerebral perfusion in the preterm newborn and are associated with an increased risk for cerebral palsy.

The border zone concept implies that blood supply is lost first, when perfusion pressure falls, at the places where arterial sources do not penetrate fully. Cerebral perfusion pressure in the preterm newborn is particularly likely to fall when systemic blood pressure falls. This may be because the range of autoregulation (the range of blood pressures over which cerebral blood flow remains constant) is narrower than in the infant, child, or adult, or it may be because under certain conditions autoregulation fails. Autoregulation fails in all species studied when significant hypoxia is induced.

Diagnostic tests performed frequently in newborns thought to have been asphyxiated include electroencephalography, cranial sonography, arterial blood gases, and serum calcium determinations. Brain stem auditory evoked response testing is used less frequently than the EEG but is used relatively frequently because the results have been shown to have some prognostic significance.

In general, the treatment of the infant with hypoxic-ischemic encephalopathy is supportive: ventilatory therapy when necessary; fluid restriction to lessen the degree of cerebral edema and effects of inappropriate secretion of antidiuretic hormone; maintenance of normal glucose and calcium levels, acid-base and electrolyte balance, and serum osmolality; provision of calories; and treatment of seizures. Many infants with hypoxic-ischemic encephalopathy have elevated ammonia levels as well as elevated serum glutamic oxaloacetic transaminase values, probably secondary to impaired liver function and increased protein breakdown. Brain-specific creatine kinase (CK-BB) seems to be an indicator of brain injury when measured in spinal fluid early in the course of hypoxic-ischemic encephalopathy.

Lumbar puncture is helpful for diagnosis of subarachnoid or intraventricular hemorrhage; to rule out meningitis in certain cases; and for determination of CSF pressure, lactate, hydroxybutyrate dehydrogenase, or CK-BB. Ultrasound and CT scans are useful for determining if structural brain injury is present early in the course of the encephalopathy (sometimes suggesting intrauterine brain injury) and for determining the progression of CNS lesions, such as hemorrhage, hydrocephalus, periventricular leukomalacia, atrophy, and multicystic encephalomalacia. Although ultrasound scans are useful and probably sensitive in the early postnatal period for changes in brain water content, in general they lack both sensitivity and specificity and should be followed by CT or MRI scans.

The EEG is useful and can correlate with specific types of brain injury. Burst suppression, voltage suppression, or an isoelectric tracing can be seen with diffuse cortical necrosis; rolandic sharp waves are frequently present in infants with periventricular leukomalacia or periventricular hemorrhagic infarction. Localized periodic lateralized epileptiform discharges imply the presence of focal cerebral infarction.

At present, glutamate receptor antagonists, inhibitors of nitric oxide synthesis, calcium channel blockers, free radical scavengers and inhibitors, monosialogangliosides, hypothermia, and higher dose barbiturates are being used only experimentally, mainly in animal studies.

INTRAVENTRICULAR HEMORRHAGE

Intraventricular hemorrhage (IVH) is mainly a lesion of the premature brain. In 1980 intraventricular hemorrhage was diagnosed in close to 40% of infants with birth weights less than 1501 g. Incidence rates in 1999 average close to 25%, with and without various preventive treatment modalities, but higher incidences are found in the lowest-birth-weight infants. The outlook for the very-low-birth-weight infant with intraventricular hemorrhage remains an important issue because the incidence of problems such as hydrocephalus, seizures, static encephalopathy, blindness, mental retardation, and learning disabilities is higher in those with symptomatic hemorrhages. The severity of neurologic sequelae is not always due just to intraventricular hemorrhage, however, because additional lesions are frequently found at autopsy in infants who succumb.

Intraventricular hemorrhage is usually diagnosed during the first 72 postnatal hours in very preterm infants and is infrequently diagnosed later in the 1st postnatal week. Most affected infants are less than 32 weeks' gestational age, are mechanically ventilated, and have had some degree of asphyxia or hemodynamic instability (or both). Although about 25% of newborns with IVH are asymptomatic, the other 75% can have symptoms of varying degrees. The classic, but infrequent, presentation is one of sudden deterioration with a bulging fontanel, decrease in blood pressure, drop in hematocrit, and seizure activity. Neurologic manifestations in these infants include flaccidity, loss of pupillary reactions, loss of extraocular movements, respiratory abnormalities, and coma. Some infants manifest a more protracted course, however, that is often described as *saltatory* because symptoms wax and wane over a period of time. These infants usually show a change from alertness to irritability or stupor, with a decrease in activity, hypotonia, and other neurologic abnormalities. They may recover for periods of time, only to become symptomatic again later. It is thought that this course reflects episodes of intermittent bleeding. Metabolic problems may also herald the onset of intraventricular hemorrhage. Some infants become hypoglycemic or hypothermic, or both. Decreased CSF glucose is frequently associated with intraventricular hemorrhage.

Prospective ultrasound scans on 33 very-low-birth-weight infants were performed during the first 48 postnatal hours. Sixteen of the infants developed intraventricular hemorrhage, and in four infants the hemorrhage occurred during the ultrasound scanning. Clinical events occurring at the time of the hemorrhages in three of the infants included (1) manual ventilation in an infant with primary pulmonary hypertension; (2) infusion of calcium gluconate and sodium bicarbonate for correction of hyperkalemia; and (3) administration of surfactant for respiratory failure secondary to pulmonary hemorrhage. In the fourth infant, the presence of hypertension (relative to the admission blood pressure) was noted at the time of the hemorrhage, and compared with the blood pressures of infants without hemorrhages, the other three infants also had persistent or rapid increases in blood pressure at the time of the IVH (after previous hypotension). Several studies have documented that the lower an infant's birth weight, the greater the likelihood that IVH will occur during the 1st postnatal day.

Intracerebral hemorrhages in the preterm infant usually originate in the subependymal germinal matrix region with extension into the ventricular system and from there into the aqueduct, cisterns, and subarachnoid spaces. Armstrong and colleagues have shown that extension into surrounding white matter does not occur unless white matter damage is already present. It has been suggested that periventricular hemorrhagic infarction occurs after substantial intraventricular hemorrhage has occluded periventricular venous return.

The grading system of Papile and colleagues reported in 1978 is used most frequently, and grading of hemorrhages can be accomplished by either ultrasound visualization or by CT scan. Grade I is a subependymal hemorrhage only; Grade II is intraventricular hemorrhage without ventricular dilation; Grade III is intraventricular hemorrhage with ventricular dilation; and Grade IV is intraventricular hemorrhage and the presence of intraparenchymal blood. It should be cautioned that ventricular dilation described for Grade III hemorrhage in the original study reflected obstructive hydrocephalus secondary to intraventricular blood; it may be difficult to distinguish between this situation and that of intraventricular hemorrhage with pre-existing cerebral atrophy and ventriculomegaly. Also, although Grade IV hemorrhage indicates the presence of parenchymal blood, the blood does not have to be adjacent to the ventricles.

Numerous prophylactic regimens, including prenatal administration of vitamin K, phenobarbital, and corticosteroids, have been shown to have some beneficial effects on the incidence of postnatal intraventricular hemorrhage. Of all the prenatal regimens, antenatal corticosteroids have had the most consistently positive effects. Postnatal regimens have included various strategies for administration of phenobarbital, indomethacin, paralysis, ethamsylate, fresh frozen plasma, vitamin E, and minimal stimulation protocols. Each of these prevention strategies has supporting and detracting data in the literature. Indomethacin is increasingly used for IVH prophylaxis in the United States. General prevention measures also include avoidance of bolus infusions, continuous monitoring of blood pressure and avoidance of hypotension or hypertension; prevention and rapid treatment of pneumothorax; careful regulation of intake of sodium and glucose; avoidance of hyperosmolar states; and careful management of the open ductus arteriosus. For the most part, however, treatment of infants once IVH has occurred has been supportive, with control of ventilation, seizures, metabolic and fluid status, temperature, and nutritional state. Attention is also paid to coagulation status to reduce the likelihood of extension of bleeding (all infants in the United States receive prophylactic vitamin K at birth). Minimal stimulation protocols are continued because hemodynamic instability may be even more severe after IVH has occurred.

Once hydrocephalus is diagnosed, medical therapy to reduce production of CSF by the choroid plexus can be instituted by using isosorbide, glycerol, or acetazolamide. If the infant is symptomatic because of increased intracranial pressure, mannitol can be given acutely, followed by decompression of the ventricles by lumbar puncture or by insertion of an external ventricular drain. In such infants, with open fontanels, lumbar puncture has not been associated with herniation.

SUPERFICIAL CRANIAL TRAUMATIC INJURY

A frequent superficial cranial traumatic injury is hemorrhagic edema of the scalp. This is termed *caput succedaneum* and usually resolves quickly. It is frequently associated with molding of the head and overriding sutures as a result of pressure during delivery. Subgaleal hemorrhage, occurring under the scalp aponeurosis but external to the periosteum, can be more severe, with extensive bleeding sometimes necessitating a blood transfusion. It occurs sometimes after vacuum assisted deliveries. A cephalhematoma occurs under the periosteum of a skull bone and does not cross suture lines. Large cephalhematomas may calcify and persist for a period of time, giving the skull an asymmetric appearance. It is useful to obtain radiologic studies in some cases to determine if a skull fracture is present, especially if there appears to be a skull depression in association with the cephalhematoma. Compound depressed fractures require surgical reduction; simple depressed fractures may be elevated in some cases by nonsurgical means.

TRAUMATIC BRAIN INJURY

Subdural hemorrhages can also occur after traumatic injury. Because the bleeding is less rapid, however, the symptoms may be delayed for several hours. Posterior fossa subdural hemorrhages can be particularly ominous because of brain stem compression. Symptoms associated with posterior fossa subdural hemorrhage can also be delayed up to several days and can include lethargy, bulging fontanel, seizures, eye deviation, facial weakness, trunk and limb hypotonia, and respiratory abnormalities. This is a critical situation.

When subdural hemorrhage is present over the convexities, there may be minimal symptoms or signs such as hemiparesis, eye deviation, and pupillary abnormalities. Subdural hematomas may become chronic, with subacute symptoms becoming apparent as the infant exhibits seizures, developmental delay, and anemia (sometimes severe enough to cause heart failure). Detection of subdural hematomas is accomplished best by using CT scanning; ultrasound is not reliable for the diagnosis of subdural hemorrhage.

TRAUMATIC NERVE INJURIES
Facial Nerve Injury

Damage to peripheral nerves can also occur during labor and delivery, with the facial nerve, brachial plexus, and phrenic and laryngeal nerves noted in descending frequency. Facial nerve injury is the most common peripheral nerve injury in the newborn, with incidences of between 2 and 8 per 1000 births. Most cases of facial nerve injury resolve spontaneously. The clinical findings of complete facial nerve injury include drooping of the mouth, flattening of the nasolabial fold, and widening of the palpebral fissure on the side of the injury; there is also paucity of movement of the side of the face and inability to wrinkle the forehead or to close the eye (lower motor neuron lesion). The injury can occur to varying degrees, with some cases involving only weakness in a small group of muscles. When there is difficulty in closing the eye, the eye of the newborn should be protected with artificial tears and covered. If the facial palsy does not begin to resolve within a few weeks, the infant should be referred to a pediatric neurologist.

Congenital unilateral facial paralysis can also be due to a developmental hypoplasia or absence of the facial nerve. In such cases, the paralysis does not resolve, and electroneurography reveals diminished or no responses from homolateral facial muscles. In cases of traumatic facial nerve injury, electroneurography usually shows normal facial nerve function within 48 hours of injury, despite traumatic compression or transection injury (the distal portions of the nerve can still function early in the course of the injury). The degree of decrease in facial nerve function that occurs for a period of time after traumatic injury is predictive of eventual recovery; however, in congenital developmental defects of the facial nerve, recovery of function does not occur.

When one corner of the mouth fails to move downward and outward during crying but all other facial movements are normal, the infant has congenital hypoplasia or absence of the angularis oris muscle. About 20% of infants with this minor anomaly have other associated congenital anomalies, with cardiac anomalies the most frequent association.

Brachial Plexus Injury

Injury to the brachial plexus has great social and practical implications, and thus, pediatricians should have knowledge of its natural history and treatment. At the present time, surgical repair is available for infants whose injuries do not heal spontaneously. Brachial plexus injury consists of weakness or paralysis of upper extremity muscles innervated by the cervical nerve roots C5 to C8 and thoracic root T1 (i.e., the roots supplying the brachial plexus). The reported incidence of brachial plexus birth injuries varies greatly, from 0.3 to 2 per 1000 live births. The true incidence has to be derived from delivery room data because many infants are "cured" of subtle and transient deficits before being seen by consultants.

Traumatic delivery causes stretch damage to the brachial plexus, with injury occurring in descending order from the suprascapular nerve through C5, C6, and C7. The brachial plexus, with its roots anchored to the cervical cord, is thought to be damaged by severe lateral traction during delivery. The upper roots are most vulnerable to injury, but with greater degrees of traction, the lower roots of the plexus are more likely to undergo avulsion (spinal cord–nerve rootlet disconnection) resulting in total paralysis.

Lesions may occur at any point from the spinal canal where nerve rootlets leave the spinal cord, to nerve roots, trunks, and divisions and cords of the brachial plexus and its peripheral nerves. The most common form of brachial plexus injury is that involving Erb point—the point where C5 and C6 join to form the upper trunk of the brachial plexus—resulting in the typical upper plexus lesion known as *Erb palsy*. A lesion at the juncture of C8 and T1, as they form the lower trunk of the brachial plexus, produces weakness of the distal upper extremity known as *Klumpke palsy*.

METABOLIC AND DEGENERATIVE DISEASES AND THE NEWBORN NERVOUS SYSTEM

Recognition of metabolic and degenerative diseases in the newborn is sometimes difficult but important: difficult because the signs and symptoms can seem nonspecific and can be confounded by the presence of drugs, infection, or hypoxia, but important because although a number of metabolic diseases cannot be treated effectively, some can be, and the window of time during which neurologic injury can be averted may be narrow.

Categories of metabolic diseases that present in the newborn period can be divided into five major types with typical presentations. This scheme is a helpful approach to diagnosis and is presented in an abbreviated form here:

Type I: Neurologic distress: intoxication, with ketosis. The cardinal disease represented here is maple syrup urine disease, in which a newborn becomes symptomatic with feeding difficulties and encephalopathy leading to coma after an initial symptom-free period.

Type II. Neurologic distress: intoxication, with ketoacidosis and hyperammonemia. These disorders have an earlier onset than Type I, with symptoms beginning frequently during the 1st postnatal day. The infants are acutely ill and may develop coma within hours. Many of the organic acidurias are included in Type II, and many of these disorders also have marked hyperammonemia. Organic acidurias frequently diagnosed include methylmalonic, propionic, and isovaloric acidemia; less frequently diagnosed are glutaric aciduria type II (multiple acyl-CoA dehydrogenase deficiency) and hydroxymethylglutaryl-CoA lyase deficiency (in these, ketosis is absent, and hypoglycemia is frequent).

Type III: Energy deficiency. This category is different from the previous two in that the infants are not as acutely ill, although they are acidotic and may have lactic acidosis. Biotin-responsive multiple carboxylase deficiency can present with lactic acidosis, and thus physicians are urged to treat all patients with lactic acidosis of unknown cause with biotin after blood and urine samples have been obtained for studies. Diseases grouped in this category include pyruvate carboxylase deficiency, pyruvate dehydrogenase deficiency, respiratory chain disorders, and multiple carboxylase deficiency.

Type IVa: Neurologic distress, intoxication, with hyperammonemia but without ketoacidosis. This category is represented by the urea cycle defects, and infants with such defects usually have a short symptom-free interval followed by rapid development of neurologic symptoms and coma. Blood ammonia is extremely high, and respiratory alkalosis and moderate lactic acidemia may be present. There is no ketonuria, which is an important diagnostic distinction between this class of diseases and the organic acidurias with hyperammonemia.

The two main urea cycle disorders are ornithine transcarbamylase deficiency (sex-linked) and carbamyl phosphate synthetase deficiency. These two diseases cannot be diagnosed by amino acid analyses, and liver biopsy is required for enzyme diagnosis. Other urea cycle defects (citrullinemia, argininosuccinic aciduria, and argininemia) can be diagnosed by amino acid analyses, which show elevated concentrations of citrulline, argininosuccinate, and arginine. Significant hyperammonemia can also be seen in some of the fatty acid oxidation disorders in the neonatal period. Ammonia determinations should be done in any infant with the rapid onset of neurologic symptoms because delay can mean permanent neurologic sequelae or death, and rapid treatment can mean reversal of some or all symptoms.

Type IVb: Neurologic distress: energy deficiency, no ketoacidosis and no hyperammonemia. This group is characterized by nonketotic hyperglycinemia. Infants with this disorder present at birth or within a few hours with hypotonia, myoclonic jerks, and coma and have a burst-suppression pattern on the EEG. This disorder is diagnosed by finding elevated plasma glycine levels and elevated CSF/plasma glycine ratio. Other disorders in this spectrum of disease include sulfite oxidase deficiency and sulfite and xanthine oxidase deficiencies, which present with hypotonia, seizures, myoclonic jerks, dysmorphic features, and microcephaly. These deficiencies are also present in molybdenum cofactor deficiency. Included in this category are the peroxisomal disorders, Zellweger syndrome, and neonatal adrenoleukodystrophy because they also have no symptom-free interval, presenting with dysmorphic features, hypotonia, and early-onset seizures. Pyridoxine-dependent seizures are also listed in this category; these seizures are resistant to anticonvulsants, and improvement in the EEG tracing can be seen as pyridoxine (vitamin B_6) is administered.

Type IVc: Storage disorders without metabolic disturbances. Storage disorders that have been diagnosed during the newborn period include GM_1 gangliosidosis, Gaucher disease, mucopolysaccharidosis Type VII, sialidosis, galactosialidosis, sialuria, and Niemann-Pick disease Type C. Two other degenerative diseases that are not as well understood, neuronal ceroid lipofuscinosis and neuroaxonal dystrophy, are discussed subsequently.

Type V: Hypoglycemia with hepatomegaly and liver dysfunction. The diseases in this category that present with hypoglycemia (often with hypoglycemic seizures), hepatomegaly, ketosis, and lactic acidosis include glucose-6-phosphatase deficiency (Type I glycogen storage disease), glycogenosis Type III, and fructose-1,6-diphosphatase deficiency. Other disorders in this category present mainly with hepatic dysfunction and jaundice (hypoglycemia may be present but usually not marked). The disorders in this group include tyrosinemia Type I, galactosemia, hereditary fructose intolerance when the diet contains fructose, alpha$_1$-antitrypsin deficiency, Wilson disease, and neonatal hemochromatosis.

Craniosynostoses

Craniosynostosis (premature closure of the sutures) is relatively common, occurring in 0.4 per 1000 infants. Sagittal synostosis is familial in 2% of cases, and coronal synostosis is familial in 8%. When premature fusion of one or more sutures occurs, brain growth forces other parts of the cranium to enlarge, leading to cranial deformities. When the sagittal suture closes prematurely, scaphocephaly or dolichocephaly occurs; coronal synostosis results in brachycephaly or plagiocephaly. Metopic synostosis causes trigonocephaly. Other, more complicated forms of craniosynostosis can also occur. Sagittal synostosis is the most common form. Certain teratogens have been associated with craniosynostoses (phenytoin, valproic acid, aminopterin, methotrexate, retinoic acids, and oxymetazoline). Numerous syndromes, including Crouzon disease and Apert disease, have craniosynostosis as one of a number of abnormalities. It is important to document other problems that might be associated with craniosynostosis, such as midfacial retrusion, septo-optic dysplasia, or ventriculomegaly, before surgery is initiated.

Three-dimensional reconstructions after neuroimaging studies are often helpful in planning surgery for complicated craniofacial abnormalities. In sagittal craniosynostosis, various procedures have been used, including removal of the fused suture followed by parasagittal craniectomies, with and without placement of some form of plastic to prevent reanastomosis of the bony edges. Experience with these patients has led to the conclusion that surgery should be carried out relatively early—within the first few postnatal weeks—to ensure a good cosmetic result.

Intracranial and Epidural Abscesses

Brain abscess does not occur frequently in newborns, although the incidence may be increasing because of the survival of susceptible very-low-birth-weight infants. Abscesses seem to occur either during meningitis or as a result of sepsis or contiguous bone infection (cranial osteomyelitis).

SEIZURES AND OTHER PAROXYSMAL DISORDERS

The reported incidence of neonatal seizures has varied, owing to definitions and methods of seizure identification and surveillance. Early studies reported that seizures occurred in 0.15% to 0.5% of all live births. More recent studies suggested a higher incidence in higher-risk groups: 1.5% in premature newborns older than 30 weeks' conceptional age and 3.9% in those less than 30 weeks' conceptional age. Lanska and colleagues determined an overall risk of seizures to be 4.4 per 1000 live births, varying inversely with birth weight (57.5 per 1000 live births with birth weights less than 1500 g; 4.4 per 1000 live births with birth weights 1500 to 2499 g; 2.8 per 1000 live births with birth weights 2500 to 3999 g; and 2.0 per 1000 live births with birth weights greater than or equal to 4000 g). The clinical manifestations of seizures in the newborn differ from those of older infants or children primarily because of the rapid rate of brain development near term and the types and number of etiologic factors that may be responsible for brain injury during the neonatal period.

All of the clinical types of motor and behavioral

seizures were characterized in studies using time-synchronized, EEG/polygraphic/video monitoring of newborns. Clonic seizures were observed to be unifocal, multifocal, alternating, migratory, or hemiconvulsive. Tonic seizures were observed to be either generalized or focal. Generalized seizures were observed to be either symmetric or asymmetric. Ocular signs were characterized as either random movements or sustained tonic deviation. Movements of progression included stepping or pedaling of the legs and swimming or rowing movements of the arms. Myoclonic seizures were described as generalized, focal, or fragmentary (multifocal). Clinical events resembling generalized spasms were also noted.

There is still no clear consensus as to whether there are long-term neurologic or cognitive sequelae of neonatal seizures per se. It does appear, however, that the most important determinant of outcome is the degree of brain injury associated with seizure occurrence. The factors that caused the seizures and concomitant brain disturbance are the most likely factors that determine long-term outcome rather than the seizures themselves.

Objectives in the therapy of neonatal seizures include maintenance of systemic homeostasis, treatment of etiologic factors underlying the seizures, and cessation of seizures. Despite these clear goals, their achievement may be difficult: Causative factors are not always identifiable, and their precise relationship to the seizures themselves may not be readily apparent. Some clinical seizure types may not warrant drug therapy, and when given, antiepileptic drugs may incompletely control seizures.

Several factors should ideally be considered in the development of a plan of therapy for neonatal seizures: cause or associated risk factors, characterization and classification of seizure type, determination of pathophysiology, assessment of duration and severity of the seizures, understanding of the natural history of the seizure disorder, and assessment of the expected effects of the seizures and drugs on the developing brain. Information concerning all of these factors, however, may not be complete. Despite this lack of complete data, consideration of each factor may provide the basis for rational management decisions at the bedside.

Three phases of therapy can be individualized to each infant: (1) initial medical management, (2) cause-specific therapy, and (3) antiepileptic drug therapy. Adequate ventilation and circulatory perfusion should be ensured because changes in respirations, heart rate, and blood pressure may occur in association with seizures, as a consequence of causative factors, or in association with drug therapy. The therapy of identified specific causative factors is essential. Treatable causes include CNS and systemic infections and metabolic factors, such as hypocalcemia, hypomagnesemia, and hypoglycemia. Pyridoxine deficiency is often cited as a treatable cause of medically refractory neonatal seizures, although it is exceedingly rare.

The antiepileptic drugs traditionally used for neonatal seizures are phenobarbital, phenytoin, and diazepam in the following dosages. phenobarbital 20 mg/kg as a loading dose, followed by additional dosages of 10 mg/kg to achieve serum levels between 20 and 40 μg/mL; phenytoin 20 mg/kg as a loading dose to achieve serum levels between 15 and 20 μg/mL; diazepam 0.1 to 0.3 mg/kg in repeated dosages. Lorazepam has been reported to be safe and efficacious. Other agents reported to be useful include carbamazepine, primidone, paraldehyde (now unavailable in the United States), and lidocaine. These agents have been used as additional therapy when first-line antiepileptics have failed to control seizures.

No specific practice guidelines have been established to assist in the decision to discontinue antiepileptic medication after a period of clinical seizure control. Thus, in clinical practice, this is highly individualized. The probable natural history of the treated disorder should be the most significant factor in this clinical decision, although it has not been well characterized. If seizures represent a short-lived phenomenon produced in reaction to an acute injury, long-term antiepileptic therapy might be maintained for a period beyond which seizures might have resolved. Reported maintenance schedules range from 1 week up to 12 months after the last seizure, although specific clinical and EEG predictors of recurrent seizures after drug withdrawal have not been identified. There has been increasing clinical interest in short-term therapy, however, with withdrawal of drugs 2 weeks after the infant's last clinical seizure.

NEUROMUSCULAR DISORDERS
Central Hypotonia

Hypotonia is a frequent symptom in newborns that may reflect an abnormality of the CNS; a systemic toxic, metabolic, infectious, or degenerative disease; a disorder of ligaments or connective tissue; or a neuromuscular disorder. Hypotonia implies decreased resistance to passive muscle stretch and decreased resting tone, and it may or may not be associated with muscle weakness.

It is useful to determine if the hypotonic newborn has a central disorder that is responsible. In these cases, there may be other neurologic signs, but usually hypotonia is greater than the degree of muscle weakness. Examples include hypoxic-ischemic encephalopathy, cerebral hemorrhage, systemic infection, toxic encephalopathy, hypothyroidism, Down syndrome, Prader-Willi syndrome, degenerative or metabolic diseases, endocrine diseases, or connective tissue diseases. Spinal cord injury or malformation can be associated early in the course with hypotonia and severe muscle weakness. Normal preterm infants are hypotonic at birth and develop increasing tone with maturity. The most common causes of central hypotonia in newborns are hypoxic-ischemic encephalopathy and dysgenetic syndromes.

Motoneuron Diseases

Spinal muscular atrophy (SMA) (anterior horn cell disease) is the most common form of neurogenic hypotonia in early infancy and is second only to the muscular dystrophies as a cause of neuromuscular disease in childhood. Autosomal recessive in inheritance, the gene locus has been mapped to the long arm of chromosome 5. SMA occurs in about 8 per 100,000 live births, with SMA Type I (Werdnig-Hoffmann disease) symptomatic before 6 months of age, not infrequently in utero or in the newborn period. Infants with SMA Type I do not sit independently and have a life expectancy of 2 years or less. SMA Types II and III are less severe forms of SMA with longer life expectancies.

After birth, the clinical picture is of an infant with symmetric severe weakness and flaccidity that is greater in lower limbs than in upper limbs and is greater proximally than distally. Head control is poor in both the prone and the supine positions. Respiration is impaired because of weakness of the intercostal muscles; relative sparing of the diaphragm causes abdominal breathing, resulting in a bell-shaped appearance to the chest. The bulbar muscles are weak causing poor cry, weak suck and swallow, pooling of secretions, and aspiration; tongue fasciculations are frequently present (although sometimes difficult to distinguish from tremor of the tongue in very young infants). Because upper cranial nerves are spared, however, the infant usually has an alert expression and normal eye movements. There may be spontaneous movements of the ankles, toes, hand, and fingers, but there is no ability to raise the limbs against gravity. Cardiac muscle is not affected, and the infants do not have arthrogryposis (multiple congenital contractures of limbs); deep tendon reflexes are absent.

CHAPTER 9

Gastrointestinal and Nutritional Conditions

DISORDERS OF THE INTESTINE AND PANCREAS

OBSTRUCTIONS

Vomiting, particularly of bile-stained material, with abdominal distention or the failure to pass meconium are symptoms highly suggestive of the presence of intestinal obstruction. If the obstruction is high or complete, symptoms start soon after birth. Vomiting of bile suggests that the lesion is located distal to the ampulla of Vater, whereas sporadic vomiting may be seen in patients with partial obstruction caused by malrotation, duplications, or annular pancreas. Abdominal distention may be present soon after birth, reaching a peak at 24 to 48 hours with visible perstaltic waves. Failure to pass meconium within 24 hours after birth suggests the presence of a colonic lesion. Infants with high obstruction or even those with obstruction as low as the ileum pass meconium, so this finding by itself does not exclude obstruction.

Atresias

Atresia, complete obstruction of the lumen of the bowel, should be distinguished from stenosis, which is a narrowing of the lumen. Atresias account for one third of all intestinal obstructions in the newborn, occurring in 1 of every 1500 live births. Sites of occurrence, in order of frequency, are jejunoileal, duodenal, and colonic. Failure of the gut to recanalize during the 8th to 10th weeks of gestation seems to be the most likely cause for duodenal atresia. In the jejunum, ileum, and colon, vascular compromise early in gestation may be responsible for bowel atresias.

Thirty percent of all atresias occur in the duodenum and most are distal to the ampulla. Approximately 70% of infants with duodenal atresia also have other associated anomalies including, in order of frequency, Down syndrome, annular pancreas, cardiovascular malformations, malrotation, esophageal atresia, small bowel lesions, and anorectal lesions. Because of the high incidence of multiple atresias (15%), inspection of the entire bowel is carried out before constructing a duodenojejunostomy or, more recently, a duodenoduodenostomy.

Duodenal Stenosis

Duodenal stenosis may be secondary to an intrinsic defect or the result of compression by extrinsic lesions. These include annular pancreas, peritoneal bands, aberrant superior mesenteric artery, or a preduodenal portal vein. Depending on the degree of obstruction, vomiting may begin at any time after birth. Because most lesions involve the second or third portion of the duodenum, the vomiting is bilious. Plain films are usually not diagnostic, but on upper gastrointestinal series the area of stenosis can be delineated; differentiation of the cause may not be possible before surgery.

Meconium Ileus

Meconium ileus refers to an intraluminal intestinal obstruction produced by thick inspissated meconium. Ninety percent of patients with meconium ileus have cystic fibrosis (CF). Indeed, 10% to 15% of CF patients present with meconium ileus. Recently, DNA markers for the CF gene have been identified and localized on chromosome 7.

Severe pancreatic involvement is not a consistent finding in CF patients presenting with meconium ileus. In utero, some CF fetuses produce exceptionally viscid secretions from the mucous glands of the small intestine. The meconium formed is dry and contains higher than usual concentrations of protein, including albumin. The abnormal meconium adheres firmly to the mucosal surface of the distal small bowel creating an intraluminal obstruction.

Prenatal diagnosis of CF is possible. A family history of CF should alert the clinician to the possibility of meconium ileus. In the simple form in which obstruction occurs in the middle and distal ileum without perforation and peritonitis, signs of obstruction appear within the first 48 hours in an otherwise healthy infant. Abdominal distention is noticed between 12 and 24 hours, after which vomiting occurs. No meconium is passed. Physical examinations may reveal hard palpable masses throughout the abdomen that are freely movable in any direction. Meconium ileus complicated by volvulus, atresias, meconium peritonitis, or pseudocyst formation is found in one third of the patients. Newborns with these complications present earlier than those with simple meconium ileus, usually within the first 24 hours of life. They appear sicker, with severe vomiting, signs of neonatal sepsis, and more marked distention causing respiratory distress.

All newborns with meconium ileus should be evaluated for CF. The identification and cloning of the primary CF gene and the ability to identify mutations causing CF have advanced the clinician's ability to provide accurate diagnosis as well as counseling.

In simple meconium ileus, approximately 60% of the infants have their obstructions successfully relieved by a hyperosmolar enema. Before the hyperosmolar enema is given, other complications, such as perforation, volvulus, or atresia, must be excluded. The hypertonic enema draws water into the intestinal tract, dislodging and breaking up the meconium. Because of rapid fluid shifts, great care must be taken to maintain fluid and electrolyte balance. Failure of the infant to pass meconium within several hours after the enema is an indication for surgical intervention, not another enema. If the enema is successful, meconium passage continues for 24 to 48 hours. Acetylcysteine, 5 mL every 6 hours for 5 days, is given via a nasogastric tube. Broad-spectrum antibiotics should also be given. Complicated meconium ileus always requires surgical intervention. The operative procedure depends on the pathologic findings.

Anorectal Malformations

Anorectal anomalies occur in 1 of every 5000 births and are slightly more common in males. Associated anomalies occur in more than half of these infants and are more frequent in cases in which the rectal pouch lies above the puborectalis sling. Vertebral malformations are the most common, followed by genitourinary malformations (28%) and gastrointestinal malformations (13%). Inspection of the perianal area will reveal abnormal anatomy in cases of anorectal anomaly.

Anal Stenosis

Anal stenosis accounts for approximately 8% of anorectal anomalies. The lesion represents a narrowing of a normally formed anorectum at its lowermost extremity. The onset of symptoms varies depending on the size of the opening. Defecation is difficult and the stools may be ribbon-like. Treatment consists of dilation but in some cases it may be necessary to excise the fibrous tissue and mobilize the rectum, suturing it to the lower part of the anal canal. The prognosis is good inasmuch as the anorectal region is basically normal.

Imperforate Anal Membrane

An imperforate anal membrane accounts for 6% of all anorectal anomalies. The newborn fails to pass meconium. On inspection of the perineum, a greenish bulging membrane of epithelium is seen overlying the anal orifice. Excision of the membrane relieves the problem, and sphincter function is usually normal.

Anal Agenesis

Anal agenesis without fistulas accounts for 7% of the lesions and is seen almost exclusively in males. Normal bowel descends through the levator sling, but because of abnormal anal development, only an anteriorly placed dimple is present externally. These infants fail to pass meconium. Anoplasty is the procedure of choice.

Rectal Agenesis

Rectal agenesis lesions make up 47% of anorectal anomalies. In the female, these high supralevator lesions occur both with and without fistula. Meconium is either not passed at all or is passed through the fistula, which is not visible on the perineum. The fistula opens either into the vagina or into the urogenital sinus, which is a common passageway for the urethra and vagina. Males may also have rectal agenesis with or without fistula formation. Fistulas in the male are rectourethral or rectovesical and can be detected by examining the urine for meconium in an infant who fails to pass meconium rectally.

Enteric Duplications

Duplications of the gastrointestinal tract are relatively rare. Sixty-five percent are located in the small bowel with more than half of these occurring in the ileum. Thirty percent of instances are associated with other anomalies, the most common being intestinal atresias. Spherical duplications are more common than tubular ones. Duplications are generally located on the mesenteric side of the lumen, are lined by intestinal mucosa, and share a common wall and mesenteric blood supply with the adjacent intestine, but usually do not communicate with the gut lumen. The diagnosis is made in at least half of the patients in the neonatal period. Presenting symptoms include vomiting and signs of obstruction with the presence of a palpable mass. Plain films of the abdomen may show displacement of adjacent viscera by a mass.

Malrotation with Volvulus

Anomalies of intestinal rotation occur in 1 per 6000 live births. Malrotation of the gut occurs between the 8th and 10th week of gestation when the elongating intestine returns to the abdominal cavity. If the mesenteric attachments do not develop properly, the midgut lies free, attached to the posterior abdominal wall at only two points: the duodenum and the proximal colon. It may therefore twist in either direction, but when volvulus occurs it is usually in the clockwise direction. The twisting may make several complete turns, resulting in obstruction of the duodenojejunal junction. Compromise of the circulation gangrene.

Of symptomatic patients, 80% are seen with evidence of high intestinal obstruction during the 1st month of life. Bilious vomiting, once it begins, occurs after each meal. Because the obstruction is often incomplete, all gradations of distention are seen. Interruption of blood flow leads to peritonitis, sepsis, and shock. Plain film of the abdomen may show dilated stomach and duodenum with little air in the distal bowel.

Annular Pancreas

Annular pancreas is an uncommon lesion that arises from a persistence of the dorsal pancreatic bud, which develops into its own lobe, grows around the left side of the duodenum, and then entraps the duodenum when it fuses to the bilobate ventral pancreatic bud. In 10% to 20% of cases, there are associated anomalies including duodenal atresia, malrotation, duodenal diaphragm, and Down syndrome. Most cases, however, are not diagnosed until adulthood. Symptoms in the newborn are those of partial obstruction.

Intussusception

Intussusception is the invagination of one loop of bowel into a loop distal to it. Although intussusception is a relatively common cause of intestinal obstruction in infants 6 to 18 months old, it is extremely rare in the 1st month of life.

Hirschsprung Disease

Hirschsprung disease is a lower intestinal obstruction caused by agenesis of ganglion cells in the Auerbach and Meissner plexuses. The lesion originates in the rectum and extends proximally over a variable distance. In 80% to 90% of the patients, involvement does not extend more proximally than the sigmoid colon. With involvement limited to the rectosigmoid, males predominate 4:1 Both sexes are equally affected in long-segment disease. Aganglionic megacolon occurs in 1 in 5000 live births and accounts for 5% of neonatal intestinal obstructions.

Delay in the passage of meconium beyond 24 hours occurs in 95% of newborns with this disease. Other clinical findings include evidence of lower intestinal obstruction (abdominal distention and vomiting), obstipation, and failure to thrive. Definitive treatment for Hirschsprung disease is operative. Most pediatric surgeons defer definitive repair until the patient is 8 to 12 months of age, temporizing by performing a colostomy. A number of definitive procedures are available, including the Swenson pull-through, the Duhamel operation, and the Soave endorectal pull-through.

Meconium Plug Syndrome

Meconium plug syndrome was initially described as an intestinal obstruction in the newborn that is relieved by the passage of an inspissated gray plug of meconium from the distal colon. It was initially thought that the meconium itself was abnormal. However, this syndrome has come to be considered a form of colonic dysmotility without an abnormality of intramural ganglion cells.

Infants pass no meconium for the first 24 to 48 hours of life and eventually symptoms of distal intestinal obstruction develop. Contrast enema may be both diagnostic and therapeutic. Because Hirschsprung disease is diagnosed in half of these patients eventually, careful follow-up is necessary.

Pseudo-Obstruction Syndrome

The chronic idiopathic intestinal pseudo-obstruction syndrome comprises a group of motility disorders of both muscular and neurogenic origin. Patients may become symptomatic at any time, including during the neonatal period. Symptoms include abdominal distention and vomiting. With onset in the newborn period, there is unlikely to be a "resolution" of the obstruction, as is seen in older patients. Pharmacologic agents such as metoclopramide, cisapride, bethanechol chloride, prostaglandins, cholecystokinin, pentagastrin, ceruletide, and acetylcholine have been tried without success. Surgical intervention is usually not successful and should be avoided. Treatment consists of long-term parenteral nutritional support.

DISORDERS OF THE PANCREAS
Cystic Fibrosis

The usual presentation of cystic fibrosis (CF) in the newborn period is meconium ileus. However, this diagnosis should be considered in the young infant with failure to thrive and hypoalbuminemia, even in the absence of respiratory disease. Incidence figures for whites vary from 1 in 600 to 1 in 2500 and for American blacks, 1 in 17,000. CF is an autosomal recessive disorder. In addition to being concerned about failure to thrive and hypoalbuminemia, parents may complain that the infant is constipated or passes large, malodorous stools. The diagnosis can be made on a sweat test.

Nesidioblastosis

Nesidioblastosis is a relatively rare cause of severe neonatal hypoglycemia. The cause is unknown, but histologically there is diffuse proliferation of nesidioblasts, the immature pancreatic cells that differentiate to form the pancreatic islets. There is a genetic predisposition of the disease inasmuch as an autosomal recessive pattern of appearance has been described, but not all patients have a familial history. Hyperinsulinemic hypoglycemia typically presents early postnatally. Aggressive glucose administration is required to maintain normoglycemia. The diagnosis is made by confirming the presence of hyperinsulinemia when hypoglycemia is present.

DISORDERS OF THE LIVER

HEPATITIS

Numerous viral agents cause neonatal hepatitis. At least five major hepatitis viruses have been described and include hepatitis A, hepatitis B, hepatitis C, hepatitis D, and hepatitis E. Other viral causes of hepatitis include infection with cytomegalovirus, Epstein-Barr virus, herpes simplex, varicella zoster, adenovirus, enterovirus, rubella, and arbovirus.

Of the five hepatitis viruses, hepatitis B virus (HBV) causes the most concern for neonatologists. HBV is a 43-nm virion that contains an outer shell, which contains the surface antigen (HBsAg), an inner shell, which contains the core antigen, and the inner contents, which contain the e antigen (HBeAg) and the double-stranded DNA. Temporally, the surface antigen is detected early in the disease, followed by the core antigen and the e antigen. When e antigen is present, DNA is also present in the serum, indicating that active viral replication is occurring. Fewer than 5% of fetuses whose mothers have hepatitis acquire HBV in utero, inasmuch as 95% have no evidence of HBV at birth. Approximately 60% of these infants, however, acquire HBV perinatally. The rate of perinatal acquisition depends on the presence of the hepatitis B e antigen. If mothers are HBsAg positive but HBeAg negative, the rate of neonatal infection is less than 20%. However, the rate of transmission increases to 90% if the mother is HBeAg positive.

Most infants who acquire hepatitis B infection

are asymptomatic. Most HBeAg-positive infants exhibit a long period of immune HBV tolerance with high serum HBV DNA but minimally elevated serum alanine transferase levels and minimal histologic changes on liver biopsy. In the third decade of life, however, there is a transition in viral immunity, because serum HBV DNA decreases. By that time, many women may have already delivered infants of their own to whom they have passed along hepatitis infection. At the time of transition, chronic active hepatitis develops in approximately half of the patients. The risk of chronic disease development is inversely related to the age at which infection occurs, such that chronic disease develops in 20% to 50% of persons who are infected in early childhood and in 80% to 90% of those infected in infancy. Of those in whom chronic disease develops, hepatocellular carcinoma will develop in a substantial number of the individuals when they reach their 60s. Chronic HBV is responsible for 80% of all cases of hepatocellular carcinoma. Thus, reduction of perinatal acquisition of HBV is done, not out of concern for the neonatal disease, which is mild, but as a public health measure based on concerns for the high rate of chronic active hepatitis and risk for hepatocellular carcinoma.

Passive immunity against HBV can be provided by hepatitis B immune globulin, which is prepared from humans with high serum concentrations of HBsAg. Although passive prophylaxis prevents perinatal acquisition of HBV, its effect is transient and 20% to 50% of infants can become carriers by 1 year of age. Active prophylaxis using inactivated virus vaccine given three or four times during infancy elicits protective serum concentrations of HB surface antibodies. When passive and active immunization is combined there is 90% efficacy among infants born to mothers who are HBsAg and HBeAg positive.

Although perinatal transmission of hepatitis C is reportedly rare, the transmission rate is high among mothers who are human immunodeficiency virus (HIV) positive. Most infants who acquire hepatitis C virus are asymptomatic until early childhood when the use of interferon alfa-2b has held some promise for treatment.

Hepatitis resulting from syphilis is being seen more frequently. Newborns present with hepatosplenomegaly and jaundice during the 1st month of life. Serum transaminase levels may reach 500 IU. Liver biopsy shows a picture consistent with giant cell hepatitis. Even after penicillin therapy, liver dysfunction may persist for up to 2 months.

Bacterial hepatitis may produce cholestasis by two mechanisms. The first is associated with generalized sepsis with bacterial invasion of the liver and markedly elevated transaminase levels, hepatomegaly, and liver necrosis. Treatment and prognosis are the same as for neonatal sepsis. The second mechanism is a "toxic cholestasis." No direct invasion or destruction of the hepatocytes occurs. Therefore, transaminases are usually seen with severe urinary tract infections caused by *Escherichia coli* or *Proteus* or with pneumonia and generalized sepsis from *Pneumococcus*. The mechanism is thought to be caused by a toxin that inhibits hepatic excretory function. Successful treatment of the infection results in resolution of the cholestasis.

INHERITED AND METABOLIC LIVER DISORDERS
Alpha$_1$-Antitrypsin Deficiency

Alpha$_1$-antitrypsin deficiency is caused by accumulation of alpha$_1$-antitrypsin in the hepatocyte with subsequent hepatocellular necrosis. Alpha$_1$-antitrypsin is an alpha$_1$-globulin and is a major serum protease inhibitor. It is inherited as an autosomal recessive trait. Although there are several phenotypes, only the homozygous Pi (protease inhibitor) ZZ and, rarely, the MZ types have been associated with liver disease in infancy. The ZZ phenotype occurs in 1 in 2000 live births, but cholestasis develops in only 10% in the neonatal period, typically by 8 to 10 weeks. Of those in whom cholestasis develops, it remains permanent and complete in 50%. However, if spontaneous remission occurs, it characteristically occurs by 6 months of age. Thereafter, the course is highly variable among those who do not have remission, and hepatic failure does develop in some infants who require transplantation. The absence of the alpha$_1$-globulin fraction seen on serum electrophoresis is highly suggestive of the disorder. Definitive diagnosis depends on finding a reduced serum alpha$_1$-antitrypsin level, Pi typing, and liver biopsy that shows periodic acid–Schiff (PAS)-positive cytoplasmic granules with variable degrees of hepatic necrosis and fibrosis. There is no specific treatment.

Cystic Fibrosis

Cholestasis in early infancy can be an initial presentation of CF. Half of such infants also have meconium ileus. Liver disease eventually occurs in up to 50% of CF patients. Cirrhosis develops in 5% but only 2% have clinical findings. Liver biopsy in the infants shows evidence of excessive biliary mucus with mild periportal inflammation and fibrosis.

Galactosemia

Galactosemia is an autosomal recessive disorder of carbohydrate metabolism that results from deficient galactose-1-phosphate uridyltransferase activity. Accumulation of galactose-1-phosphate results in cholestasis, hepatomegaly, hypoglycemia, cataracts, vomiting, and failure to thrive. The diagnosis is made by demonstrating low levels of erythrocyte galactose-1-phosphate uridyltransferase activity. Treatment consists of removing all sources of galactose (lactose) from the diet.

Hereditary Fructose Intolerance

Hereditary fructose intolerance is a congenital deficiency of fructose-1-phosphatase that results in the accumulation of fructose and fructose-1-phosphate in body tissues. Introduction of fructose into the diet results in vomiting, hepatomegaly, and jaundice.

Tyrosinemia

Tyrosinemia is a rare autosomal recessive disorder characterized by decreased activity of *p*-hydroxyphenylpyruvic acid oxidase, methionine-activating enzyme, and cystathionine synthetase. Both acute and chronic forms have been described. The acute form presents with vomiting, failure to thrive, liver failure, and renal tubular dysfunction, usually within the first 3 to 6 weeks of life. Plasma and urine aminograms reveal elevated levels of tyrosine and its metabolites. Dietary restriction of tyrosine and phenylalanine may slow the progress of the liver disease, but without a liver transplant, most infants die during the 1st year of life.

Lipid Storage Diseases

Niemann-Pick disease, Gaucher disease, Wolman disease, and cholesterol ester storage disease are rare genetic disorders of lipid metabolism. They present with hepatosplenomegaly and varying degrees of liver dysfunction, including cholestasis.

Familial Recurrent Cholestasis

Familial recurrent cholestasis is an autosomal recessive disorder characterized by episodic cholestasis. The initial presentation is within the first 6 months of life. The cholestatic episodes may last weeks to months. Cirrhosis eventually develops. Death from liver failure occurs between 2 and 15 years of age.

Recurrent Cholestasis with Lymphedema

Recurrent cholestasis with lymphedema (Aagenaes syndrome) is a rare genetic disorder characterized by cholestasis and lymphedema of the lower extremities. Cirrhosis develops in some patients.

Cerebrohepatorenal Syndrome

Cerebrohepatorenal (Zellweger) syndrome is one of a group of disorders of peroxisomal dysfunction.

Inherited as an autosomal recessive trait, it presents in the neonatal period with cholestasis, hepatomegaly, profound hypotonia, and dysmorphic features. The diagnosis is made by demonstrating abnormal very-long-chain fatty acid levels in the serum.

TOTAL PARENTERAL NUTRITION–ASSOCIATED CHOLESTASIS

Cholestasis develops in 50% of infants with birth weights less than 1000 g after 2 weeks of parenteral nutrition. In newborns with birth weights between 1000 and 2000 g, the incidence is 15%. The incidence increases with the duration of parenteral nutrition. Cholestasis develops in up to 90% of low-birth-weight infants after 13 weeks of total parenteral nutrition.

No precise cause has been found, but a number of factors appear to be important. These include immaturity of biliary excretion, lack of oral feedings, toxicity of certain amino acid components of the parenteral nutrition solution, and inadequate intake of certain nutrients such as taurine. Lipid infusion does not appear to play a role. The final common pathway may be the accumulation in the serum and bile of toxic bile acids, such as glycolithocholate.

Serum bile salt concentrations increase before clinical jaundice becomes obvious. After 2 weeks or more on total parenteral nutrition, there is a gradual increase in the conjugated bilirubin with a modest increase in the serum transaminases and alkaline phosphatase. Physical findings are limited to jaundice and hepatomegaly. In some infants the gallbladder becomes hydropic and is palpable. The diagnosis is made by excluding other causes of cholestasis. Histologic changes on liver biopsy are nonspecific.

Treatment consists of the introduction of enteral alimentation and the discontinuation of intravenous nutrition. If total parenteral nutrition must be used, sufficient protein (at least 8% of the total calories) should be provided to prevent hepatic steatosis.

After discontinuation of the parenteral nutrition, liver function abnormalities usually resolve after 4 to 12 weeks. Gallbladder hydrops also resolves with the institution of feedings. Gallstones that necessitate cholecystectomy do develop in some infants. Progressive cirrhosis may develop in a small number of infants despite discontinuation of the parenteral nutrition. Deaths have been reported from liver failure. Liver transplantation may be required.

PARENTERAL AND ENTERAL NUTRITION

The goals for nutritional support of the healthy full-term infant are to provide nutrient deposition and body composition to match that of the infant who is breast-fed exclusively. The Recommended Dietary Allowances (RDA) for the first 6 months after birth assume that the breast-fed infant receives 750 mL milk per day. In the second 6 months, approximately 600 mL are ingested daily with other foods.

BREAST-FEEDING

Breast-feeding is recommended for term infants because of its acknowledged benefits with respect to infant nutrition and host defense. Contraindications are maternal illness, including HIV, if alternatives are available.

The total nitrogen content in human milk declines with postpartum age, and the protein quality (proportion of whey and casein) of human milk (30% casein and 70% whey) differs from that in bovine milk and milk-based formula (82% casein and 18% whey). The whey fraction provides lower concentrations of phenylalanine, tyrosine, and methionine and higher concentrations of taurine than the casein fraction of milk. These differences may be significant because infants have a relative inability to process phenylalanine and methionine and have a relative inability to form taurine compared with adults.

The constituents of the whey fraction differ between human and bovine milks. Human whey proteins include alpha-lactalbumin, which serves as a nutritional protein for the infant, as well as lactoferrin, lysozyme, and secretory immunoglobulin A (sIgA), which serve important roles in host defense. These three latter proteins are present only in trace quantities in bovine milk, and the major whey protein in bovine milk, beta-lactoglobulin, is thought to cause milk protein allergy and colic. The whey fraction in human milk also contains nonprotein nitrogen-containing compounds, such as free amino acids, taurine, and urea, which may contribute to nitrogen utilization in the infant.

Lipids in human milk are comprised of organized milk fat globules, containing fatty acids (high in palmitic 16:0, oleic 18:1, linoleic 18:2n-6, and linolenic 18:3n-3) distributed on the triglyceride molecule (16:0 at the 2-position of the molecule). The mixture of fatty acids in commercial formulas differs from that in human milk. Generally, commercial formulas have a greater quantity of medium chain–length fatty acids. Arachidonic acid (20:4n-6) and docosahexaenoic acid (22:6n-3), derivatives of linoleic and linolenic acids, are found in human but not bovine milk. These fatty acids are precursors of prostaglandins as well as components of phospholipids found in brain and red cell membranes. Their presence has been associated with improved cognition, growth, and vision. Human milk also contains bile salt–stimulated lipase, which contributes significantly to the digestion of fats present in human milk.

Human milk contains approximately 7% lactose. Lactase absorption may not be fully present in the newborn. Thus, a softer stool consistency, more nonpathogenic bacterial fecal flora, and improved absorption of minerals have been attributed to the presence of small quantities of unabsorbed lactose from human milk feeding. Oligosaccharides, including the glycoproteins and mucins, are important in the host defense of the infant.

Data from numerous studies suggest that there is decreased morbidity in breast-fed versus formula-fed full-term infants. The presence of specific factors such as sIgA, lactoferrin, lysozyme, oligosaccharides, growth factors, and cellular components in human milk may contribute to the improved host defense of the breast-fed infant. When the mother is exposed to foreign antigens, her gastrointestinal plasma cells produce sIgA antibody, which circulates to mucosal surfaces, one of which is the mammary gland. Thus, specific antibody is present in her milk. When the infant ingests the milk, the infant receives specific passive immunity. This system is active in infants against a variety of antigens. The complex interplay among the immune components results in a reduced incidence of gastrointestinal and respiratory diseases and otitis media among breast-fed infants.

Numerous drugs and viruses may be excreted in human milk. Human milk may contain hepatitis B virus, cytomegalovirus, herpes simplex if lesions are localized to the breast, and HIV. The World Health Organization and the American Academy of Pediatrics currently do not recommend discontinuing breast-feeding for the HBsAg-positive mother. The infant, however, should be given hepatitis B immunoglobulin and hepatitis B vaccine. Although it is common practice in the United States to avoid breast-feeding by HIV-positive mothers, it is not a World Health Organization policy because of the immune protection it provides. Although most drugs ingested by the mother are excreted in human milk, interruption of nursing currently is indicated only occasionally.

In general, the healthy, breast-fed, full-term infant receiving adequate sunlight exposure does not require vitamin and mineral supplements. The breast-fed infant, however, should receive vitamin K at birth. Moreover, the physician should be aware that the vitamin D concentration in human milk may be insufficient to prevent rickets. Although most breast-fed infants do not require vitamin D supplements, those who do not receive sunlight exposure and who also have dark skin pigmentation may need vitamin D supplementation of 400 IU per day. Because the concentration of iron declines during lactation, the breast-fed infant needs an iron supplement by 6 months of age.

ENERGY NEEDS OF THE LOW-BIRTH-WEIGHT INFANT

Because the parenterally nourished low-birth-weight (LBW) infant has less fecal energy loss, fewer episodes of cold stress, and less activity, the actual energy needs for growth are lower for the preterm infant than for the term infant and range from 80 to 120 kcal/kg per day. In chronic disease, such as bronchopulmonary dysplasia, the resting energy expenditure may rise significantly.

PARENTERAL NUTRITION

The use of parenteral nutrition containing glucose and amino acids reverses the negative nitrogen balance characteristic of the first days after birth, increases the serum concentration of essential amino acids, and increases the rate of protein synthesis. Several amino acid solutions are available, and the percentage of essential total amino acids is variable among them, ranging from 40% to 53%. Evidence indicates that histidine, tyrosine, cysteine, and taurine may be conditionally essential amino acids. Tyrosine and cysteine are not present in all amino acid preparations, principally because of difficulties in solubility. Taurine and glutamic acid are not present in all solutions, although their need is unclear.

There is a direct relationship between the quantity of nitrogen (amino acids) provided in total parenteral nutrition (TPN) and nitrogen balance or retention. In addition, specific amino acids may affect nitrogen balance. The addition of cysteine hydrochloride to TPN increases plasma free and total cyst(e)ine and urinary cyst(e)ine concentrations, but increasing cysteine intake does not increase nitrogen balance or weight gain. Therefore, cysteine hydrochloride is added to TPN solutions to meet presumed cysteine needs and to enhance the solubility of the calcium and phosphorus salts because it can lower the pH of the TPN solution.

Nitrogen retention can be increased in infants receiving TPN in one of three ways: by changing the mixture of essential/nonessential amino acids, increasing the nitrogen intake, or increasing the energy intake. There is a positive relationship between energy intake and nitrogen balance for any given nitrogen intake, in that nitrogen balance (retention) increases as energy intake increases from 50 to 90 kcal/kg per day.

Intravenous lipid emulsions containing soybean oil (with or without safflower oil) with glycerin and egg yolk phospholipid emulsifiers are available in 10% or 20% concentrations to supplement parenteral nutrition regimens. Intravenous lipid emulsion can be used in sick LBW infants as early as the day of birth without short-term adverse effects. Early administration of intravenous lipid reverses essential fatty acid deficiency, provides needed energy for tissue healing and growth, and equalizes the distribution of nonprotein calories.

Intravenous lipid may theoretically affect lung function adversely through a variety of mechanisms, although none have been found to be clinically important.

The concentration of the lipid emulsion (10% versus 20%) may affect the infant's tolerance of the preparation. For example, LBW infants receiving the 20% solution at the same or even greater lipid intakes had lower serum concentrations of triglycerides, cholesterol, and phospholipids than similar infants receiving the 10% solution. It is postulated that the excess phospholipid, cholesterol, and liposomes contained in the 10% solution accumulate to form lipoprotein X. These lipoprotein X particles then compete with lipoprotein lipase to reduce the clearing of triglycerides. Thus, regardless of the dose of lipid or the age of the infant, most LBW infants should receive the 20% solution.

The method of lipid infusion also is a concern. Intermittent infusion may produce higher serum triglyceride concentrations than continuous infusion of the same dose. Intermittent infusions and lipid-free intervals do not appear to be justified in routine circumstances.

Several conditionally essential nutrients are being evaluated for inclusion in TPN solutions for newborns, including carnitine, inositol, choline, and glutamine. Data conflict concerning the need for carnitine supplementation of TPN for LBW infants.

Supplementation of TPN with inositol in the first week after birth has been reported to reduce the incidence of chronic pulmonary disease in LBW infants with respiratory distress syndrome. No data exist concerning the inclusion of glutamine in parenteral solutions for LBW infants. The use of choline to prevent hepatic cholestasis also is speculative.

Although there is a direct relationship between intake and net retention of calcium and phosphorus, the delivery of optimal intakes is often limited by the lack of solubility of calcium and phosphorus in intravenous solution. It is generally agreed that calcium/phosphorus ratios of 1:1 (molar) or greater are appropriate for LBW infants. The parenteral needs for calcium, phosphorus, and magnesium were derived in a longitudinal study evaluating serial balance studies using TrophAmine 2.2% (130 mL/kg/day) and Intralipid 20% (20 mL/kg/day). Intrauterine accretion rates were most closely approximated in parenteral nutrition solutions containing 80 mg calcium, 80 mg phosphorus, and 7 mg magnesium per 100 mL.

Generally the parenteral needs for sodium and potassium are determined by the infant's clinical circumstance, with a range of intakes recommended. The majority of sodium intake is derived from common medications received by the LBW infant. Mild acidosis may occur when infants are receiving parenteral nutrition because the LBW infant has decreased renal reabsorption of bicarbonate. Moreover, the use of amino acid solutions with low pH and the use of cysteine hydrochloride further reduce the pH. The addition of acetate to the solution, as either the sodium or potassium salt, has been reported to correct the acidosis. The small quantity of acetate, 1 to 2 mEq/kg per day, has not been observed to affect the solubility of the minerals in TPN solutions containing TrophAmine and cysteine hydrochloride.

Suggested parenteral intakes of copper and zinc for LBW infants have been evaluated from serial balance studies conducted during the first 3 weeks postnatally. Estimated parenteral intakes of zinc range from 350 to 450 μg/kg per day. A greater dose may be indicated in LBW infants with ongoing intestinal losses of zinc. Differences in recommendations for trace elements may arise because of the various sources of amino acids used and medical conditions of the infants studied.

Vitamin A circulates in association with retinol-binding protein, which is synthesized in the liver and bound to the vitamin before secretion. As much as 70% to 80% of vitamin A is lost in the delivery system because it is adsorbed to plastic and degraded by light exposure. The addition of vitamin A to intravenous lipid solutions results in greater delivery of the vitamin. When retinal palmitate is used, the losses in vitamin A delivery are minimized. The substitution of retinal palmitate for retinol in parenteral nutrition solutions also appears to maintain the greater plasma retinol concentrations that are achieved if retinol is mixed and infused with intravenous lipid. An association between deficient vitamin A status and the development of bronchopulmonary dysplasia has been reported. High doses of intramuscular vitamin A (averaging 1500 to 2000 IU/kg/day) resulted in greater plasma vitamin A and retinol-binding protein concentrations and a lower incidence of bronchopulmonary dysplasia. The recommended parenteral intakes of vitamin A approximate this dose.

The need for vitamin E is directly related to the content of polyunsaturated fatty acids (PUFA) in the diet. This is particularly important in parenteral nutrition because the proportion of PUFA in intravenous fat emulsions is high. Vitamin E doses of 2.1 versus 4.6 mg per day have been evaluated during 3 to 4 weeks of parenteral nutrition therapy. The higher dose resulted in a large proportion of elevated plasma vitamin E concentrations (greater than 3.5 mg/dL) in infants less than 1000 g birth weight. A vitamin E dose of 3.5 mg per day reportedly produced adequate plasma vitamin E concentrations at 7 days' postnatal age in infants 1000 g birth weight or less. In neither study were lipid intakes reported. A dose of 2.8 mg/kg per day administered in intravenous lipid, however, resulted in appropriate plasma vitamin E concentrations.

Current formulations generally provide more water-soluble vitamins than are needed by LBW infants. Plasma ascorbate (vitamin C) and vitamin B_2 (riboflavin) concentrations reportedly were elevated in LBW infants receiving parenteral nutrition. The elevated riboflavin concentrations appear paradoxical in view of the known degradation of the vitamin under infusion and nursery lighting conditions. Thus, significantly lower doses of some water-soluble vitamins are indicated. When used in a dose of 2 mL/kg per day (40% of the vial M.V.I. Pediatric), no deficiencies of thiamine or riboflavin were detected, and plasma concentrations of folate and vitamin B_{12} indicated sufficient status.

ENTERAL NUTRITION

The quality of protein (e.g., the greater proportion of whey to casein) in human milk is particularly suitable for the LBW infant. The quantity and quality of protein needed for LBW infants have been investigated longitudinally. Infants were fed one of five preparations: formulas that provided protein intakes of 2.25 or 4.50 g/kg per day (containing whey or casein) or pasteurized human milk that provided a protein intake of 1.6 g/kg per day. LBW infants who received 4.5 g/kg per day and infants given casein-dominant milk had greater plasma amino acid concentrations of phenylalanine, tyrosine, and methionine during the 8-week study. Infants fed whey-dominant formulas had higher plasma threonine concentrations and improved retention of cyst(e)ine and taurine compared with infants fed casein-dominant formula. Because elevations of particular amino acids may be toxic to brain development, there is a potential concern that feeding LBW infants a high-protein intake, especially of a casein-dominant milk, may be harmful.

After the first 2 weeks of feeding, human milk may not provide adequate protein intake for the LBW infant. Protein intakes of 2.2 and 2.8 g/kg per day result in lower serum indices, weight gain, and nitrogen retention, whereas protein intakes of 3.8 g/kg per day appeared somewhat excessive. It is recommended that preterm infants receive 3.5 g/kg per day of protein with energy intakes of 120 kcal/kg per day. Thus, protein intakes from unfortified human milk or full-term infant formulas are inadequate for feeding LBW infants. The protein contents of human milk and various preterm formulas are summarized in Table 9–1.

Manufacturers of infant formulas modify their fat blends to mimic the fat absorption in human milk. Generally, commercial formulations have a greater quantity of medium chain–length fatty acids to compensate for the absence of the lipid system in human milk. In addition, the saturated fatty acids, especially palmitic acid, may not be absorbed as readily because of the differences in intrinsic packaging of human milk compared with commercial fat preparations. The malabsorbed palmitic acid, therefore, has a greater tendency toward soap formation, which could potentially interfere with mineral absorption.

Research has focused on the respective derivatives of linoleic and linolenic acids, arachidonic acid (20:4n-6), and docosahexaenoic acid (22:6n-3). These very long-chain fatty acids, which are found in human but not bovine milk, are components of phospholipids found in brain and red cell membranes. When supplemented with marine oil, formula-fed LBW infants had red blood cell concentrations of 22:6n-3 that parallel those of similar infants fed human milk. Follow-up studies of supplemented infants suggest improvements in visual acuity. These data indicate that human milk may be suitable for LBW infants not only for the ability to promote fat absorption in the immature infant, but also because of the profound metabolic functions attributed to this particular pattern of essential fatty acids. Recommendations for the supplementation of preterm formulas with marine oil have been published.

The proportion of medium-chain fatty acids, here defined as carbon length 6:0 to 12:0, is below 12% of total fatty acids in human milk but approaches 50% in preterm formulas. There are no compelling data to suggest that a high proportion of medium-chain fatty acids is needed for preterm formulas.

One can capitalize on the variability in the fat content of human milk in feeding the LBW infant.

The fat content of human milk varies among women, changes during the day, rises slightly during lactation, and increases dramatically within a single milk expression. The fat content of hindmilk may be 1.5-fold to 3-fold greater than that of foremilk. No differences between foremilk and hindmilk are reported for the contents of nitrogen, calcium, phosphorus, sodium, or potassium. Thus, the use of hindmilk can be recommended for LBW infants whose rate of weight gain is low (less than 15 g/kg/day).

Because it is not homogenized, on standing, the fat separates out of human milk. Care should be taken that continuous milk infusion systems use a short length of tubing.

Although mucosal lactose levels are low until 32 to 34 weeks' gestation, LBW infants have the capacity to absorb more than 90% of the lactose present in human milk. Artificial formulas for LBW infants contain a mixture, usually 50:50, of lactose and glucose polymers. In general, the replacement of some lactose with glucose polymers reduces the osmolality compared with a formulation based entirely on lactose as the carbohydrate source. No beneficial effect on mineral absorption was reported when a formulation containing a mixture of lactose and glucose polymers was compared with lactose alone. Improved mineral absorption was reported when an exclusive lactose-containing formula was used compared with a formula containing sucrose and corn syrup solids (glucose polymers) as the carbohydrate source.

A linear relationship exists between calcium (or phosphorus) intake and net retention in enterally fed LBW infants. LBW infants who are fed unfortified human milk never achieve intrauterine accretion rates for calcium and phosphorus. Intakes of calcium and phosphorus greater than 3.5 and 3.0 mmol/kg per day can be achieved by feeding specialized preterm cow milk–based formulas (see Table 9–1). Full-term infant formulas and specialized formulas, however, provide inadequate quantities of calcium and phosphorus to meet the needs of LBW infants.

The benefits of feeding LBW infants human milk

TABLE 9–1
Nutrient Composition of Preterm Human Milk, Fortified Human Milk, Preterm Formulas, and Specialized Formulas

	Preterm Human Milk 1 week	Mature Human Milk (MM) 1 month	EHMF* + MM	SNC† + MM	EPF‡ 24	SSC§ 24	Pregestimil**	Similac 27††	PediaSure‡‡
Volume, mL	100	100	100	100	100	100	100	100	100
Energy, kcal	67	70	84	76	81	81	67	91	100
Protein, g	2.4	1.8	2.5	2.0	2.4	2.2	1.9	2.5	3.0
% Whey/casein	70/30	70/30	70/30	65/35	60/40	60/40	0/100	18/82	18/82
Fat, g	3.8	4.0	4.0	4.2	4.1	4.4	2.7	4.8	4.9
% MCT/LCT	2/98	2/98	2/98	25/75	40/60	40/60	55/45	8/92	20/80
Carbohydrate, g	6.1	7.0	9.7	7.8	9.0	8.6	6.9	9.6	11.2
% Lactose	100	100	72	72	40	50	0%	100%	0%
Calcium, mg	25	22	112	116	134	146	63	82	96
Phosphorus, mg	14	14	59	60	67	73	42	64	79
Magnesium, mg	3.1	2.5	3.5	6.1	5.5	9.7	7.3	6.4	20

Sodium, mg	50	37	33	32	35	26	31	38
Potassium, mg	70	75	82	83	104	73	120	129
Chloride, mg	90	78	63	69	66	58	74	100
Zinc, µg	500	1030	770	1215	1215	630	683	1167
Copper, µg	80	120	130	100	200	63	82	100
Vitamin A, IU	560	1350	475	1013	550	255	273	254
Vitamin D, IU	4	214	63	219	122	50	55	50
Vitamin E, mg	1.0	4.9	1.8	5.1	3.2	2.5	2.7	2.3
Vitamin C, mg	5.4	17.2	17.8	16	30	7.8	8	10

*Enfamil Human Milk Fortifier (EHMF) (Mead Johnson Nutritionals, Evansville, IN), 4 packets + 100 mL mature milk.
†Similac Natural Care (SNC) 24 (Ross Laboratories, Columbus, OH) diluted 1:1 with mature milk.
‡Enfamil Premature Formula (EPF) 24 (Mead Johnson).
§Similac Special Care (SSC) 24 (Ross Laboratories).
**Mead Johnson.
††Ready To Feed (Ross Laboratories).
‡‡With fiber (Ross Laboratories).
MCT, medium-chain triglyceride; LCT, long-chain triglyceride.
Data from Butte et al, 1984; Gross et al, 1980; Litov and Combs, 1991; Moran et al, 1983; Newman, 1994; Schanler, 1988; Slagle and Gross, 1988.

are beginning to be recognized. Specific factors such as sIgA, lactoferrin, lysozyme, oligosaccharides (including mucins), growth factors, and cellular components may affect the host defense of the LBW infant. The quantity of host defense factors in preterm milk is greater than in term milk. Lactoferrin, lysozyme, and sIgA are specific human whey proteins that are particularly resistant to hydrolysis and, as such, line the gastrointestinal tract to play a primary role in host defense. The enteromammary immune system is the mechanism through which the human milk–fed infant receives a portion of its host protection. To what extent the enteromammary immune system functions in the LBW infant–mother dyad is unknown. Protocols that encourage skin-to-skin contact between the LBW infant and mother may affect milk protective antibody concentrations.

CHAPTER 10

Bilirubin

PHYSIOLOGIC JAUNDICE

Jaundice is the visible manifestation in skin and sclera of elevated serum concentrations of bilirubin. Most adults are jaundiced when serum bilirubin levels exceed 2.0 mg/dL (34 µM/L). Neonates, however, may not appear jaundiced until the serum bilirubin concentration exceeds 5.0 to 7.0 mg/dL (119 µM/L).

Chemical hyperbilirubinemia, defined as a serum total bilirubin level of 2.0 mg/dL (34 µM/L) or more, is virtually universal in newborns during the 1st week of life. Bilirubin concentrations in premature babies are even higher, persist longer, and are more likely to be associated with neurologic injury than those in term neonates. Debate and controversy remain in efforts to define either normal or physiologic ranges of serum bilirubin concentration in newborns, because the data are influenced by such variables as length of gestation, birth weight, nutritional status, mode of feeding, race, and even geographic location. Even within a single racial group, genetic variation may affect the intensity and duration of physiologic jaundice. At issue is whether the normal range should be determined by rate of increase in serum bilirubin concentration, a level for a specific postpartum age, or the maximum level attained.

Traditionally, a distinction has been made between this physiologic jaundice and hyperbilirubinemia, which is either pathologic in origin or severe enough to be considered deserving of further evaluation and intervention. If the total serum bilirubin concentration exceeds 5 mg/dL on the 1st day of life in a term neonate, 10 mg/dL on the 2nd day, or 12 to 13 mg/dL thereafter, the bilirubin is considered not physiologic.

Distinctive aspects of normal newborn physiology that contribute to neonatal hyperbilirubinemia include (1) increased bilirubin synthesis, (2) less effective binding and transportation, (3) less efficient hepatic conjugation and excretion, and (4) enhanced absorption of bilirubin via the enterohepatic circulation.

INCREASED BILIRUBIN SYNTHESIS

In neonates, hemoglobin breaks down at twice the adult rate, and there is an increased rate of red cell degradation in the marrow even before release. In addition, bilirubin synthesis in healthy neonates results from a greater erythrocyte mass at birth and a shorter half-life of neonatal red blood cells. Normal term newborns have a hemoglobin level of approximately 19 g/dL, and a hematocrit of approximately 50% to 55%. Polycythemia, defined as a hematocrit greater than 65%, occurs in 1.4% to 1.8% of infants born at sea level and in 4% of those born at altitude.

The life span of erythrocytes is less than 70 days for premature babies. It is estimated to be approximately 70 to 90 days in healthy term infants compared with 120 days in adults.

BINDING AND TRANSPORTATION

The full-term newborn infant has a significantly lower plasma albumin level than an adult and, therefore, correspondingly fewer bilirubin binding sites. The albumin level is dependent on gestational age, and the more premature an infant is, the lower the level. Plasma albumin level increases rapidly over the first few days after birth, resulting in a mean increase over the first 7 days of almost 30%. Adult levels are reached by about 5 months of age.

CONJUGATION AND EXCRETION

During intrauterine life, removal of bilirubin from the fetus is accomplished by way of the placenta and maternal-fetal circulation, and the bilirubin in cord blood is virtually all unconjugated. At birth, blood supply to the right lobe of the liver changes from the high oxygen content of the umbilical vein to portal venous flow. Blood flow through the hepatic arteries develops only in the 1st week of extrauterine life. In addition, the ductus venosus may remain partially patent for several days, allowing blood to bypass the liver altogether. All these factors can contribute to a delay in plasma clearance of bilirubin.

The conjugating capacity of normal infants varies greatly; delayed conjugation and excretion may in some cases be related to immaturity of the liver cell itself. The activity of the glucuronyl transferase system in the newborn liver must be induced. Evidence that it can be induced prenatally in cases of severe fetal hemolysis suggests that elevated bilirubin levels may be necessary to induce the conjugating enzymes.

ENHANCED ENTEROHEPATIC CIRCULATION

Conjugated bilirubin, as either the monogluronide or diglucuronide, is unstable and can be spontaneously or enzymatically hydrolyzed to unconjugated bilirubin, which is easily absorbed through the mucosa. In addition, absorption is enhanced by the sterility of the intestinal contents; older children and adults have intestinal flora that can metabolize conjugated bilirubin to break down products, such as urobilin and stercobilin, which are water soluble and relatively easy to excrete. Newborns have no such advantage; instead, the neonatal intestinal mucosa has a greater concentration of beta-glucuronidase than does the adult. This enzyme can deconjugate bilirubin, resulting in more unconjugated bilirubin that can be absorbed via the enterohepatic circulation, adding to the unconjugated bilirubin load.

EPIDEMIOLOGY

The knowledge that racial groups differ in the peak bilirubin levels could have important implications for management of these infants. Using criteria for intervention based on Caucasian and African populations might lead to overtreatment of significant numbers of infants from other races.

Controversy exists regarding the influence of breast-feeding on serum bilirubin levels. The question has been asked, "Is physiologic jaundice in the newborn exaggerated in breast-fed babies?" Many studies have attempted to answer this question, and results are conflicting. The consensus of practitioners and investigators in the past decade is that breast-feeding is indeed associated with statistically significant elevations of serum bilirubin concentrations.

BREAST-FEEDING JAUNDICE

Two separate patterns of jaundice in breast-feeding infants have been described. The first has been termed *breast-feeding associated jaundice,* or simply *breast-feeding jaundice,* a condition that occurs in the 1st week of life; the second is less common and is called *breast milk jaundice* and presents as prolonged hyperbilirubinemia lasting into the 3rd week of life or beyond. Several reports suggesting that the cause of breast-feeding jaundice may be nutritional show that this condition can be prevented by encouraging frequent (e.g., nine times daily) breast-feeding in the first 3 days of life and by avoidance of supplementation with water or glucose solutions. Breast milk jaundice is considered by some researchers to be an extension of physiologic hyperbilirubinemia beyond the first 5 or 6 days of life and continuing for weeks. This entity was first described in 1963 and was considered to be a disease that occurred in less than 1% to 2% of the breast-feeding population. Epidemiologic studies suggest it is much more frequent, affecting as many as 10% to 30% of the breast-fed infants in the 2nd to 6th week of life, with some experiencing hyperbilirubinemia into the 3rd month. With the realization that the prolongation of jaundice in breast-fed infants is so common, the view of this condition has changed from that of a disorder to perhaps a normal extension of physiologic jaundice.

One hypothesis regarding this prolonged jaundice associated with breast-feeding suggests that it results from enhanced enterohepatic absorption of unconjugated bilirubin related to the presence of an unidentified factor in human milk. This theory holds that breast-fed infants who do not have prolonged jaundice either do not respond to this factor in their mother's milk or their mother's milk lacks it. Another possibility is that breast-fed infants are able to metabolize and excrete the resulting increase in bilirubin load, successfully accommodating for the enhanced intestinal absorption of bilirubin. No specific factor has been identified and etiologic theories are still considered speculative.

BILIRUBIN TOXICITY, ENCEPHALOPATHY, AND KERNICTERUS

Bilirubin neuropathy does not usually become overt until high bilirubin levels have been established for several hours. A prodrome of reversible signs has been described which includes decreased activity, loss of interest in feeding, changes in the infant's cry, lethargy, irritability, and possibly apnea. If the bilirubin level is rapidly decreased (e.g., by way of exchange transfusion), these findings can often be reversed.

If hyperbilirubinemia persists, however, these more subtle findings are followed within a few hours by rigid extension of all four extremities, tight-fisted posturing of arms, crossed extension of the legs, and a high pitched irritable cry. Sometimes these changes are accompanied with opisthotonos or seizure activity. After several months in patients who survive, reduced muscle tone, difficulty feeding, and spastic or choreoathetoid cerebral palsy usually develop, with tremors, fine motor clumsiness, and poor visual tracking or a fixed upward gaze. High-frequency hearing loss and mental retardation are also part of this syndrome. The most common findings later in childhood are choreoathetosis, ocular paralysis, and eighth nerve deafness; severe mental retardation and spastic cerebral palsy occur in a minority. In general, the motor findings are the most obvious abnormalities in long-term survivors.

Classic findings of kernicterus are not often seen in neonatal follow-up clinics for premature and low-birth-weight infants, because most affected infants do not survive into childhood. However, a spectrum of mild neurologic disabilities and subtle developmental delays has been associated with moderate elevation of serum indirect bilirubin concentration. Because developmental delays related to other factors of prematurity, neonatal illness, or environmental situations are commonly associated with neonatal intensive care, there is controversy regarding the reversibility or long-term implications of the subtle neurologic damage attributed to bilirubin in low-birth-weight babies. Debates about the need for aggressive or conservative treatment for mild to moderate hyperbilirubinemia in infants persist.

EXCHANGE TRANSFUSION

Although the first successful exchange transfusion performed on an infant with familial icterus gravis was reported in 1925, this mode of intervention was not accepted until hemolytic disease of the newborn was conceptually understood in the 1940s. Exchange transfusion decreases the risk of bilirubin encephalopathy by reducing the total bilirubin load, increasing the binding sites of plasma albumin, and shifting bilirubin out of tissue into the plasma as well as providing erythrocytes less apt to hemolyze. Early attempts at exchange transfusion involved removing blood from the sagittal sinus or radial artery and infusing blood into the saphenous vein. With the development of polyethylene tubing, Diamond and coworkers in 1946 introduced the technique of alternate removal and administration of blood for each transfusion via umbilical vein catheterization.

Before exchange transfusion came into common usage in the 1950s, kernicterus affected 15% of live born infants with erythroblastosis. Seventy percent of patients with kernicterus died within 1 week of birth, and many of the remainder died during the 1st year of life. Survivors had permanent neurologic sequelae and were thought to account for 10% of all cases of cerebral palsy. Considering the severe morbidity of this condition, the major contribution provided by exchange transfusion can be appreciated, even though the procedure was recognized as having inherent risks of its own.

With the publication describing congenital familial nonhemolytic jaundice with kernicterus in 1952, a new family of diseases, currently understood to be hereditary deficiencies of bilirubin uridinediphosphoglucuronyl transferase, was discovered. Our understanding of kernicterus as a process related more to elevated unconjugated bilirubin levels rather than to specific blood group incompatibilities or even hemolysis was established.

PHOTOTHERAPY

The next major advances in the management of neonatal jaundice involved prevention of isoimmunization and a simpler method to reduce the peak serum bilirubin concentration—phototherapy. Although Native Americans had long been aware of the beneficial effects of the sun in reducing the yellow color of babies exposed to its light, phototherapy for neonatal hyperbilirubinemia was first proposed in 1958 by Cremer and colleagues in England. Subsequently this therapy has been used for the reduction of elevated serum bilirubin levels and for the "prophylactic" prevention of hyperbilirubinemia in premature infants. With the development of Rh-immune globulins to prevent maternal isoimmunization and the introduction of phototherapy, the need for exchange transfusions in healthy term babies was reduced significantly.

The progress in preventing maternal-fetal blood group incompatibility and in reducing bilirubin concentration coincided with the development of neonatology as a specialty and the ability to rescue sick premature babies. Kernicterus was reappearing in the autopsies of sick low-birth-weight infants, particularly in those with severe respiratory distress, acidosis, and sepsis. It was evident in neonates whose serum bilirubin level was never elevated to the extremes reported earlier, suggesting that bilirubin toxicity in low-birth-weight babies might be in some way different from that in full-term infants with erythroblastosis fetails. Even though kernicterus is mainly seen in premature babies with respiratory distress, acidosis, and moderately elevated bilirubin levels, the same questions are being asked as they were decades earlier.

UNCONJUGATED HYPERBILIRUBINEMIAS

In a recent review of 88,000 live born infants in Melbourne, Australia, from 1971 to 1989, it was determined that 12.4% of all the infants had hyperbilirubinemia, defined as total bilirubin levels over 9 mg/dL. Correlates of jaundice were determined in 32% of the infants. Most often these were prematurity (20%) followed by isoimmunization (7%), with sepsis, bruising, and glucose-6-phosphate dehydrogenose (G6PD) deficiency accounting for less than 2% each. Of the infants defined as having hyperbilirubinemia, the maximum levels exceeded 20 mg/dL in 2% (212 of 10,944), representing 0.25% of all the births. Nearly 60% of these infants had some determined cause of jaundice, with the hemolysis of isoimmunization (54 of 212) being the most common identifiable cause of the severe hyperbilirubinemia. The largest single group with high bilirubin levels, however, comprised babies with no known cause of jaundice (90 of 212).

In the newborn period, unconjugated hyperbilirubinemia is common, multifactoral, and associated with a variety of physiologic and pathologic conditions.

EXCESSIVE PRODUCTION OF BILIRUBIN (HEMOLYSIS)
Rh Isoimmunization

The most common identified pathologic cause leading to hyperbilirubinemia is hemolytic disease of the newborn. The first understanding of hemolytic disease in the newborn resulted from the studies of erythroblastosis fetalis resulting from presence of Rh antibody. The Rh antibody in the mother is produced in response to the presence of Rh antigen of the fetal red blood cell membrane. Initially, maternal response to this antigenic stimulus is production of IgM antibodies, which do not cross the placenta in significant amounts. Later, IgG antibodies are formed which cross into the fetus and attach to antigenic sites on the red blood cell membrane. Although small volumes of fetal red cells may enter the maternal circulation throughout pregnancy, the major sensitizing event is delivery, during which a greater amount of fetal blood may enter the maternal circulation. For this reason, blood group incompatibility is less likely to cause hemolysis or hyperbilirubinemic complications with the first pregnancy. Mothers are frequently sensitized by transplacental hemorrhage of only 0.5 mL, an amount not uncommon in active labor or during obstetric complications or procedures such as amniocentesis and therapeutic abortions. The development of maternal sensitization can be identified by the *indirect antiglobulin (Coombs) reaction in the mother,* which identifies the presence of IgG antibody in her circulation or from spectrophotometric examination of amniotic fluid. Because the placenta efficiently transports bilirubin to the mother, affected infants do not appear significantly jaundiced at birth, but the hemolysis experienced may result in severe anemia, hydrops, and intrauterine death. After delivery of the infant, the hemolysis resulting from Rh sensitization may result in rapid development of hyperbilirubinemia reaching levels requiring intervention. Presence of the Rh antigen in an infant is identified by blood typing; isoimmunization, which is the attachment of maternal antibody to fetal red blood cells, can be identified with a positive *direct antiglobulin (Coombs) reaction in the infant*. Red cells coated with maternal antibodies are destroyed in the fetal or newborn liver and spleen, resulting in excessive amounts of hemoglobin being catabolized to bilirubin. The severity of the Rh-induced hemolysis depends on several factors including the antigenicity of the fetal erythrocytes (e.g., males in general are more antigenic than females), degree of sensitization, the specific Rh antigen involved, and the amount of maternal-fetal transfusion. Fifteen percent to 20% of Rh-positive infants born to Rh-negative sensitized mothers show no clinical signs of illness, whereas 25% have severe disease with fetal death, hydrops, or severe anemia at birth.

ABO Incompatibility

Hemolytic disease caused by maternal anti-A or anti-B antibodies reacting with fetal A or B antigens on the erythrocyte surface, a process similar to Rh incompatibility, is more common but generally milder than hemolytic disease caused by Rh incompatibility. This condition occurs almost exclusively in type O mothers, in that the relevant antibodies produced by A mothers or B mothers are mostly IgM antibodies that do not cross the placenta. The jaundice of ABO heterospecificity usually appears within the first 24 to 72 hours after birth, later than that of Rh incompatibility.

Minor Blood Group Incompatibility

Traditionally, less than 2% of infants with hemolytic disease have isoimmunization caused by minor blood group antibodies. However, because the cases resulting from Rh incompatibility have dramatically declined since the use of blocking antibodies (Rho-GAM) was instituted, there is a higher percentage of contribution from minor blood group incompatibilities.

Red Blood Cell Enzyme Abnormalities

Congenital nonspherocytic hemolytic anemia has been associated with a group of red blood cell enzymopathies that result in chronic spontaneous hemolysis of early onset that persists throughout life. In the newborn period, marked hyperbilirubinemia can occur as a result of the severe hemolysis. The two most studied of these defects, G6PD deficiency and pyruvate kinase (PK) deficiency, may be associated with hemolytic anemia and jaundice even in the absence of a recognized trigger agent or event in the neonatal period.

Glucose-6-Phosphate-Dehydrogenase Deficiency

G6PD deficiency is a sex-linked recessive trait whose occurrence in several forms has a geographic distribution, with increased prevalence in African, Mediterranean, and Asian regions. Some of the clinical manifestations of this condition, such as favism and hemolytic reactions to certain drugs, were well recognized long before the deficiency of the enzyme was recognized. Although severe neonatal jaundice is the most common clinical manifestation of G6PD deficiency, the relationship between hyperbilirubinemia and the hemolytic anemia was recognized only when the enzyme deficiency was identified in the late 1950s. Since then, it has become apparent that the situation in the neonatal period is special, because severe jaundice rather than the anemia may predominate in the clinical presentation. Moreover, severe neonatal jaundice develops apparently spontaneously in some G6PD-deficient babies. G6PD-deficient red cells cannot activate the pentose phosphate metabolic pathway and therefore they are unable to defend adequately against oxidant stresses. Because of this phenomenon, severe hyperbilirubinemia can result from hemolysis associated with sepsis, exposure to chemicals such as naphtha in mothballs, or administration of pharmaceutical agents. Even though some of these agents and stresses have received public attention, others represent generally unsuspected dangers, such as the intramuscular injection of vitamin K analogues (but not when vitamin K_1 oxide is administered orally), or the inhalation of paradichlorobenzene, which is used in many countries in moth repellents, car and carpet fresheners, and bathroom deodorizers. Exposure of the newborn to a hemolytic agent can occur transplacentally, via breast milk, or directly by inhalation, ingestion, or injection.

Understanding of the processes leading to the clinical manifestations of G6PD deficiency has come from studies examining the intracellular events following exposure of red blood cells to naphthoquinones. In these studies, oxidation of hemoglobin to methemoglobin and Heinz body formation and growth stimulating hormone depletion were described even in normal erythrocytes. All these phenomena are exaggerated in red blood cells deficient in G6PD, because the pentose phosphate pathway is essential to the defense against such oxidative stress. The data in these studies suggest that neonates with G6PD deficiency may be particularly susceptible to the hemolytic action of vitamin K analogues.

Different genetic forms of the enzyme deficiency have characteristic risks, with the Mediterranean region exhibiting a more severe type of deficiency, called Gd^{Mediterranean}, than the type found in West Africa, termed Gd A−. The initial association between G6PD deficiency and neonatal hyperbilirubinemia and kernicterus was reported from Greece. Reports from other Mediterranean countries followed. A similar relationship between G6PD deficiency and hyperbilirubinemia was reported in neonates in China and in ethnic groups of other east Asian countries, and it appears that the Asian forms of this condition have a severe reduction in enzyme activity similar to the Mediterranean forms. Reports from Africa associating G6PD deficiency of the Gd A− type with neonatal hyperbilirubinemia and kernicterus in infants in Nigeria, Senegal, Ghana, and South Africa were significant because the earlier reports had suggested that only the Gd^{Mediterranean} form of the enzyme deficiency was severe enough to cause kernicterus. Early reports suggesting that black infants with G6PD deficiency exhibit no increased incidence or severity of hemolysis and jaundice have been shown to be incorrect, although their enzyme deficiency, the GD A− form of the disease, is less severe than the others. The susceptibility to hemolysis is not dependent only on the level of enzyme deficiency but also on the amount of oxidant stress or degree of exposure to an offending agent. Normal erythrocytes can be similarly affected if the stress or exposure is severe enough.

Between 200 and 400 million people are estimated to carry the G6PD deficiency gene. In Greece, for example, the prevalence is estimated at 2% to 4%. Even though the distribution of this genetic trait has historically been centered in the tropics where malaria has flourished, several centuries of migration have led to worldwide dissemination of the gene. Therefore, physicians in all countries need to be familiar with the clinical manifestations and risks of G6PD deficiency.

Severe jaundice develops in approximately 5% of Caucasian or Asian infants with this disorder, usually after 24 to 48 hours of life and sometimes only after some trigger event. Maximum bilirubin level is reached between the 3rd and 5th days of life after exposure to a triggering agent or event.

Also, red cells deficient in G6PD are unable to reduce methylene blue to leukomethylene blue; therefore, exposure to even normally acceptable levels of methylene blue causes hemolytic anemia and hyperbilirubinemia when the dye accumulates and functions as a hemoglobin oxidizing agent. Thus, severe hyperbilirubinemia, and even kernicterus, have resulted from the use of methylene blue in patients with unsuspected G6PD deficiency.

Pyruvate Kinase Deficiency

Pyruvate kinase (PK) deficiency is an autosomal recessive disorder occurring uncommonly in all ethnic groups. PK is a key enzyme in the production of adenosine triphosphate in red blood cells. Its deficiency leads to shortened red blood cell survival, resulting in excess hemolysis. Unexplained jaundice in a newborn, with no isoimmunization or no sepsis or drug administration, but with evidence of hemolysis (excessive CO production, anemia, reticulocytosis) raises the possibility of this disorder. Although it occurs much less frequently than G6PD deficiency, this disease represents a classic example of a specific enzyme deficiency leading to a series of events resulting in a major effect on overall health of the individual.

Septicemia

Sepsis is one of the important treatable problems associated with bilirubin overproduction. From the earliest studies of septicemia in newborns, it was observed that 25% to 30% had clinical jaundice early in the illness, sometimes reaching extreme levels. The hyperbilirubinemia in septic neonates is thought to be a consequence of rapid hemolysis, although there are several theories regarding the mechanism of occurrence. Neonatal erythrocytes are susceptible to cell injury and Heinz body formation in response to oxidative stress. In addition, heme oxygenase (HO) is known to be induced by oxidants, and its induction could lead to increased catabolism of heme to bilirubin. Unstable hemoglobins are known to precipitate to form Heinz bodies when exposed to certain chemicals (e.g. methylene blue), resulting in production of erythrocytes that tend to lyse. It is possible that some aspect of sepsis has similar effects.

Recent data suggest that bilirubin is a protective antioxidant and that initially in infection bilirubin levels may be decreased as a result of its consumption. However, the predominant view that sepsis results commonly in hyperbilirubinemia suggests that this protective mechanism is overwhelmed in septicemia, which manifests with increased levels of unconjugated bilirubin.

Red Blood Cell Membrane Defects
Hereditary Spherocytosis

Hereditary spherocytosis is characterized by spherocytic erythrocytes that are abnormally fragile under osmotic stress. This condition is inherited as a mendelian dominant trait, but in 10% to 25% of cases, neither parent is found to have spherocytes.

Jaundice develops in approximately 50% of infants with spherocytes and is usually misdiagnosed as physiologic jaundice. Because isoimmunization is not involved as an etiologic factor, the direct Coombs test in the infant is negative. The diagnosis is made by examination of a peripheral smear of blood and recognition of the abnormal shape of erythrocytes. Red cell fragility tests are also abnormal.

Hereditary Elliptocytosis

Even less common than hereditary spherocytosis is hereditary elliptocytosis, which usually is found as a red blood cell morphologic abnormality without significant anemia.

However, occasionally in homozygous individuals, there is enough hemolysis resulting from increased osmotic fragility to cause hyperbilirubinemia. The peripheral smear in these cases demonstrates many budding erythrocytic forms similar to those seen in pyropoikilocytosis.

Extravascular Blood

Blood that has been swallowed or that remains entrapped after a hemorrhagic event commonly leads to hyperbilirubinemia because of the excess bilirubin production resulting from the breakdown of hemorrhagic red blood cells. The common sites for such substantial collections of blood in term infants are cephalhematomas and the space beneath the galeal aponeurosis. Intracranial hemorrhages are more frequent in ill premature infants, and they may be more subtle than other sites of blood sequestration.

Polycythemia

Because neonatal erythrocytes have a shorter life span and increased fragility compared with those of older infants and children, any excess in the number or concentration of erythrocytes at birth can be associated with increased heme degradation and bilirubin production. For this reason, any baby who is plethoric or polycythemic runs some risk of development of hyperbilirubinemia. Because polycythemia is regularly associated with newborns with specific clinical entities (e.g., trisomy 21, maternal diabetes), these entities are associated with increased risks of neonatal jaundice.

Infants of diabetic mothers have factors, in addition to polycythemia, that may contribute to their risk for hyperbilirubinemia. For example, hypoglycemia can be associated with high levels of unconjugated bilirubin. In this instance, the cause is not excess bilirubin production, but rather limitation of conjugation. Glucose is a substrate that participates in the synthesis of the bilirubin–glucuronide conjugate; its absence may reduce the capacity to conjugate bilirubin, accentuating jaundice in young infants.

Hypothyroidism

Congenital hypothyroidism can be accompanied by prolonged hyperbilirubinemia (unconjugated), presumably on the basis of delay in maturation of the bilirubin conjugating enzymes. First recognized in 1954, this association has been documented in approximately 10% of all newborns with hypothyroidism. Several mechanisms may be involved in this process because only a portion of hypothyroid patients with jaundice demonstrate rapid resolution of the problem after hormonal therapy. Clinically a similar picture is seen in infants with congenital hypopituitarism, although this condition is much less common than hypothyroidism.

CHAPTER 11

Hematologic System

HEMOSTATIC DISORDERS IN NEWBORNS

HEMORRHAGIC DISORDERS

All infants with clinically significant bleeding should be evaluated for a hemostatic deficit. Although acquired problems are more frequent, severe forms of congenital factor deficiencies often first present in early infancy and should be seriously considered in otherwise healthy infants. Evaluation of any infant with hemorrhagic complications includes a careful history of family bleeding problems, outcome of previous pregnancies, maternal illnesses (especially infections), drug administration (maternal and neonatal), and documentation that vitamin K (VK) was given at birth.

Simple observations on physical examination, such as localized versus diffuse bleeding and healthy or sick appearance of the infant, have tremendous importance for the classification of hemorrhagic disorders. Healthy infants frequently have petechiae over presenting parts secondary to venous congestion and the trauma of delivery. These petechiae are seen shortly after birth but gradually disappear and are not associated with bleeding. Infants with isolated platelet disorders generally appear healthy except for progressive petechiae, ecchymoses, and mucosal bleeding. Hemorrhages due to VK deficiency or inherited coagulation defects characteristically occur in apparently healthy children with large ecchymoses or localized bleeding (large cephalhematomas, umbilical cord bleeding, or gastrointestinal hemorrhage). Bleeding due to disseminated intravascular coagulation (DIC) or liver injury is generally seen in sick infants with diffuse bleeding from several sites.

The clinical presentation of bleeding disorders differs in newborns compared with children or adults. Severe congenital factor deficiencies commonly present with bleeding from the umbilicus, from mucous membranes, following circumcision, from peripheral blood sampling sites, into the scalp forming large cephalhematomas, and into the skin. Hemarthrosis, a common presentation of severe congenital factor deficiencies in older children, rarely occurs in newborns. A small but important proportion of infants presents with an intracranial hemorrhage as the first manifestation of their bleeding tendency.

In otherwise healthy infants, the most common causes of bleeding are thrombocytopenia secondary to transplacental passage of a maternal antiplatelet antibody, VK deficiency, and less commonly, a congenital coagulation factor deficiency. Although sick infants may have an underlying congenital deficit, acquired disorders such as DIC and liver failure are more common.

The initial laboratory evaluation of infants with bleeding complications should include a prothrombin time (PT), activated partial thromboplastin time (APTT), thrombin clotting time (TCT), fibrinogen level, platelet count, and on rare occasion, a bleeding time. Abnormalities in these tests usually guide the selection of additional tests such as specific factor assays and paracoagulation tests. For a male child in whom hemophilia A or B is suspected, specific factor assays should be performed regardless of the APTT value. Deficiencies of FXIII and alpha$_2$-antiplasmin (α_2-AP) do not prolong the screening tests and must be measured directly if they are suspected. Differentiation of congenital and acquired deficiencies from physiologic values can be difficult for some coagulation proteins, a problem unique to newborns.

The appropriate management of an infant with a hemorrhagic disorder is dependent on the current identification of the hemostatic defect. Options for replacement therapy consist of specific factor concentrates, fresh-frozen plasma, stored plasma, platelet concentrates, and cryoprecipitate. Other problems to consider are technical access, particularly if an exchange transfusion is planned, and the risk of graft-versus-host disease.

Congenital Factor Deficiencies

For most congenital coagulation factor deficiencies, both a severe and a milder form occur. Most of the genetic coagulation disorders that present in newborns are the sex-linked defects, FVII (hemophilia A) and FIX deficiency (hemophilia B). Factors II, VII, V, and XI, are rare, autosomal inherited disorders, with consanguinity present in many families. Combined deficiencies of FII, FVII, FIX, and FX; or FV and FVIII are extremely rare but frequently present in the neonatal period. Prenatal diagnosis of most congenital factor deficiencies is available at a molecular level.

An otherwise healthy newborn with unexplained bleeding should be carefully investigated for a severe congenital coagulation factor deficiency. The most common sites of bleeding include circumcision, umbilical, intracranial hemorrhage (ICH), scalp, and peripheral heel sticks. Massive bleeding may occur, resulting in concurrent DIC, which can mask the underlying factor deficiency. Full-term infants with unexplained ICH should be carefully evaluated for congenital or acquired hemostatic defects. All severe congenital coagulation protein deficiencies can present with ICH at birth. The widespread use of ultrasonography during pregnancy has resulted in the detection of ICH in utero and has provided a safe modality for monitoring fetuses at risk. In utero factor replacement also has been accomplished in a few infants.

The diagnosis of a previously unexpected inherited coagulation protein deficiency is usually initiated by abnormal coagulation screening tests and completed by subsequent specific factor assays. Plasma concentrations of any coagulation protein must be interpreted in the context of age-specific physiologic values. Severe deficiencies of FV, FVIII,

FIX, and FXIII result in levels less than 0.01 U/mL, which are easily distinguishable from physiologic values. In contrast, homozygous deficiencies of FII, FX, and FXI are defined by levels less than 0.20, 0.10, and 0.15 U/mL, respectively, which all overlap with physiologic levels. Although it seems probable that patients with severe factor deficiencies would have values outside the physiologic range, this has not been confirmed.

The fundamental principle of treatment in the presence of active bleeding or a planned hemostatic challenge is to increase the plasma concentration of the deficient coagulation protein to a minimal hemostatic level. A minimal hemostatic level of a particular coagulation protein varies and is dependent on the protein and the nature of the hemostatic challenge.

ACQUIRED HEMOSTATIC DISORDERS
Disseminated Intravascular Coagulation

Historically, the term *disseminated intravascular coagulation (DIC)* has referred to diffuse fibrin deposition in the microvasculature. Subsequently, a relationship among fibrin deposition, clinical bleeding, and decreased concentrations of some coagulation factors was observed. Currently, the term *DIC* includes patients with in vivo activation of the coagulation and fibrinolytic systems as detected by sensitive assays of thrombin and plasmin generation.

DIC is not a primary diagnosis but a secondary process related to a variety of primary disease states. Common etiologies in the neonatal period include asphyxia and shock (usually related to pathologic disorders involving the fetal-placental unit), infection, hypothermia, meconium aspiration, and disorders related to prematurity.

Unlike bleeding due to VK deficiency or inherited factor deficiencies, DIC occurs in sick infants, most commonly premature infants. The clinical spectrum of DIC is changing, reflecting the ever-improving perinatal care of sick infants. Intensity and duration of activation of the hemostatic system, degree of impaired blood flow, and liver function all influence the clinical severity of DIC. In the past, infants who clinically manifested hemorrhagic or thrombotic complications from DIC frequently died. Currently, most infants with DIC survive, and for some, DIC is of little immediate clinical significance.

The laboratory diagnosis of severe DIC is characterized by prolonged PT and APTT, depletion of certain coagulation factors (fibrinogen, FV, FVIII), increased fibrin degradation products (FDPs), thrombocytopenia, and a microangiopathic hemolytic anemia. Pathologic decreases in fibrinogen FV and FVIII are readily identifiable because physiologic concentrations of these proteins at birth are similar to those of adult values. In practice, no single laboratory test can be used to confirm or exclude DIC.

The cornerstone of management of DIC remains the successful treatment of the underlying problem. The decision to treat the hemostatic disorder is often difficult to make. In the absence of clinical manifestations, newborns probably do not require therapy for the hemostatic disorder itself. In the presence of clinically significant bleeding, therapeutic intervention with plasma products is indicated and often improves hemostasis. For infants between these two ends of the spectrum, treatment is dictated by the severity of the hemostatic impairment and the underlying problem. In general, the more pronounced the laboratory abnormalities, the greater the risk of bleeding or thrombotic complications. The argument that replacement therapy may "fuel the fire" is theoretical and not proven to occur.

Therapeutic interventions in infants with DIC include fresh-frozen plasma, cryoprecipitate, factor concentrates (i.e., antithrombin concentrates and prothrombin complex concentrates [PCCs]), anticoagulants, and exchange transfusions. Fresh-frozen plasma is extensively used because it contains all the coagulation proteins present in adult concentrations. Cryoprecipitate provides high concentrations of fibrinogen and FVIII, two proteins that are frequently depleted in DIC. Exchange transfusions are occasionally used in severe DIC, but their effects are transient unless the underlying problem resolves. PCCs have been used in newborns but are not generally recommended because of the potential thrombotic and infectious side effects.

Respiratory Distress Syndrome

In 1999 neither fibrinolytic agents or anticoagulants can be recommended for the treatment of respiratory distress syndrome (RDS). However, the biology of RDS and the results of early clinical trials support further investigation with antithrombotic agents in neonatal RDS.

Vitamin K Deficiency

The discovery of VK and its important role in hemostasis was intertwined with the role of VK in the treatment and subsequent prevention of hemorrhagic disease of the newborn (HDN). HDN consists of bleeding from multiple sites in otherwise healthy infants in the absence of trauma, asphyxia, or infection on days 1 to 5 of life. The link between VK deficiency and spontaneous hemorrhaging was first seen in chicks by Dam in 1929. The association between VK deficiency and HDN quickly followed with subsequent treatment of infants with HDN. The original term *HDN* has been changed to *VK-dependent bleeding* (VKDB) because the original term *HDN* included many infants with bleeding from other causes.

Infants are at greater risk for VKDB than are similarly affected adults because plasma concentrations of VK-dependent factors are physiologically decreased. The clinical presentation of VKDB can be classified into three patterns (early, classic, late) based on the timing and type of complications. The classic form of VKDB presents on days 2 to 7 of life in breast-fed, healthy full-term infants. Etiologies include poor placental transfer of VK, marginal VK content in breast milk, inadequate milk intake, and a sterile gut. VKDB rarely occurs in formula-fed infants because formula is supplemented with VK (approximately 4 to 100 µg/L). The frequency of classic VKDB, without VK prophylaxis, depends on the population studied, the supplemental formula, and the frequency of breast-feeding. In the absence of prophylactic VK, the frequency of VKDB ranges from 1.7% to 0.25%.

The early form of VKDB presents in the first 24 hours of life and is linked to maternal use of specific medications that interfere with VK stores or function. The late form of VKDB presents between weeks 2 and 8 of life and is linked with disorders that compromise the supply of VK.

Laboratory tests used to detect VK deficiency include screening tests, factor assays, detection of decarboxylated forms of VK-dependent factors (protein induced by vitamin K antagonists [PIVKA]), and direct measurements of VK. Clinically, a prolonged PT is usually the first laboratory test to indicate that VK deficiency is present.

Most of the controversy concerning the prophylactic use of VK can be explained by the design of the trials and subsequent interpretations. There are two well-controlled studies that assessed the benefits of VK prophylaxis, using clinical bleeding as the outcome measure. Both trials showed a significantly positive result for prophylactic VK administration. In addition, numerous laboratory studies showed biochemical evidence of VK deficiency in infants who did not receive VK at birth.

Further support for prophylactic VK comes from cohort studies reporting biochemical indices of VK deficiency at birth. Population-based studies generally show that VKDB rarely occurs when VK prophylaxis is used, but it does occur when prophylactic VK is withdrawn.

Daily requirements of VK for newborns are approximately 1 to 5 µg/kg of body weight. Recommendations for VK prophylaxis are similar in most countries and consist of a single dose of 0.5 to 1 mg intramuscularly or an oral dose of 2 to 4 mg at birth, with subsequent dosing for breast-fed infants.

Certain risk groups require, in addition to general prophylaxis at birth, further VK prophylaxis (i.e., infants with alpha$_1$-antitrypsin deficiency, chronic diarrhea, cystic fibrosis, or celiac disease). Pregnant women receiving oral anticonvulsant therapy should receive about 5 mg of VK daily during the third trimester to prevent overt VK deficiency in their infants at birth.

An infant suspected of having VKDB should be treated immediately with VK pending laboratory confirmation. VK should not be given intramuscularly to infants with VKDB, because large hematomas may form at the site of the injection. The absorption of subcutaneous VK is rapid, and its effect is only slightly slower than systematically administered VK. Intravenous VK should be given slowly because it may induce an anaphylactoid reaction. Infants with major bleeding secondary to VK deficiency should also be treated with plasma products to rapidly increase levels of VK-dependent proteins. Plasma is the product of choice for treatment of a non–life-threatening hemorrhagic event, and PCCs should be considered for life-threatening bleeding.

THROMBOTIC DISORDERS
Congenital Prethrombotic Disorders

Patients with single gene defects for recognized inherited prethrombotic disorders rarely present with their first thromboembolic event during infancy, unless there is another pathologic event that unmasks the defect. In contrast, patients who are homozygotes or double heterozygotes for a congenital prethrombotic disorder usually present in the neonatal period.

Homozygous Prethrombotic Disorders

The classic clinical presentation of homozygous protein C–protein S deficiency consists of cerebral and ophthalmic damage that occurred in utero, purpura fulminans within hours or days of birth, and, on rare occasions, large-vessel thrombosis. Purpura fulminans is an acute, lethal syndrome of DIC with rapidly progressive hemorrhagic necrosis of the skin due to dermal vascular thrombosis. The skin lesions start as small ecchymotic sites that increase in a radial fashion, become purplish black with bullae, and then necrotic and gangrenous. The lesions occur mainly on the extremities but can occur on the buttocks, abdomen, scrotum, and scalp. They also occur at pressure points, at sites of previous punctures, and at previously affected sites. Affected infants also have severe DIC with secondary hemorrhagic complications.

The diagnosis of infants with homozygous protein C/S deficiency depends on the appropriate clinical picture, a protein C/S level that is usually undetectable, a heterozygous state in the parents and, ideally, the identification of the molecular defect. The presence of very low levels of protein C/S in the absence of clinical manifestations and family history cannot be considered diagnostic because physiologic plasma levels can be as low as 0.12 U/mL. Homozygous forms of antithrombin or heparin cofactor II (HCII) deficiencies have not been confirmed in newborns, but one would anticipate that they would present with severe life-threatening thromboembolic complications.

The diagnosis of homozygous protein C/S deficiency is usually unanticipated and is made at the time of the clinical presentation. Although numerous forms of initial therapy have been used, 10 to 20 mL/kg of FFP every 6 to 12 hours is usually the form of therapy immediately available. Replacement therapy should be continued until all of the clinical lesions resolve, which is usually 6 to 8 weeks. In addition to the clinical course, plasma D-dimer concentrations may be useful for monitoring the effectiveness of protein C replacement.

The modalities used for long-term management of infants with homozygous protein C/S deficiency include oral anticoagulation therapy, replacement therapy with protein C concentrate, and liver transplantation.

Venous Catheter–Related Thrombosis

Umbilical venous catheters (UCs) and other forms of central venous catheters (CVLs) are associated with a significant risk of thrombosis. Based on autopsy studies, 20% to 65% of infants who die with UC in place have an associated thrombus. Short-term consequences of venous catheter thrombi include loss of access, pulmonary embolism (PE), superior vena cava syndrome, and organ impairment, if the catheter is improperly placed (i.e., hepatic vein thrombosis).

Arterial Catheter–Related Thrombosis

Seriously ill infants require indwelling arterial catheters, which incur a risk for thrombosis, regardless of the vessel and type of catheter. Catheter-related thrombosis not only occludes catheters, resulting in loss of patency, but may also obstruct major arterial vessels. In a retrospective examination of approximately 4000 infants who underwent umbilical artery catheterization, severe symptomatic vessel obstruction was observed in 1% of infants. Asymptomatic catheter-related thrombi occur more frequently, as evidenced by postmortem (3% to 59% of cases) and angiographic studies (10% to 90% of cases).

For arterial thrombosis, contrast angiography is considered the reference test. Noninvasive techniques such as Doppler ultrasonography offer advantages, but their sensitivity and specificity are unknown. A review of 20 neonates with aortic thromboses treated in one institution revealed that ultrasonography failed to identify thrombi in four patients, three of whom had complete aortic obstruction.

The sequelae of catheter-related thrombi can be immediate or long term. Acute symptoms reflect the location of the catheter and include renal hypertension, intestinal necrosis, and peripheral gangrene. The long-term side effects of symptomatic and asymptomatic thrombosis of major arteries have not been studied but are probably significant.

A low-dose, continuous heparin infusion (3 to 5 U per hour) is commonly used to maintain arterial catheter patency. The effectiveness of heparin was assessed in seven studies using three outcomes: patency, local thrombus, and ICH. Patency, which is likely linked to the presence of a local thrombus, is prolonged by the use of low-dose heparin.

Renal Vein Thrombosis

Renal vein thrombosis (RVT) occurs primarily in newborns and young infants. The incidence in males and females is similar, and the left and right sides are equally at risk. It is bilateral in 25% of cases. Infants of diabetic mothers are predisposed to venous thromboses.

Presenting symptoms and clinical findings differ between neonates and older patients and are influenced by the extent and rapidity of thrombus formation. Neonates usually present with a flank mass, hematuria, proteinuria, thrombocytopenia, and nonfunction of the involved kidney. Clinical findings suggestive of acute inferior vena cava thrombosis include cold, cyanotic, and edematous lower extremities. RVT results from pathologic states characterized by reduced renal blood flow, increased blood viscosity, hyperosmolality, or hypercoagulability.

The most common coagulation abnormality is thrombocytopenia, which is usually mild, with average values of $100,000 \times 10^9$/L. Coagulation screening tests may be prolonged and fibrin/fibrinogen degradation products increased. Infants with RVT should be evaluated for a congenital prethrombotic disorder.

Ultrasonography is the radiographic test of choice because of ease of testing and sensitivity to an enlarged kidney. Treatment options include supportive care, anticoagulation, and thrombolytic therapy. In the 1990s, there is uniform agreement that aggressive supportive care is indicated. One approach is to use supportive care to unilateral RVT in the absence of uremia and extension into the inferior vena cava. Heparin therapy should be considered for unilateral RVT that does extend into the inferior vena cava or bilateral RVT because of the risk of PE and complete renal failure. Average doses of heparin required in newborns to achieve adult therapeutic APTT values are bolus doses of 75 to 100 U/kg, and average maintenance doses of

28 U/kg per hour. The usual duration of treatment is 10 to 14 days. Thrombolytic therapy should be considered in the presence of bilateral RVT and pending renal failure. Thrombectomy, although a common therapeutic choice in the past, is rarely indicated.

The outcome of RVT has changed from a frequently lethal complication to one in which more than 85% of children survive. Unfortunately, there are no recent studies assessing long-term morbidity, such as hypertension and renal atrophy.

QUANTITATIVE PLATELET DISORDERS

Thrombocytopenia in newborns is defined as a platelet count less than 150×10^9/L and requires investigation but not necessarily treatment. Postnatally, mean platelet volumes increase slightly over the first 2 weeks of life, concomitant with an increase in platelet count.

Thrombocytopenia is the most common hemostatic abnormality in neonatal intensive care units (Table 11–1). Nearly 25% of sick infants develop thrombocytopenia, which is trivial for some infants with a platelet count between 100 and 150×10^9/L. However, in more than 50% of affected infants platelet counts fall below 100×10^9/L and 20% of infants have platelet counts less than 50×10^9/L. The natural history of thrombocytopenia in sick newborns is remarkably consistent. It is present by day 2 of life in 75% of infants, reaches a nadir by day 4, and recovers to more than 150×10^9/L by day 10 of life in nearly 90% of infants. Although mild thrombocytopenia may not be clinically relevant, it is indicative of an underlying pathologic process.

The pathogenesis of neonatal thrombocytopenia can be considered to be the result of decreased platelet production, increased platelet destruction, platelet pooling in an enlarged spleen, or a combination of these mechanisms. Determining the mechanism responsible for thrombocytopenia is important because the risk of bleeding and management is dependent on the mechanism. Increased

TABLE 11-1
Disease States Associated with Neonatal Thrombocytopenia

I. Increased destruction
   A. Immune mediated
       Maternal ITP
       Maternal SLE
       Maternal hyperthyroidism
       Maternal drugs
       Maternal preeclampsia
       Neonatal alloimmune thrombocytopenia
   B. Nonimmune—likely related to DIC
       Asphyxia
       Perinatal aspiration
       Necrotizing enterocolitis
       Hemangiomas
       Neonatal thrombosis
       Respiratory distress syndrome
   C. Unknown
       Hyperbilirubinemia
       Phototherapy
       Polycythemia
       Rh hemolytic disease
       Congenital thrombotic thrombocytopenic purpura
       Total parenteral nutrition
       Inborn error of metabolism
       Wiskott-Aldrich syndrome
       Multiple congenital anomalies
II. Hypersplenism
III. Decreased production of platelets
   A. Bone marrow replacement disorders
       Congenital leukemia
       Congenital leukemoid reactions
       Neuroblastoma
       Histiocytosis
       Osteopetrosis
   B. Bone marrow aplasia
       Thrombocytopenia absent radii
       Amegakaryocytic thrombocytopenia
       Fanconi's anemia
       Other marrow hypoplastic or aplastic disorders

ITP, idiopathic thrombocytopenic purpura; SLE, systemic lupus erythematosus; DIC, disseminated intravascular coagulation.

platelet destruction is the mechanism responsible for thrombocytopenia in most infants. Splenic sequestration contributes to thrombocytopenia in some infants.

The evidence for increased platelet consumption consists of increased mean platelet volumes (MPVs), the presence of megakaryocytes in the bone marrow, and short platelet survivals. Although the MPV is similar to that of adults at birth, it increases by day 7 of life in both thrombocytopenic infants and sick nonthrombocytopenic infants. The increase in MPV parallels a decrease in platelet count, suggesting that increased consumption of platelets occurs in many sick infants. Similar numbers of megakaryocytes are present in bone marrow biopsies from thrombocytopenic infants and nonthrombocytopenic infants. Finally, the strongest evidence of platelet consumption comes from uniformly short platelet survivals in thrombocytopenic infants. Hypersplenism also contributes to thrombocytopenia in some infants.

Increased Platelet Destruction

Increased platelet destruction causing thrombocytopenia can be classified as nonimmune or immune events. For newborns, nonimmune causes of thrombocytopenia include DIC and exchange transfusion. Exchange transfusions and intrauterine transfusions cause thrombocytopenia by a dilutional effect, depending on the amount of blood transfused. After an exchange transfusion, platelet counts increase within 3 days and reach preexchange levels in about 7 days. Increased platelet-associated IgG (PAIgG) or complement causes immune thrombocytopenia. For reasons that are not clear, 50% of infants with platelet counts less than $100 \times 10^9/L$ have increased amounts of PAIgG on their platelets. Underlying diseases for these infants include sepsis, preeclampsia, maternal idiopathic thrombocytopenic purpura, and neonatal alloimmune thrombocytopenia.

Disease States Associated with Platelet Consumption.
Many pathologic states are associated with neonatal thrombocytopenia. Thrombocytopenia secondary to acute and chronic asphyxia is likely the result of concurrent DIC. Mechanisms responsible for bacterial sepsis–induced thrombocytopenia include DIC, endothelial damage, platelet aggregation secondary to binding of bacterial products to platelet membrane, immune-mediated thrombocytopenia, and decreased production due to marrow infection. Mechanisms responsible for thrombocytopenia due to viruses include loss of sialic acid from platelet membrane due to viral neuraminidase, intravascular platelet aggregation, and degeneration of megakaryocytes. Congenital rubella causes thrombocytopenia in 75% of affected infants with platelet counts ranging from 20 to 60 × 10^9/L for the first 4 to 8 weeks of life. For premature infants, thrombocytopenia frequently complicates other disorders such as RDS, persistent pulmonary hypertension, necrotizing enterocolitis, preeclampsia, and hyperbilirubinemia treated with phototherapy. Persistent pulmonary hypertension in newborns may be due to intrapulmonary platelet aggregation and release of platelet-derived vasoactive substances such as thromboxane A_2. Infants with necrotizing enterocolitis are frequently thrombocytopenic with laboratory evidence of DIC. Hyperbilirubinemia and phototherapy are associated with mild thrombocytopenia and short platelet survivals.

Giant Hemangiomas. Giant hemangiomas, or Kasabach-Merritt syndrome, cause a local consumptive coagulopathy characterized by hypofibrinogenemia, elevated fibrinogen-FDPs, microangiopathic fragmentation of red blood cells, and thrombocytopenia. The thrombocytopenia is usually severe, with platelet counts less than 50 × 10^9/L. Approximately 50% of affected infants experience systemic bleeding during the first month of life. Treatment may include glucocorticoids or interferon.

Drug-Induced Thrombocytopenia. On rare occasion, transplacental passage of drugs and drug-dependent antibodies can result in both maternal and neonatal thrombocytopenia. Agents implicated are quinine, hydralazine, tolbutamide, and thiazine diuretics. Recently, heparin has been implicated as a cause of thrombocytopenia (heparin-induced thrombocytopenia [HIT]). If HIT is suspected, heparin should be discontinued immediately, and alternative forms of anticoagulation therapy should be considered if necessary.

Decreased Platelet Production

Thrombocytopenia due to decreased platelet production accounts for less than 5% of thrombocytopenic infants. Etiologies include congenital leukemia, leukemoid reactions in patients with Down syndrome, neuroblastoma, histiocytosis, some viral infections, osteoporosis, and disorders of bone marrow failure. Aplastic disorders include thrombocytopenia absent radius (TAR) syndrome, and amegakaryocytic thrombocytopenia. Infants with aplastic disorders are at the greatest risk of serious bleeding in the first months of life. Neither splenectomy nor steroids are of benefit for infants with TAR syndrome. Platelet transfusions are highly effective but should be reserved for symptomatic infants because prophylactic platelet transfusions could result in refractoriness owing to alloimmunization. By several months of age, increased numbers of megakaryocytes usually appear in the bone marrow and platelet counts increase. A functional platelet defect may be present in some children with TAR syndrome. Isolated amegakaryocytic thrombocytopenia may present with bleeding during the newborn period.

Hypersplenism

Splenic sequestration, demonstrated by decreased recovery of ^{111}In-oxine–labeled platelets, is a contributing cause of thrombocytopenia and is usually mild, with platelet counts ranging from 50 to 100 × 10^9/L.

Clinical Impact of Neonatal Thrombocytopenia

Newborns with consumptive thrombocytopenia are less likely to bleed than are infants with decreased production of platelets. If a platelet function defect is present in addition to thrombocytopenia, the bleeding risk is increased. Choosing a platelet count at which one should intervene, although simplistic, provides a guideline for therapy. Platelet counts less than 50×10^9/L place some otherwise healthy full-term newborns at risk for intracranial hemorrhage (ICH). The importance of "moderate" thrombocytopenia (platelet counts between 50 and 100×10^9/L) in sick premature infants has been controversial. The bleeding time, which reflects platelet number and function, is prolonged in about 60% of premature infants with moderate thrombocytopenia and shortens when the platelet count increases above 100×10^9/L. However, maintaining a platelet count over 150×10^9/L with platelet concentrates did not have a beneficial effect on ICH, although it did reduce blood product requirements.

The management of thrombocytopenic infants depends in part on the underlying disorder. If the infant is bleeding, a trial of platelet concentrates (10 to 20 mL/kg) is indicated. The increased platelet count usually shortens the bleeding time and is frequently clinically effective. Autoimmune and alloimmune thrombocytopenia do not respond to random donor platelet concentrates and require specific forms of therapy.

Alloimmune and Autoimmune Thrombocytopenia

Immune thrombocytopenia should always be suspected in otherwise healthy infants with isolated severe thrombocytopenia. An IgG antiplatelet autoantibody or alloantibody is produced in mothers and crosses the placenta, causing fetal thrombocytopenia. Since the antibody is not autologous, the thrombocytopenia persists only as long as the maternal IgG antibody remains in the infant's circulation. Normally, this would be several months, because the half-life of IgG is approximately 21 days. However, since the antibody binds to platelets, its life span is dependent on the life span of the sensitized platelets and, therefore, can be very short. Therefore, immune thrombocytopenic disorders of neonates are usually short-lived but can cause serious bleeding, making the correct diagnosis and management of these disorders all the more important. The differentiation of autoimmune from alloimmune thrombocytopenia in neonates is critical, since the management and severity of these disorders are quite different.

Neonatal Alloimmune Thrombocytopenia

Neonatal alloimmune thrombocytopenia is similar to HDN and neonatal alloimmune neutropenia. All three disorders are caused by maternal IgG alloantibodies that cross the placenta into the fetal circulation, bind to specific cell antigens, and accelerate the removal of the cell type in question from the circulation. Mothers of infants with alloimmune thrombocytopenia have normal platelet counts and no bleeding history, although they may have previously delivered thrombocytopenic newborns. Maternal IgG alloantibodies are directed against specific paternally derived antigens on the infant's platelets, which are absent from the mother's platelets. The most frequently implicated alloantigen (in greater than 75% of cases) is the Pl^{A1} (Zw^a) antigen, which is present on the platelets of 98% of the general population. The second most common alloantigen is Br^a (Zav^a Hc^a). ABO and HLA alloantibodies are infrequent causes of neonatal alloimmune thrombocytopenia. One potential explanation is that maternal HLA alloantibodies do not enter the fetal circulation in sufficient quantities because they are absorbed by foreign HLA antigens on the placenta.

The clinical presentation of neonatal alloimmune thrombocytopenia is usually severe, isolated thrombocytopenia in a healthy, full-term infant. First-born infants are affected as often as subsequent infants. Minor bleeding in the form of petechiae, gastrointestinal tract hemorrhage, hematuria, or hemoptysis frequently occurs. Of great concern and serious morbidity is the occurrence of ICH in as many as 15% of infants. ICH may occur prenatally as well as postnatally. Hydrocephalus, porencephalic cysts, and epilepsy are a few of the outcomes of ICHs. The severity of bleeding in infants with alloimmune thrombocytopenia may reflect not only the severe thrombocytopenia but also an additional platelet dysfunction caused by antiplatelet alloantibody impairing aggregation by binding to the glycoprotein IIb/IIIa.

The diagnosis of alloimmune thrombocytopenia is based on the clinical presentation and the presence of severe thrombocytopenia with a platelet count frequently less than 10×10^9/L. Confirmation by serologic testing follows; however, specific therapy should be instituted immediately. The serologic testing includes typing the mother to determine which platelet alloantigen she is missing and whether an antiplatelet alloantibody is present in her serum. Not infrequently, no alloantibodies can be detected in the maternal serum. Sometimes, testing maternal serum against paternal platelets detects the alloantibody. Platelet-associated IgG is elevated on the newborn's platelets.

The cornerstone of management of affected infants is the transfusion of washed, irradiated maternal platelets. These platelets can be prepared before delivery if a planned cesarean section is the mode of delivery. Although matched platelets from an unrelated donor may also be used, maternal platelets are preferred because of their certain compatibility, availability, and safety. Most prepartum or postpartum mothers can easily tolerate the removal of 1 unit of whole blood and subsequent reinfusion of their red blood cells. Maternal platelets must be washed to remove maternal alloantibody and irradiated to prevent graft-versus-host disease caused by maternal lymphocytes. Frozen maternal platelets have also been used successfully. Random donor platelets should be used in an infant with significant hemorrhage while awaiting maternal platelets. The infusion of random donor platelets may transiently help the bleeding infant, and the lack of increase in platelet number confirms the diagnosis. Intravenous IgG may also be effective in raising the platelet count in affected infants in the absence of, or in addition to, maternal platelets. Other forms of therapy that have been previously used include corticosteroids and exchange transfusions to remove maternal alloantibody. Such approaches are no longer indicated and probably are not effective.

Autoimmune Neonatal Thrombocytopenia

Newborns with thrombocytopenia secondary to maternal autoimmune disorders present with a milder clinical course compared with that in newborns affected with alloimmune disorders. Usually the mother has idiopathic thrombocytopenic purpura (ITP), but autoimmune platelet consumption can also be associated with other maternal disorders such as systemic lupus erythematous (SLE), lymphoproliferative disorders, and hyperthyroidism. Serologically, the antibody is directed against antigens common to maternal and neonatal platelets. The management of the fetus and infant of a mother with ITP is controversial. First, maternal ITP must be distinguished from the frequent occurrence of mild thrombocytopenia in healthy pregnant women at term. The latter appears to have no adverse effect on either the mothers or their infants and does not necessitate any specific treatment or delivery by cesarean section.

QUALITATIVE PLATELET DISORDERS

Pathologic impairment of platelet function may occur in some pathologic states in both mothers and infants. In mothers, conditions that have been implicated include some drugs, diabetes, diet, smoking, and ethanol. For infants, implicated conditions include some drugs, perinatal aspiration syndrome, hyperbilirubinemia, phototherapy, renal failure, and hepatic failure.

Indomethacin

Indomethacin is an antiplatelet agent used for nonsurgical closure of a patent ductus arteriosus in premature infants. Indomethacin, like salicylate, has a longer half-life in newborns (21 to 24 hours) compared with adults (2 to 3 hours) and probably results from underdevelopment of hepatic drug metabolism, renal excretory function, or altered protein binding. Indomethacin inhibits platelet function in newborns, as evidenced by prolonged bleeding times. Randomized, controlled trials have provided conflicting conclusions on the effect of indomethacin on intraventricular hemorrhage in premature infants.

Maternal Diabetes

The reactivity of platelets from diabetic mothers and their infants is increased, with enhanced thromboxane B_2 production, enhanced platelet aggregation, and a lower threshold to many aggregating agents. The enhanced platelet function in diabetes is associated with an increased synthesis of a prostaglandin E–like material that crosses the placenta and can affect the fetus.

Diet

Alterations in the diet of mothers or infants during the postnatal period can affect newborn platelet function. Increasing the ratio of polyunsaturated to saturated fatty acids in the diet of mothers breast-feeding their infants results in an increased concentration of linoleic acid and enhanced thromboxane B_2 production. Infants receiving a diet deficient in essential fatty acids may have arachidonic acid depletion and platelet dysfunction. Vitamin E functions as an antioxidant and an inhibitor of platelet aggregation and release in humans. There are case reports of vitamin E–deficient infants with increased platelet aggregation that reversed following vitamin E supplementation.

Amniotic Fluid

Amniotic fluid contains procoagulant activity that enhances the generation of thromboxane A_2 by platelets. Infants who develop a perinatal aspiration syndrome have pulmonary hypertension characterized by platelet thrombi in the pulmonary microcirculation. The exact mechanisms leading to persistent pulmonary hypertension in these infants are unknown, although alterations in prostaglandin synthesis have been suggested, in addition to thrombocytopenia, hypoxia, and acidosis.

Nitric Oxide

Nitric oxide prevents adhesion of platelets to endothelial cells and inhibits aggregation of cord platelets induced by adenosine phosphate, similar to results in adults.

CHAPTER 12

Renal and Genitourinary Systems

RENAL INSUFFICIENCY AND ACUTE RENAL FAILURE

Severe perinatal blood loss, perinatal asphyxia, respiratory distress syndrome, dehydration of the extremely immature preterm infant owing to increased transepidermal free water loss, necrotizing enterocolitis, hydrops, septic shock, and the use of certain pharmacologic agents (see later) are the most frequent conditions associated with absolute or relative decreases of intravascular volume or renal hypoperfusion (or both) resulting in the development of prerenal acute renal failure (ARF) in the newborn. In addition, acute decreases in cardiac output during cardiac surgery or placement on extracorporeal membrane oxygenation may also lead to the development of prerenal ARF.

INTRINSIC ACUTE RENAL FAILURE

Approximately 6% to 8% of newborns admitted to neonatal intensive care units have intrinsic ARF with severe perinatal asphyxia being the most common cause. In contrast to in prerenal ARF, the renal functional abnormalities in intrinsic ARF are not immediately reversible. The severity of intrinsic ARF ranges from mild tubular dysfunction to acute tubular necrosis with or without oliguria and anuria and to renal infarction and corticomedullary necrosis with irreversible renal damage. It is of great clinical importance that untreated and sustained prerenal or obstructive ARF can eventually develop into intrinsic ARF.

The term *acute tubular necrosis* has been used interchangeably with ARF. Although extensive tubule injury is a frequent pathologic finding in ARF, acute tubular necrosis should be used only for cases of intrinsic ARF secondary to renal ischemia or nephrotoxic substances in which tubular necrosis is always one of the main mechanisms causing the renal failure.

The course of intrinsic ARF may be subdivided into initiation, maintenance, and recovery phases. The initiation phase includes the original insult and the associated events. The sustained low glomerular filtration rate (GFR), tubular dysfunction, and azotemia represent the maintenance phase. The duration of the maintenance phase depends, at least in part, on the severity and duration of the initial insult. The recovery phase is characterized by the gradual restoration of GFR and tubular functions. Recognition of the different phases of neonatal intrinsic ARF is helpful in the diagnosis, clinical management, and prognostication of the disorder.

Ischemic-Hypoxic Injury

Despite being the best oxygenated organ, the kidney is susceptible to ischemic-hypoxic injury because of the redistribution of its blood flow under pathologic circumstances as well as because of the unique vascular supply of the renal medulla. The presentation and course of the renal damage depend on the severity and duration of the insult. Mild ischemia results in transient loss of renal concentrating capacity owing to the extreme sensitivity of the medullary thick ascending limb to tissue hypoxia. This loss may be difficult to detect, however, in immature preterm newborns with the underlying and developmentally regulated immaturity of their renal concentrating capacity.

The primary cause of ischemic-hypoxic intrinsic ARF is the damage to the renal tubular epithelium resulting in backleak of the glomerular filtrate and intraluminal obstruction with necrotic cellular debris. The latter results in an elevation of the pericapillary hydrostatic pressure in the Bowman space leading to further decreases in GFR. The tubuloglomerular feedback mechanism may also be activated by the compensatory increases in the delivery of sodium and water to the distal parts of the nephron in the unobstructed tubules resulting in a further loss in GFR. In addition, abnormalities in the ultrastructure of the glomerulus and decreases in the total filtering surface area occur. The cumulative effect of these changes in the most severe cases of intrinsic ARF is the complete cessation of glomerular filtration.

The use of some medications, including captopril or enalaprilat and tolazoline, may also lead to the development of ischemic intrinsic ARF in the sick newborn. The angiotensin-converting enzyme inhibitors (captopril and enalaprilat) may induce unpredictable decreases in systemic blood pressure so that renal perfusion pressure drops below the autoregulatory range leading to tissue hypoperfusion with subsequent hypoxic-ischemic damage to the renal epithelium. Tolazoline, in addition to causing systemic hypotension, may also induce severe renal vasoconstriction, which further compromises renal perfusion.

Nephrotoxic Injury

The predominant lesion in nephrotoxic ARF is the damage to the proximal tubule cells. In clinical practice, aminoglycoside administration to the newborn is one of the most common conditions in which such damage can occur. Aminoglycosides inhibit lysosomal phospholipases leading to tubule cell phospholipidosis and subsequent necrosis. Changes in the ultrastructure of the glomerulus also occur. The immature kidney appears to be less susceptible to aminoglycoside toxicity than that of the adult. The clinician must also remember that aminoglycoside toxicity is usually *nonoliguric,* and therefore serial monitoring of serum creatinine values is necessary, especially during prolonged administration of these antibiotics, to detect their potential nephrotoxicity in the newborn. The mechanisms of aminoglycoside toxicity appear to be activated even when serum levels are in the accepted range for toxicity in the newborn. The potential long-term consequences of this observation on neonatal renal function are unknown.

Combined Ischemic and Nephrotoxic Injury

Other medications, including amphotericin B and indomethacin, exert their renal side effects by causing both ischemic and direct nephrotoxic renal injury. Amphotericin B alters renal function by reducing renal blood flow (RBF) and GFR and by directly affecting tubular function resulting in renal tubular acidosis and increased urinary potassium excretion. Although these renal toxic effects are most often reversible, cases of fatal neonatal renal failure owing to amphotericin B toxicity have also been reported.

Severe, although usually transient, nephrotoxicity can occur with indomethacin administration. The potentiation of the vasoconstrictive and sodium-retaining and water-retaining effects of angiotensin II, norepinephrine, and vasopressin by the indomethacin-induced inhibition of renal prostaglandin production is the mechanism of the renal actions of the drug. Because neonatal renal function is more dependent on local prostaglandin production than that of the euvolemic adult (especially when intravascular volume is decreased owing to fluid restriction and increased capillary leak in the preterm infant with patent ductus arteriosus), indomethacin administration is almost always associated with elevated serum creatinine concentrations, decreased urine output, and hyponatremia. In addition, indomethacin may also exert a direct aldosterone-like effect on the distal tubule. Because the renal side effects of indomethacin are mostly transient, some clinicians prefer to wait until spontaneous recovery of renal function occurs while maintaining a restricted fluid intake without additional sodium supplementation. Alternatively, concomitant low-dose dopamine infusion may be used to aid in the recovery from the renal tubular side effects of indomethacin treatment. If severe oliguria and anuria develops in the preterm infant, however, furosemide administration may become necessary to prevent the persistence of the ARF caused by indomethacin. If gentamicin or other nephrotoxic medications are being concomitantly administered, the dose interval of these medications should be prolonged when increases in serum creatinine occur.

A less common form of neonatal intrinsic ARF associated with hypoxia, perinatal asphyxia, or polycythemia is uric acid nephropathy. In such cases, precipitation of uric acid or monosodium urate crystals results in obstruction of the renal tubules causing intrinsic ARF. Because newborns normally excrete more uric acid, they may be prone to the development of uric acid nephropathy if severe and prolonged hyperuricemia develops. In addition, intrinsic ARF, partly as a result of intratubular obstruction, may develop with cases of rhabdomyolysis in severe perinatal asphyxia or with massive hemoglobinuria resulting from intravascular hemolysis. Finally, radiopaque contrast agents may also cause intrinsic ARF, especially in newborns who already have compromised renal function, such as those with congenital heart disease undergoing cardiac catheterization.

TREATMENT OF NEONATAL ACUTE RENAL FAILURE
Prerenal Acute Renal Failure

The approach of diagnosing prerenal ARF with the provision of fluid boluses and diuretic treatment (if appropriate) also serves as the initial management of the condition. Most newborns admitted to neonatal intensive care units with ARF have the prerenal form of ARF and respond to fluid therapy. If systemic hypotension develops despite adequate volume administration, early initiation of dopamine with the subsequent normalization of blood pressure ensures appropriate renal perfusion. Other management goals include the maintenance of normoxemia and normal pH to avoid the recurrence of renal vasoconstriction and to improve capillary integrity as well as the replacement of blood and free water losses as needed.

Intrinsic Acute Renal Failure

Whenever possible, newborns presenting with conditions potentially associated with the development of intrinsic ARF should be monitored closely and, if available, preventive measures applied before the onset of renal injury. In established intrinsic ARF of the newborn, management centers around providing appropriate *supportive care* until renal function recovers. Additional *nonspecific therapy* includes the use of furosemide and dopamine. Although there is no conclusive evidence that the attempt to provide selective renal vasodilation and diuresis improves renal function or prognosis in intrinsic ARF, patients who respond to diuretic management with an increase in urine output early in the course of renal failure are more likely to survive. In addition, the use of these medications may aid in ensuring an appropriate fluid and electrolyte balance. If dopamine is used, it should be started early in the course of the disease and at low doses (1 to 4 $\mu g/kg$ per minute) to avoid unnecessary increases in systemic blood pressure and possible renal vasoconstriction. The combined use of dopamine and furosemide may have a synergistic effect on inducing diuresis even in the preterm newborn. The potential toxicity of long-term and aggressive furosemide therapy, including ototoxicity, interstitial nephritis, osteopenia, nephrocalcinosis, hypotension, and persistence of patent ductus arteriosus, should be taken into consideration, especially in the preterm newborn.

CLINICAL COURSE OF NEONATAL ACUTE RENAL FAILURE

Derangement of glomerular and tubular function may last for up to 3 to 6 weeks in newborns with ARF. In the case of oliguric ARF, recovery is usually heralded by a gradual increase in the urine output over the course of several days and, in some cases, by the appearance of a polyuric phase. The free water and electrolyte losses associated with the polyuric phase of recovery mandate monitoring of serum electrolytes and appropriate replacement therapy with sodium, potassium, and free water if indicated. Serum creatinine and blood urea nitrogen usually start decreasing later in the course of polyuria.

OUTCOME OF NEONATAL ACUTE RENAL FAILURE

The mortality rate of newborns with ARF caused by congenital malformations or acquired diseases is around 50% for the oliguric form, whereas newborns with nonoliguric ARF have a much better prognosis. The long-term sequelae of neonatal ARF include reduced GFR in cases with excessive nephron losses and tubular dysfunction. GFR remains decreased in approximately 40% of newborns in both acquired oliguric and nonoliguric ARF. Newborns with the history of ARF secondary to congenital malformation have the worst long-term prognosis; close to 80% of such infants later develop chronic renal failure.

With regard to renal tubular dysfunction, a permanent decrease in the concentrating capacity owing to injury to the epithelium of the thick ascending limb is the most frequent finding on follow-up. Other abnormalities include chronic hypertension; renal tubular acidosis; impaired renal growth; and, mostly in cases of renal cortical necrosis, nephrocalcinosis.

CHAPTER 13

Endocrine Disorders

DISORDERS OF CALCIUM AND PHOSPHORUS METABOLISM

NEONATAL HYPOCALCEMIA

Neonatal hypocalcemia has been variously defined as a serum calcium level of less than 8 mg/dL, less than 7.5 mg/dL, or less than 7.5 mg/dL and as a Ca^{2+} level of less than 4.0 mg/dL. Under conditions of normal acid-base status and normalbuminemia, the serum calcium level and Ca^{2+} are linearly correlated, so that total serum calcium measurements remain useful as a screening test. However, because Ca^{2+} is the physiologically relevant fraction, in sick infants it is preferable directly to determine Ca^{2+} in freshly obtained blood samples. A precise definition of hypocalcemia, like hypoglycemia, in preterm infants is particularly difficult and is probably best defined with reference to Ca^{2+}.

A useful approach to the classification of neonatal hypocalcemia is by the time of onset. "Early" and "late" occurring hypocalcemias have different causes, usually occur in different clinical settings, and prompt different strategies of evaluation and patient management.

Early Neonatal Hypocalcemia. Hypocalcemia occurring during the first 3 days of life, usually between 24 and 48 hours post partum, is termed "early neonatal hypocalcemia." It is a pathologic exaggeration of the normal decline in circulating calcium that is part of physiological transition to the extrauterine environment. Characteristically, early neonatal hypocalcemia is seen in one of four circumstances, namely, preterm infants, asphyxiated infants, infants of diabetic mothers, and infants with significant intrauterine growth restriction. Typically, in preterm infants, the postnatal decline in serum calcium level is steeper and occurs more rapidly than in term infants, the magnitude of the depression being inversely proportional to the gestation. Many low-birth-weight infants, and essentially all extremely low-birth-weight infants (ELBWs), exhibit total calcium levels of less than 7.0 mg/dL by day 2. However, the fall in Ca^{2+} is not proportionate to the fall in total calcium concentration and the ratio of ionized to total Ca is higher in these infants. The reason for the maintenance of Ca^{2+} is uncertain but is probably related to the low serum protein concentration and pH associated with prematurity. The sparing effect of the Ca^{2+} may, in part, explain the frequent lack of signs in preterm infants with low total calcium levels.

The neonatal parathyroid glands, regardless of degree of prematurity, appear capable of mounting an appropriate physiologic response to hypocalcemia. Hypocalcemia in extremely preterm newborns or infants undergoing cardiac bypass has been shown to provoke increases in intact parathyroid hormone (PTH) levels that are at least as great as those reported in adult subjects during citrate-induced hypocalcemia. Refractoriness to PTH action plays an uncertain role in early neonatal hypocalcemia. A several-day delay in the phosphaturic and renal cyclic adenosine monophosphate (cAMP) responses to PTH in preterm and term infants has inconsistently been reported, suggesting that there might be a maturational delay in response to PTH by the nephron. High renal sodium excretion in preterm infants also probably aggravates calciuric losses. The preterm infant's exaggerated rise in calcitonin may promote hypocalcemia. Currently, there is no convincing evidence that abnormalities in 25-hydroxyvitamin D [25(OH)D] metabolism play a pathogenic role in the hypocalcemia of preterm infants and, like fetuses, even extremely preterm newborns efficiently synthesize 1,25 dihydroxyvitamin D [1,25(OH)$_2$D] if vitamin D stores are adequate.

Infants of diabetic mothers (IDMs) also demonstrate an exaggerated postnatal drop in circulating calcium levels when compared to gestational age controls. The natural history usually is similar to that of early neonatal hypocalcemia in preterm infants, but hypocalcemia sometimes persists for several additional days. Maternal and neonatal hypomagnesemia and low fetal PTH and parathyroid-related protein (PTHrP) biological activity may be causative factors. The greater bone mass with relative undermineralization typical of macrosomic IDMs also may increase the neonatal demand for calcium, producing a more profound and prolonged decline in postnatal serum calcium levels. Similar mechanisms may come into play in the transient hypocalcemia often observed in small-for-gestation (SGA) infants. Hypercalcitonemia, hypoparathyroidism, abnormalities in vitamin D metabolism, and hyperphosphatemia all have been implicated, but none has been consistently found.

Historically, symptomatic neonatal hypocalcemia in IDMs has been associated with the severity of maternal diabetes (White classification) and inadequate glycemic control. Preterm IDMs who have sustained intrauterine growth restriction and asphyxia secondary to uteroplacental insufficiency invariably develop very low serum calcium levels. In recent years, improved metabolic control for pregnant diabetic women has markedly diminished the occurrence and severity of early neonatal hypocalcemia in IDMs. In our experience, healthy IDMs who are able to begin milk feedings on the first day do not require serum calcium monitoring unless suggestive signs (e.g., jitteriness, stridor) occur.

Late Neonatal Hypocalcemia. Late neonatal hypocalcemia, or hypocalcemia occurring after 3 to 5 days of life, occurs more frequently in term than in preterm newborns and is not correlated with maternal diabetes, birth trauma, or asphyxia. Historically, it has been associated with cow's milk or cow's milk formula feedings, but occasionally does occur in breast-fed infants. The entity of "late infantile tetany" seen in infants fed whole cow's milk has become a rarity in the United States with adjustment of phosphorus content in humanized cow's milk and soy infant formulas. Human milk contains 150 mg/L of phosphorus as compared with over 500 mg/L in infant formulas prepared from cow's milk, whey, or soy protein. Therefore, a relatively low-phosphate "humanized" formula preparation is recommended for the first 2 weeks of life for full-term newborns who are not breast-fed, as well as for any infant with hyperphosphatemic renal failure.

The hyperphosphatemia that is a prominent feature of late neonatal hypocalcemia may result from varying combinations of dietary phosphate load, immaturity of renal tubular phosphate excretion, transiently low levels of circulating PTH, hypomagnesemia, or marginal maternal vitamin D intake. The ingestion of a relatively high phosphate load coupled with a low glomerular filtration rate leads to an increase in serum phosphate levels and a reciprocal decline in serum calcium levels. However, the normal response to hypocalcemia is an increase in PTH secretion leading to an increase in both urinary excretion of phosphate and tubular resorption of calcium. It is relevant, therefore, that low circulating PTH levels have sometimes been observed in infants with late neonatal hypocalcemia. Serum calcium levels frequently increase when these infants are placed on a lower phosphate formula and calcium supplements. After several days to weeks, the serum PTH usually increases and the infants are able to tolerate higher dietary phosphate loads. The pathogenesis of this "transient hypoparathyroidism" in late neonatal hypocalcemia is poorly understood. Some of these infants have a persistent or recurrent inability to mount an adequate PTH response to a hypocalcemic challenge and, therefore, may have a forme fruste congenital hypoparathyroidism. In other affected infants, hypoparathyroidism may not be contributory. Maternal vitamin D deficiency also is an important cause of late (and occasionally of an "early") neonatal hypocalcemia. It is investigated by assay of maternal and neonatal serum 25(OH)D levels. A role for maternal vitamin D deficiency role is also implicated by the increased occurrence of late neonatal hypocalcemia in winter and the high incidence of enamel hypoplasia of incisor teeth reported in these infants, which indicates a defect in mineralization during the third trimester of pregnancy.

Low serum calcium and hyperphosphatemia after the first 1 to 2 days should prompt a thorough investigation for underlying cause(s). Hypocalcemia in this setting usually implies some primary or secondary dysregulation of the parathyroid-renal [PTH-1,25(OH)$_2$D] axis, hypomagnesemia, or renal insufficiency. The earlier observations of a universally favorable neurologic outcome in newborns with hypocalcemic or hypomagnesemic seizures (which may be valid for those who have a nutritional cause for the metabolic disturbance) may be less relevant to the neonatal population in whom hypocalcemia or hypomagnesemia from dietary phosphate overload is seldom observed. In this group, neurologic prognosis may be more related to associated medical conditions.

Neonatal Hypocalcemia Associated with Hypomagnesemia or Renal Tubular Acidosis

Hypomagnesemia may produce hypocalcemia by impairing parathyroid function. Hypomagnesemia interferes with PTH secretion and it also blunts the end-organ response to PTH. Depression of serum magnesium levels in newborns is either due to (1) chronic congenital low serum magnesium levels or primary hypomagnesemia with secondary hypocalcemia, or (2) transient hypomagnesemia.

Primary familial hypomagnesemia with secondary hypocalcemia presents in infancy with persistent hypocalcemia and seizures that cannot be controlled with anticonvulsants and/or calcium gluconate. It is a rare, probably autosomal recessive disorder resulting from primary defects in intestinal and/or renal tubular transport of magnesium. The clinical spectrum includes polyuria, hyposthenuria, a moderate degree of metabolic acidosis with an inappropriately high urine pH and a positive urine anion gap, low citrate excretion, renal wasting of magnesium and calcium, secondary renal potassium wasting, nephrocalcinosis, muscle weakness, persistent tetany, seizures, and sometimes abnormal facies and sensorineural hearing loss. The partial distal acidification defect, which is probably a secondary effect of a medullary interstitial nephropathy, can be functionally distinguished from that present in primary distal renal tubular acidosis (RTA I). The serum magnesium is frequently less than 0.8 mg/dL (normal 1.6 to 2.8 mg/dL), and circulating levels of PTH are low despite the presence of hypocalcemia. The administration of magnesium to these infants leads to spontaneous parallel increases in serum PTH levels, serum calcium levels, and renal phosphate clearance.

Transient hypomagnesemia in newborns often occurs in association with hypocalcemia. Less commonly, the serum calcium level may be normal. In transient hypomagnesemia, the decrease in serum magnesium level typically is less severe (0.8 to 1.4 mg/dL) than it is in magnesium transport defects. In many infants with transient hypomagnesemia, the serum magnesium level increases spontaneously as the serum calcium level returns to normal following the administration of calcium supplements. However, in other cases the hypocalcemia responds poorly to calcium therapy, but when magnesium salts are given, both serum calcium and magnesium levels rise.

Treatment

The mainstay of treatment for neonatal hypocalcemia is intravenous administration of calcium salts. Calcium gluconate is preferred over calcium chloride (which, in sufficient doses, can produce hyperchloremic acidosis) or calcium lactate. A 10% solution of calcium gluconate contains 9.4 mg Ca/mL. A constant infusion of approximately 45 to 75 mg/kg per day usually produces a sustained increase in serum calcium level (7 to 8 mg/dL). Bolus infusions are hazardous and only transiently effective.

The risks associated with calcium infusions can be minimized by paying attention to detail. Rapid intravenous infusion of calcium can cause sudden elevation in serum calcium level, leading to bradyarrhythmias. Bolus infusion of calcium should be reserved for treatment of hypocalcemic tetany and seizures. Extravasation of calcium solutions into subcutaneous tissues may cause necrosis and subcutaneous calcifications. Therefore, scrupulous attention to peripheral intravenous catheter sites is particularly important when calcium-containing solutions are infused. Inadvertent intrahepatic injection of calcium through an umbilical venous catheter (owing to failure to reach the inferior vena cava) can cause hepatic necrosis. Rapid intra-aortic infusion via the umbilical artery can cause arterial spasm and, at least experimentally, intestinal necrosis.

For emergency treatment of hypocalcemic crisis with seizures, tetany, or apnea, 1 to 2 mL/kg of a 10% solution of calcium gluconate should be administered over 5 to 10 minutes. The initial serum calcium level may be less than 5.0 mg/dL. Careful observation of the infant and the infusion site is essential, and the infusion should be discontinued if there is bradycardia, or when the desired clinical result is obtained. The intravenous dose of calcium gluconate necessary to stop convulsions is usually 1 to 3 mL/kg. Toxic reactions may be avoided if the maximum intravenous dose of calcium gluconate administered at any one time does not exceed 2 mL/kg; doses above 3 mL/kg should be administered with caution. If necessary, intravenous calcium therapy may be repeated 3 or 4 times in 24 hours to help control acute symptoms.

After acute symptoms have been controlled, calcium therapy should be continued as needed to maintain the serum calcium level above 7.0 mg/dL. In part, the level of serum calcium to be achieved depends on the level of serum total protein, particularly serum albumin. In hypoalbuminemic infants, lower levels of total serum calcium are normally present. In preterm and sick infants in whom the oral intake is limited, 5 to 8 mL/kg of 10% calcium gluconate (45 to 75 mg Ca/kg) may be infused with intravenous fluids over a 24-hour period. The lower dose range is preferred whenever there is hyperphosphatemia. If oral feedings are tolerated, 10%

calcium gluconate may be given in the same daily dose divided into four to six feedings. Alternatively, Neo-Calglucon (calcium glubionate), which contains 23.6 mg Ca/mL, may be given in a dose of 2 mL/kg/day divided into feedings. Oral calcium gluconate is better tolerated by young infants because the high sugar content and osmolality of Neo-Calglucon may cause gastrointestinal irritation or diarrhea. Intravenous or oral calcium supplements are continued until the serum calcium level stabilizes.

In late neonatal tetany, dietary factors and hypoparathyroidism are important, and the goals of therapy are to reduce the phosphate load and to increase the calcium/phosphorus ratio of feedings to 4:1. This can be accomplished by the use of low phosphorus feedings such as human milk or formulas with low phosphorus and reduced iron in conjunction with calcium supplements. These measures will inhibit intestinal absorption of phosphorus. Phosphate binders are generally not necessary. The serum calcium and phosphorus levels should be monitored once to twice weekly and the calcium supplements discontinued in a stepwise fashion after several weeks.

When hypomagnesemia contributes to (or causes) the hypocalcemia, administration of magnesium salts is indicated. Magnesium may be administered intramuscularly as a 50% solution of magnesium sulfate (50% $MgSO_4 \cdot 7H_2O$ contains 4 mEq/mL of magnesium). The suggested intramuscular or intravenous dose of 50% magnesium sulfate is 0.1 to 0.2 mL/kg. Intravenous infusions should be administered slowly with electrocardiographic monitoring to detect acute rhythm disturbances, which may include prolongation of atrioventricular conduction time and sinoatrial or atrioventricular block. The magnesium dose may be repeated every 12 to 24 hours, depending on clinical response and monitoring of serum magnesium levels. Serum magnesium levels should be carefully monitored to guard against hypermagnesemia. Many infants with transient hypomagnesemia will respond sufficiently to one or two injections of magnesium. Infants with primary hypomagnesemia have permanent magnesium wasting and low serum magnesium levels and require lifelong treatment with magnesium supplements.

Infants with normal intestinal absorption who develop late hypocalcemia with vitamin D deficiency rickets usually respond within 4 weeks to 1000 to 2000 IU/day of oral vitamin D. These infants should receive at least 40 mg/kg per day of elemental calcium in order to prevent hypocalcemia because the unmineralized osteoid is able to mineralize when vitamin D is provided ("hungry bones" syndrome). In the various forms of persistent congenital hypoparathyroidism, long-term treatment with vitamin D or its therapeutic natural or synthetic metabolites is indicated.

OSTEOPENIA IN PRETERM INFANTS

Osteopenia in the context of this discussion is defined as radiographic evidence of diminished bone density. Osteopenia is present in rickets, osteomalacia, and osteoporosis. *Rickets* is a disorder of mineralization of the bone matrix, or osteoid, in growing bone; it involves both the growth plate (epiphysis) and newly formed trabecular and cortical bone. Radiographic features in rickets include osteopenia and characteristic findings at the cartilage-shaft junction of growing bones, including an increase in the width of the growth plate, cupping, and fraying. In rickets, the serum phosphorus or calcium level, or both are characteristically depressed, and the serum alkaline phosphatase level is elevated. *Osteomalacia* is rickets that occurs in the presence of little or no linear growth, such as might occur in some preterm infants. Radiologically, osteomalacia is characterized by osteopenia but lacks the radiographic features of rickets at the cartilage-shaft junction. *Osteoporosis* is defined as a state of reduced bone mass per unit volume with a normal ratio of mineral to matrix. Unlike rickets and osteomalacia, in which the primary abnormality is a defect in mineralization, the primary abnormality in osteoporosis is either a decrease in matrix formation or an increase in matrix and mineral resorption. Osteoporosis may not be distinguishable from osteomalacia radiographically because both are characterized by an osteopenia without the rachitic changes at the cartilage-shaft junction. In contrast to patients with rickets and osteomalacia, patients with osteoporosis have normal serum concentrations of calcium, phosphorus, and alkaline phosphatase. In some disorders, histologic examination reveals evidence of both osteoporosis and osteomalacia.

Osteopenia with or without radiologic evidence of rickets at the cartilage-shaft junction is commonly observed between 3 and 12 weeks of age in preterm infants. The incidence and severity of this disorder increases with decreasing gestation and birth weight and are more common in infants with a complicated course. On the other hand, osteopenia usually is not a problem for the low-birth-weight, healthy preterm infant. In osteopenic very-low-birth-weight (VLBW) babies, postnatal bone mineralization lags significantly behind expected intrauterine bone mineralization. Radiologic and biochemical monitoring suggests that the pathogenesis of this disorder is increased endosteal resorption rather than decreased bone formation, that is, it is a high turnover osteopenia.

The clinical findings in preterm infants with osteopenia include a widened anterior fontanel, craniotabes (with the "ping pong ball" sign), bony expansion of the wrists, costochondral beading, and rib or long bone fractures. Respiratory distress (tachypnea) may occur secondary to demineralization and softening of the thoracic cage. Long-term effects of osteopenia in preterm infants include delays in dental maturation and linear growth.

Unlike nutritional rickets in term infants and older children, the osteopenia associated with prematurity is chiefly caused by deficiencies in dietary phosphate and calcium rather than by vitamin D deficiency. Eighty percent of bone mineralization in the fetus occurs during the third trimester when fetal calcium and phosphorus requirements are at least 100 to 120 mg/kg per day and 60 to 75 mg/kg per day, respectively. Diets that are particularly low in mineral content predispose preterm infants to osteopenia and rickets. The greatest risks for phosphate deficiency rickets result from feeding unsupplemented human milk or milk formulas not designed for use in preterm infants, and from prolonged parenteral nutrition.

DISORDERS OF THE ADRENAL GLAND

The differential diagnosis of neonatal adrenal insufficiency is summarized in Table 13–1.

ADRENAL HEMORRHAGE

The large adrenal glands of the newborn are vulnerable to mechanical trauma during labor and delivery. Focal hemorrhage at the junction of the fetal zone and the permanent cortex is a common finding in infants dying of other causes. Minor bleeding into the adrenal cortex may not produce symptoms

TABLE 13–1

Causes of Neonatal Adrenal Insufficiency

Adrenal hemorrhage
Transient adrenal insufficiency
Congenital adrenal hypoplasia
   Primary: X-linked, autosomal recessive
   Secondary: Adrenocorticotropic hormone (ACTH) deficiency
Congenital adrenal hyperplasia
   21-Hydroxylase deficiency (P450 C21)
   11-Beta-hydroxylase deficiency (P450 C11/C18)
   17-Hydroxylase deficiency (P450 C17)
   3-Beta-hydroxysteroid dehydrogenase deficiency (3-HSD)
   20,22-Desmolase deficiency (P450 SCC)
Isolated aldosterone deficiency
   18-Hydroxylase deficiency (P450 C11/C18)
Pseudohypoaldosteronism
Congenital adrenal ACTH resistance
Neonatal adrenoleukodystrophy
Infantile glycerol kinase deficiency

but may be associated with adrenal calcifications noted incidentally later in life. To result in adrenal insufficiency, hemorrhage must involve both adrenals and at least 90% of the adrenocortical tissue must be destroyed. Massive adrenal hemorrhage is an uncommon but life-threatening event. Predisposing factors include large birth weight, prolonged or difficult labor, placental bleeding, and perinatal anoxia. Adrenal hemorrhage may occur in premature infants without obvious trauma. The adrenal may be a site of hemorrhage in infants with sepsis or with primary coagulopathies. In most published series, affected male infants outnumber females by 3:1.

The affected infant may show signs of hypovolemic shock, but commonly presents with pallor, apnea, and hypothermia accompanied by a falling hematocrit and jaundice. A large flank mass may be palpated, more commonly on the right side. In only 5% to 10% of cases the hemorrhage is bilateral. The condition must be differentiated from renal vein thrombosis. In both conditions, there may be azotemia, proteinuria, and hematuria, but in adrenal hemorrhage the hematuria is of a lesser degree. Intravenous pyelograms typically reveal no function on the affected side when a renal vein or artery has been thrombosed. Adrenal hemorrhage typically displaces the kidney downward and rotates it laterally, with flattening of the upper calyces.

Signs of adrenal insufficiency may be subtle and delayed. Even with extensive bilateral hemorrhage, functioning islands of zona glomerulosa cells are generally preserved. Hypoglycemia is a more common finding than is salt loss.

Immediate management is directed at blood and volume replacement. Indications for steroid replacement include bilateral hemorrhage, failure to respond to volume expansion, hypoglycemia, polyuria, hyponatremia, hyperkalemia, or anticipated general anesthesia.

Within 1 to 3 weeks after the hemorrhage, a thin zone of calcification appears at the periphery of the gland. As blood and necrotic adrenal tissue are resorbed, the area of calcification shrinks and assumes the shape and size of the original gland. Such calcification may persist for life. Adrenal function generally improves with resolution of the hemorrhage. Adrenocorticotropic hormone (ACTH) stimulation with measurement of plasma or urinary corticoid responses is indicated after the acute phase of the illness; late adrenal insufficiency has been reported.

TRANSIENT ADRENAL INSUFFICIENCY

In 1946, Jaudon described a series of 14 infants with dehydration, salt loss, and failure to gain weight. All responded to steroid replacement, and in each case it was eventually possible to discontinue treatment without a recurrence of symptoms. Other researchers have reported additional infants with an apparent delay in maturation of adrenal cortical function. Bongiovanni described a premature infant with marked hyponatremia and hyperkalemia and no detectable serum cortisol or urinary corticoids. The infant did well on cortisol replacement, and at age 6 months, following discontinuation of steroid treatment, he showed normal cortisol and aldosterone responses to ACTH. Kreines and DeVaux described a similar course in an infant born to a mother with Cushing syndrome resulting from an adrenal adenoma.

The combination of hyponatremia, hyperkalemia, and polyuria may occur in acutely ill infants under a variety of other circumstances that do not involve adrenal insufficiency. Infants recovering from hypovolemic shock and acute tubular necrosis demonstrate these features, as do infants given furosemide without replacement of sodium. In doubtful cases, one may collect serum and urine specimens during a therapeutic trial of desoxycorticosterone acetate. This agent, given intramuscularly in a dosage of 0.5 mg/kg per day, provides a potent mineralocorticoid effect and does not inhibit pituitary ACTH or interfere with serum cortisol or urinary corticoid estimation. If steroid measurements do not support a diagnosis of adrenal insufficiency and if serum sodium levels do not increase and serum potassium levels decline in response to desoxycorticosterone acetate, then the medication may safely be discontinued.

ADRENAL HYPOPLASIA

In the absence of pituitary gland function, the adrenal glands fail to develop normally. The adrenal glands of anencephalic infants weigh less than 0.5 g at birth, as opposed to normal combined weights greater than 6 g. Arrested development of the adrenals has been attributed to a lack of trophic stimulation of ACTH. Pituitary hypoplasia can also occur in infants without major central nervous system malformations. In these infants, severe hypoglycemia can result in death within the first 48 hours of life. Blizzard and Alberts described a male infant who had, in addition, microphallus and cryptorchidism. The association has been noted in several other cases and probably reflects a lack of trophic hormone stimulation of both adrenals and testes. Prompt glucocorticoid replacement is required.

Adrenal hypoplasia occurs in infants with anatomically and functionally intact pituitary glands. Isolated and familial forms, with either X-linked or autosomal recessive transmission, have been described. Early recognition, cortisol replacement, and prolonged survival have permitted studies of the mechanisms that underlie familial adrenal hypoplasia. The disease is manifested in infancy or early childhood by hyperpigmentation as a consequence of elevated ACTH levels and by hypoglycemia as a consequence of glucocorticoid deficiency. In contrast to congenital adrenal hyperplasia, familial adrenal hypoplasia has no associated excess of abnormal steroid metabolites. Mineralocorticoid production is generally unimpaired. A possible defect might involve the adrenal membrane receptor for ACTH

CONGENITAL ADRENAL HYPERPLASIA

Adrenal steroid biosynthesis requires a sequence of enzymatic reactions. Studies using techniques of molecular biology have demonstrated that the synthesis of cortisol and aldosterone requires only five apoenzymes, some having more than one function. In recent years, complementary DNA probes have been cloned, permitting gene mapping and sequencing of these particular protein products. The disease states in this category have several features in common. Each condition is inherited in an autosomal recessive manner. Thus, multiple sibling involvement is common, and recurrence risk in subsequent pregnancies is 25%. Each, with the exception of 18-hydroxysteroid dehydrogenase deficiency, involves hyperplasia of the adrenal cortex under the stimulus of elevated ACTH levels. In each case, the disorder may be managed well with appropriate steroid replacement.

Clinical manifestations of adrenal hyperplasia depend on the site and severity of the enzymatic block. With a block, precursors accumulate and are diverted into alternative metabolic pathways. Laboratory confirmation of a suspected defect involves measurement of these metabolites. The pathophysiology of all of these enzyme deficiencies is related to (1) the specific enzyme involved and severity of the defect; (2) the amount and type of precursor overproduction; (3) the impact of precursors on differentiation of the external genitalia; (4) the severity of glucocorticoid deficiency; and (5) the severity of mineralocorticoid deficiency.

Deficiency of 21-Hydroxylase

The 21-hydroxylase deficiency is the most common form of congenital adrenal hyperplasia as well as the most common cause of ambiguous genitalia. The incidence of 21-hydroxylase deficiency is estimated to be 1 in 15,000 in whites in the United States and Europe. However, the gene frequency varies in different ethnic groups, and a high incidence of the disorder (1 in 490) has been reported in the Yupik Eskimos of Alaska. The gene that codes for 21-hydroxylation is located on the short arm of chromosome 6 in proximity to the locus of the histocompatibility gene HLA-B and the loci for complement factors C4a and C4b. Knowledge of this genetic linkage has led to the use of human leukocyte antigen (HLA) typing in families with affected individuals for detection of heterozygotes as well as for the prenatal diagnosis of affected fetuses. Newer techniques relying on demonstration of the specific gene defect have been successful in the prenatal diagnosis of 21-hydroxylase deficiency.

Hydroxylation at the C21 position is required for synthesis of glucocorticoids and mineralocorticoids. There are two clinical syndromes of congenital adrenal hyperplasia due to a 21-hydroxylation defect: simple virilization and virilization with salt wasting. In both forms, defective cortisol synthesis leads to increased secretion of ACTH, which, in turn, stimulates the adrenal to produce increased amounts of cortisol precursors, including androgens and androgen precursors. The plasma concentrations of 17-hydroxyprogesterone, androstenedione, and testosterone are elevated in affected patients, and the metabolites of these steroids result in increased urinary excretion of 17-ketosteroids and pregnanetriol. As a result of high levels of circulating fetal androgens, female newborns demonstrate varying degrees of virilization, ranging from mild to severe clitoral enlargement with complete labial fusion and a phallic urethra. Affected males are formed normally at birth. If the condition is untreated, both females and males show progressive virilization during infancy and early childhood with rapid linear growth and skeletal and somatic maturation. In addition to virilization, some infants show signs of salt wasting and aldosterone deficiency with failure to thrive, hyponatremia, hyperkalemia, and ultimately vascular collapse. Salt-losing crisis is uncommon before 6 days of age but occurs in approximately 50% of affected infants between 6 and 14 days of age. Patients with virilization and salt wasting are aldosterone deficient, as reflected by reduced circulating aldosterone levels and increased plasma renin activity. By contrast, patients with simple virilization have normal or elevated serum aldosterone levels and plasma renin activity in the baseline state that increase in response to sodium restriction. The reason for the increased circulating aldosterone in patients with simple virilization is uncertain.

ABNORMALITIES OF SEXUAL DIFFERENTIATION

Most of the known errors of human sexual differentiation can be provisionally explained by genetic or biochemical alterations in sexual development (see the classification scheme shown in Table 13–2).

DISORDERS OF GONADAL DIFFERENTIATION
Klinefelter Syndrome

Klinefelter syndrome is one of the most common sex chromosome anomalies, occurring in 1 in 1000 male births. The 47,XXY chromosome constitution arises during meiotic division in either parent or, less commonly, from mitotic nondisjunction in the zygote and is associated with advanced maternal age. Infants with 47,XXY karyotype as a group have lower birth weights than control subjects and have an increased incidence of major and minor congenital anomalies, especially clinodactyly. Although the testes may be noticeably small during infancy, there are seldom any genital abnormalities, and the diagnosis is seldom made during early childhood. Presenting features in older children and adolescents include low verbal intelligence quotient (I.Q.), behavioral disorders, poor gross motor control, eunuchoid habitus, gynecomastia, and variable virilization. Variants involving 46,XY/47,XXY individuals have been described. In addition 46,XX males occur with an incidence of 1 in 20,000 males. They share the endocrine manifestations of 47,XXY individuals but typically have normal stature. The biochemical basis for this defect is unknown but may involve Y chromosome translocations.

Turner Syndrome and Variants

Turner syndrome is defined as gonadal dysgenesis owing to a missing or structurally defective X chromosome. The 45,X karyotype is associated with a

TABLE 13-2
Classification of Abnormalities of Sexual Differentiation

I. Disorders of gonadal differentiation
   A. Klinefelter syndrome: 47,XXY and variants
   B. Turner syndrome (gonadal dysgenesis): 45,X and variants
   C. Pure gonadal dysgenesis: 46,XX
   D. True hermaphroditism
II. Virilization of the female fetus: 46,XX
   A. Due to maternal ingestion of drugs
   B. Due to maternal overproduction of androgens
   C. Due to congenital adrenal hyperplasia
      1. P450 C21 deficiency
      2. 3-Beta-hydroxysteroid dehydrogenase deficiency
      3. P450 C11/C18 deficiency
III. Undervirilization of the male fetus: 46,XY
   A. Anorchia, or vanishing testis syndrome
   B. Genetic defects in testosterone biosynthesis
      1. Defects common to cortisol and testosterone pathways
         a. 3-Beta-hydroxysteroid dehydrogenase deficiency
         b. P450 C17 deficiency
      2. Defects unique to androgen and estrogen synthesis
         a. 17, 20-Desmolase deficiency
         b. 17-Beta-hydroxysteroid oxidoreductase deficiency
   C. End-organ insensitivity to testosterone
      1. 5-Alpha-reductase deficiency
      2. Testicular feminization
      3. Partial testicular feminization
   D. Testicular unresponsiveness to human chorionic gonadotropin and luteinizing hormone
   E. Maternal ingestion of progestins and estrogens
IV. Anatomic abnormalities
   A. As isolated findings
      1. Hypospadias
      2. Cryptorchidism
      3. Persistence of müllerian structures
   B. Associated with other birth defects

high intrauterine mortality rate. Its frequency is 1 in 20 spontaneous abortuses but only 1 in 10,000 live newborn females. The incidence of 45,X karyotype is increased in the pregnancies of teenaged mothers. The condition should be suspected in female infants with webbing of the neck, edema of the extremities, or coarctation of the aorta. In most infants with gonadal dysgenesis, the external genitalia and internal duct structures are unequivocally female. Half the individuals with 45,X genotype also exhibit renal anomalies, some of which may not be suspected clinically. More subtle findings include low birth weight for gestational age, ptosis, hypertelorism, micrognathia, hypertension, low-set or deformed ears, cubitus valgus, and dysplasia of fingernails and toenails. In the newborn, pleural effusions and ascites that clear spontaneously are not uncommon, and pericardial effusion has been reported. In other affected girls, somatic abnormalities are minimal and the condition is suspected because of short stature, failure of breast development, and primary amenorrhea at the age of puberty. A lack of feedback inhibition in the hypothalamic-pituitary axis by the dysgenic ovary is reflected in elevated serum follicle-stimulating hormone (FSH) and luteinizing hormone (LH) levels in affected infants as early as 5 days of age.

Roughly 85% of the girls with gonadal dysgenesis have a 45,X karyotype. The remainder have either mosaicism or a structural abnormality of the X chromosome. Structural abnormalities include isochromosomes of either the short (XXpi) or long arm (XXqi), deletion of the short (XXp$^-$) or long arm, or ring chromosomes. The diagnosis is thus confirmed by chromosome analysis and banding studies.

Suspicion and confirmation of gonadal dysgenesis in a newborn confers an unusual responsibility on the physician. There is seldom any doubt about gender assignment, because these infants are females. However, their ovaries have in most instances regressed to vestigial streaks by the time of birth. Most of these girls are short and infertile as adults. The parents should be told that their child will be shorter than average and probably infertile and will require hormone replacement at the age of puberty to foster a growth spurt, breast development, and menstrual cycles. However, even though streak gonads are the rule in 45,X gonadal dysgenesis, exceptions have been documented. Primary follicles have been observed in the ridges of some 45,X individuals in adolescence, and this correlates with the rare occurrence of menarche and a variable but attenuated period of regular menses. Moreover, conceptions have been documented in some women in whom extensive karyotypic studies revealed only 45,X cell line in multiple tissues. Some fertile 45,X women may be unrecognized sex chromosome mosaics.

Mosaicism involving the Y chromosome is less common than classic Turner syndrome and produces a wider variety of phenotypes. Infants with 45,X/46,XY karyotypes commonly have ambiguous genitalia. Gender assignment should be in accordance with the expected potential for adult sexual function. Gonads in these individuals generally consists of bilateral dysgenic testis and a contralateral gonadal streak. Either or both gonads may have failed to produce müllerian-inhibiting substance, and there may be a uterus and unilateral or bilateral fallopian tubes. Depending on the extent and timing of intrauterine testosterone production, there may also be well-developed wolffian structures. Short stature and the somatic abnormalities of Turner syndrome are inconstant findings. Dysgenic gonads are predisposed to neoplasia and should be removed at an early age. Hormone replacement at the age of puberty must be concordant with the sex of rearing.

Pure Gonadal Dysgenesis

Pure gonadal dysgenesis is a term applied to phenotypic females with bilateral streak gonads who lack the somatic stigmata of Turner syndrome and who are of normal or tall stature. Karyotype may be either 46,XX or 46,XY. The internal and external genitalia of the 46,XX individuals with gonadal dysgenesis are normal female. The 46,XX patients seldom show clitoral enlargement, may show ovarian function at puberty, and are not prone to gonadal neoplasms. Familial cases are not uncommon in 46,XX gonadal dysgenesis, and transmission is consistent with an autosomal recessive trait. Deafness is an associated finding in some families with 46,XX gonadal dysgenesis. Inheritance consistent with an X-linked or male-limited dominant trait has been observed. Usually, the external and internal genital tract is completely female. However, clitoral enlargement occurs, and affected siblings may have ambiguous external genitalia and development of the genital ducts. Both H-Y antigen–positive and H-Y antigen–negative forms have been described, findings that further reflect the genetic heterogeneity of this syndrome.

True Hermaphroditism

True hermaphroditism is a rare condition that requires the presence of both ovarian and testicular tissue in the same individual. The tissue may be present in the same or opposite gonads. In almost half of the cases there is an ovotestis on one side and an ovary or testis on the other. In one fifth of cases there are bilateral ovotestes, and in one third there is an ovary on one side and a testis on the other. The external genitalia are extremely variable, but roughly three fourths of patients have phallic enlargement, generally with hypospadias, and many have been raised as males. Cryptorchidism is common, and an inguinal hernia that may contain a gonad or uterus is present in about half of the cases. A uterus is usually present and often asymmetric. Genital ducts develop in accordance with the function of the ipsilateral gonad. Most patients with an ovotestis have predominantly female development of the genital ducts. Chromosomal findings are varied and do not correlate with gonadal histology or external genital appearance. Approximately 70% of patients with true hermaphroditism are X chromatin positive. Van Niekerk reported that of 148 patients, 89 were 46,XX, 18 were 46,XY, 21 were XX/XY chimeras, and the remainder were sex chromosome mosaics. All patients with true hermaphroditism are

H-Y antigen positive. The presence of H-Y antigen in 46,XX true hermaphroditism supports the postulate that the structural gene for H-Y antigen is on an autosome and not the Y chromosome. Therefore, an autosomal mutation affecting the structural gene for H-Y antigen results in the differentiation of a testis or ovotestis in an XX individual. However, until the sites of the putative regulatory genes that may affect the expression of H-Y are determined, the pathogenesis of true hermaphroditism in relationship to H-Y antigen remains uncertain.

At puberty, breast development is common, menses occurs in more than half the patients, and virilization occurs in a large number. Although spermatogenesis is rare, ovulation is not uncommon, and pregnancy and childbirth have occurred in several patients with an XX karyotype.

True hermaphroditism should be considered in any infant or child with ambiguous genitalia in whom an alternative explanation cannot be established from chromosomal, hormonal, and radiologic contrast studies. Diagnosis requires laparotomy and biopsy of gonads. Management involves surgical removal of gonads, internal duct structures, and features of the external genitalia that are incongruous with gender assignment.

VIRILIZATION OF THE FEMALE FETUS

Virilization of the female fetus is the most common category of disorders producing ambiguity of the external genitalia. As previously stated, in the absence of androgens, external female genitalia proceed to develop along female lines. Androgens, which may be derived from either maternal or fetal sources, can cause the external genitalia of otherwise normal 46,XX girls to virilize. In some cases, this process is so complete as to mimic the external genitalia of a cryptorchid male. Fusion of the genital folds or the genital swellings is a result of androgen exposure before the 12th gestational week. Clitoral enlargement can occur with androgen exposure at any time. Buccal smears are chromatin positive, and karyotypes are 46,XX. Management of underlying pathologic processes and surgical correction of anatomic abnormalities are followed by normal pubertal development and normal adult sexual and reproductive function.

Virilization by Maternal Ingestion of Drugs

Virilization of the female fetus has been attributed to testosterone, the 19-nortestosterone progestins, progesterone, and even, paradoxically, diethylstilbestrol. In each case, a fairly small proportion of exposed infants had clinically evident virilization. There was seldom evidence of virilization in the mother. It is not known which of these compounds act directly on the external genitalia and which act indirectly through altering androgen synthesis by the mother or fetus. It seems reasonable to speculate that differences in maternal, placental, or fetal metabolism of the synthetic steroids determine which infants are affected.

The incidence of this condition has diminished as the use of synthetic estrogens and progestins for management of threatened abortion has waned. However, the condition is still seen in offspring of women who unknowingly continue to take birth control pills following conception. Severity of virilization ranges from mild clitoral enlargement to complete labial fusion with a phallic urethra. The infant does not show progressive virilization or accelerated growth and skeletal maturation after birth. Even in the presence of a positive history of maternal hormone ingestion, it is mandatory to obtain a buccal smear or a chromosome analysis and a determination of 17-ketosteroids or 17-hydroxyprogesterone to exclude other possible diagnoses.

Virilization by Maternal Overproduction of Androgens

Severe disorders of maternal androgen production generally preclude pregnancy. However, artificial induction of ovulation in a virilized woman or development of a virilizing neoplasm during pregnancy can set the stage for virilization of a female infant. In most cases, the mother has clinical signs of virilization, such as hirsutism, acne, clitoromegaly, and deepening of the voice. Virilization has been observed in a female infant born to a mother with a virilizing form of congenital adrenal hyperplasia. The clinical features of the offspring of virilized mothers are identical with those described previously for girls whose mothers received sex hormones. Diagnosis requires demonstration of elevated urinary 17-ketosteroids or plasma testosterone in the mother as well as exclusion of alternative diagnoses in the infant.

DISORDERS OF THE THYROID GLAND

CONGENITAL HYPOTHYROIDISM

Congenital hypothyroidism has been recognized for centuries and its treatment known for decades, but only recently has the link between early treatment and the prevention of sequelae been proposed. With the emphasis being placed on early screening, many conditions that lead to the syndrome of congenital hypothyroidism have been recognized. The importance of adequate neonatal screening in the management of newborn thyroid diseases must be emphasized. Before the advent of screening, less than one third of the infants found to ultimately have congenital hypothyroidism were given the diagnosis before 3 months of age, and only half by 6 months of age; irreversible brain damage developed in most of these infants.

Newborn screening programs for congenital hypothyroidism are designed to detect elevated serum thyroid-stimulating hormone (TSH) levels in blood samples collected on filter paper. Some programs measure TSH directly, and others measure TSH in samples with low or low-normal thyroxine (T_4) concentrations. In most programs in the United States, an initial T_4 measurement is conducted, and TSH is measured in samples with the lowest 10% of T_4 values. An elevated TSH level (greater than 20 µIU/mL) suggests primary hypothyroidism. Most screening programs are just that, and some infants with hypothyroidism are missed in the screening process. Thus, no infant who presents with signs or symptoms suggestive of thyroid dysfunction should be excluded from investigation on the basis of previous screening results. A determination of serum T_4 and TSH values is necessary in any infant with suspicious clinical or laboratory findings.

Thyroid Dysgenesis

The term *thyroid dysgenesis* describes infants with ectopic or hypoplastic thyroid glands (or both) as well as those with total thyroid agenesis. Thyroid dysgenesis is the etiologic factor in most infants with permanent congenital hypothyroidism detected in newborn screening programs. Some thyroid tissue probably is present in two thirds of these infants, so that they represent a spectrum of severity of thyroid deficiency. A normal or near-normal circulating level of triiodothyronine (T_3) in the face of a low T_4 value suggests the presence of residual thyroid tissue, and this can be confirmed by a thyroid scan. A measurable level of serum thyroglobulin also indicates the presence of some thyroid tissue; athyrotic infants have no circulating thyroglobulin.

Thyroid dysgenesis occurs in 1 in 4000 live born infants and is more prevalent in female than in male infants by a ratio of almost 2:1. Although thyroid dysgenesis usually is sporadic, rare familial cases have been described, and the incidence is increased in infants with Down syndrome. Seasonal variations in incidence have been observed in Japan, Australia, and Canada. In isolated instances thyroid dysgenesis has occurred in association with maternal autoimmune thyroiditis. However, this may be coincidence; there usually is no correlation between thyroid dysgenesis and the presence of maternal autoimmune thyroiditis or circulating thyroid antimicrosomal or antithyroglobulin autoantibodies.

As discussed, most newborns with thyroid dysgenesis are asymptomatic, and few infants have signs of hypothyroidism during the early weeks of life. Most affected infants have low serum T_4 and high TSH concentrations in cord blood or in filter-paper blood spots collected at 2 to 5 days of age. Ten percent to 20% of hypothyroid infants have T_4 levels in the low-normal range with increased TSH values. These infants usually have ectopic functional thyroid tissue on scanning and significant levels of circulating thyroglobulin. Another 5% have a delayed elevation of serum TSH and are missed in the screening process unless a second screening test is done. Again, thyroid function should be determined in any infant presenting with suspicious clinical signs or symptoms. Individuals with thyroid dysgenesis also show abnormalities of thyroidal C cells; calcitonin levels and responsiveness are reduced throughout infancy and childhood. Urinary calcium and hydroxyproline levels are increased, and there is a tendency toward osteopenia, but this seems of limited clinical significance.

Hypothalamic-Pituitary Defects

Congenital hypothyroidism resulting from ineffective TSH stimulation of thyroid hormone secretion can result from a variety of abnormalities in TSH synthesis and metabolism. These include anomalous hypothalamic or pituitary development, isolated or familial deficiencies in thyrotropin-releasing hormone (TRH) or TSH secretion, or TSH deficiency in association with other pituitary hormone deficiencies. Several TSH deficiency syndromes have been described: hypothalamic (tertiary) hypothyroidism with TRH deficiency or pituitary insensitivity (or both), isolated TSH deficiency, familial panhypopituitarism, congenital absence of the pituitary, and panhypopituitarism with absence of the sella turcica. The combined prevalence of these abnormalities associated with congenital hypothyroidism approximates 1 in 60,000 to 140,000 live births.

Transient Congenital Hypothyroidism

Congenital hypothyroidism may present as a transient defect persisting for a variable period after birth. Usually, transient neonatal hypothyroidism is caused by maternal ingestion of goitrogenic substances that reach the fetus via placental transfer. One frequently ingested goitrogenic drug is iodide prescribed in expectorants for the treatment of asthma or as treatment for maternal thyrotoxicosis. The mothers of these infants often have taken large doses of iodide for many years without development of large goiters and have been euthyroid during pregnancy. The fetal thyroid gland is unusually sensitive to iodide-induced hypothyroidism because of immaturity of the mechanisms that decrease thyroid iodide uptake in response to high plasma iodide levels. Urine iodine concentrations in affected infants usually exceed 1 mg/L.

Other substances that have been associated with neonatal goiter include thioureylene (antithyroid) drugs, sulfonamides, and hematinic preparations containing cobalt. Neonatal goiters resulting from antithyroid drug administration are uncommon unless large doses of the drugs are given to the mother (more than 150 mg per day propylthiouracil or equivalent near term). Amniotic injection of radiographic contrast agents used during amniofetography also can lead to transient congenital hypothyroidism.

Maternal-to-fetal transfer of TSH-receptor–blocking antibodies also can lead to transient perinatal hypothyroidism. This condition is rare but has been reported in the newborns of women with either euthyroid or hypothyroid autoimmune thyroid disease. In these infants, TSH-receptor autoantibodies are detectable in maternal and cord blood. These antibodies can be measured either as TSH-binding–inhibiting immune globulins (TBII) or TSH (cAMP) blocking antibodies (TBA). The duration of the hypothyroid state in these newborns is correlated with the initial titer of blocking antibody and the duration of its presence in newborn blood. Transient congenital hypothyroidism must be differentiated from transient hyperthyrotropinemia.

NEONATAL THYROTOXICOSIS

Neonatal Graves disease is rare, probably because of the low incidence of thyrotoxicosis in pregnancy (1 to 2 cases per 1000 pregnancies) and the fact that the neonatal disease occurs only in about one of 70 cases of thyrotoxic pregnancy. In most cases, the disease is due to transplacental passage of thyroid-stimulating antibody (TSA) from a mother with active or inactive Graves disease or Hashimoto thyroiditis. Thus, prediction of neonatal Graves disease from the maternal clinical status is not always possible. However, it is possible to predict the occurrence of Graves disease in newborns on the basis of maternal TSA titers. In one study, all women with TSA titers exceeding 500% of control values (measured by stimulation of cAMP in human thyroid slices) delivered thyrotoxic infants, whereas those with lower titers delivered euthyroid infants. In some infants, both TSH-receptor–stimulating and TSH-receptor–blocking antibodies are acquired from the mother, and the blocking antibodies have been reported to block the effect of the stimulating antibodies for 4 to 6 weeks so that late-onset neonatal Graves disease develops in a previously unrecognized infant.

Graves disease in the newborn is manifested by irritability, flushing, tachycardia, hypertension, poor weight gain, thyroid enlargement, and exophthalmos. Thrombocytopenia, hepatosplenomegaly, jaundice, and hypoprothrombinemia also have been observed. Arrhythmias, cardiac failure, and death may occur if the thyrotoxicity is severe and the treatment is inadequate. Mortality rate approaches 25% in disease severe enough to be diagnosed. In some infants the onset of symptoms and signs may be delayed as long as 8 to 9 days. This is due to the postnatal depletion of transplacentally acquired blocking doses of maternal antithyroid drugs and to the abrupt increase in conversion of T_4 to active T_3 shortly after birth in the newborn. The diagnosis is confirmed by measuring high levels of T_4, free T_4, and T_3 in postnatal blood. Cord blood values may be normal or near normal whereas levels at 2 to 5 days may be markedly increased; the serum TSH is low. Neonatal Graves disease resolves spontaneously as maternal TSA in the newborn is degraded. The usual clinical course of neonatal Graves disease extends 3 to 12 weeks.

The treatment of hyperthyroidism in the newborn includes sedatives and digitalis as necessary. Iodide or antithyroid drugs are administered to decrease thyroid hormone secretion. These drugs have additive effects with regard to inhibition of hormone synthesis; in addition, iodide rapidly inhibits hormone release. Lugol solution (5% iodine and 10% potassium iodide; 126 mg of iodine per milliliter) is given in doses of one drop (about 8 mg) three times daily. Methimazole, carbimazole, or propylthiouracil are administered in doses of 0.5 to 1 mg, 0.5 to 1 mg, or 5 to 10 mg, respectively, per kilogram daily in divided doses at 8-hour intervals. A therapeutic response should be observed within 24 to 36 hours. If a satisfactory response is not observed, the dose of antithyroid drug and iodide can be increased by 50%. Corticosteroids in anti-inflammatory doses and propranolol (1 to 2 mg/kg per day) also may be helpful. Radiographic contrast agents (ipodate, 200 mg/kg per day) also may be useful in treatment either alone or in conjunction with antithyroid drug treatment.

DISORDERS OF CARBOHYDRATE METABOLISM

HYPOGLYCEMIA
Definition and Diagnosis

In adults, brain metabolism accounts for nearly 80% of the total glucose consumption. This value may be higher in newborns in whom the brain represents a proportionally larger tissue mass. Thus, glucose utilization is highest in the preterm infant when compared with term infant and adult values. The rate of glucose utilization in preterm infants is approximately 6 to 8 mg/kg per minute, whereas adult values range from 2 to 4 mg/kg per minute. That the brain is the primary site for glucose utilization and uses glucose as a primary energy source leads to the predominance of neurologic symptoms that accompany hypoglycemia.

There is no consensus defining a blood glucose level diagnostic of hypoglycemia. Earlier data defining hypoglycemia as blood glucose levels of 30 mg/dL in term infants and 20 mg/dL in preterm infants relied on measurements in fasted infants and are probably not valid. Other concerns about the long-term effects of asymptomatic neonatal hypoglycemia have led to efforts to aggressively diagnose and treat this entity. There are limited data correlating the length of the hypoglycemic period with outcome or the relative risk of symptomatic versus asymptomatic hypoglycemia. Because of these concerns and uncertainties, it seems prudent to aggressively screen infants at risk for hypoglycemia and treat those with values less than 40 mg/dL. In most nurseries, this consists of heel stick whole blood determinations of glucose using a commercially available indicator (Dextrostix or Chemstrip). Although useful, these methods have limitations. Low glucose values as reported by the reagent strips tend to underestimate the degree of hypoglycemia present. Values close to those representing hypoglycemia (less than 40 mg/dL) or hyperglycemia (greater than 125 mg/dL) should be confirmed by actual laboratory chemical analysis. Initial therapies, especially in asymptomatic infants, should not be postponed in borderline cases, but continuation of therapy should be based on reliable laboratory glucose values. Because the onset and duration of hypoglycemia is variable in infants at risk, repeated routine screening of these infants should continue until the risk period for development of hypoglycemia has passed. Certain pathophysiologic states (infants of diabetic pregnancies or infants who are small for gestational age) may require screening over several days.

Conditions Associated with Hypoglycemia

Limited Glycogen Stores

Most hepatic glycogen accumulation occurs in the third trimester of pregnancy. Prematurity is associated with decreased hepatic stores of glycogen and thus may predispose infants to hypoglycemia. Hypoglycemia develops in as many as 15% of preterm infants in the first hours of birth. As a variety of other conditions, associated with a risk of hypoglycemia (e.g., sepsis, feeding intolerance, and hypothermia), may develop, there may be additive effects on the duration and course of their hypoglycemia. Because hypoglycemia is so prevalent in preterm infants, routine blood glucose screening while the infant is sick or until feedings are well established is critical. The onset of hypoglycemia after the immediate newborn period in an otherwise stable preterm infant should prompt an evaluation for other associated conditions (e.g., sepsis).

Perinatal Distress

Infants who are stressed in utero or intrapartum are at risk for hypoglycemia. Hypoxia and acidosis lead to increased catecholamine activity, which promotes hepatic glycogenolysis. Hypoxia also accelerates glucose utilization due to the effects of anaerobic metabolism. Roughly 18 times more glucose is required to produce comparable amounts of adenosine triphosphate (ATP) during anaerobic metabolism. There is evidence that neurologic outcome in stressed fetuses requiring resuscitation at birth is improved by early glucose administration. However, others have reported detrimental effects of hyperglycemia in association with or following fetal/neonatal asphyxia. In the absence of better data, euglycemia is the goal.

Disorders of Glycogen Metabolism

Three disorders of glycogen metabolism may present with hypoglycemia in the newborn period. Glucose-6-phosphatase deficiency, amylo-1,6-glucosidase deficiency, and phosphorylase deficiency limit either glycogen metabolism or glucose release, resulting in excess glycogen stores, hepatomegaly, and hypoglycemia. Diagnosis of these disorders ultimately rests on laboratory analysis of biopsy material in children with characteristic phenotypes (cherubic face, truncal obesity, and hepatomegaly). These disorders are inherited primarily in an autosomal recessive manner.

Hyperinsulinism

Infant of a Diabetic Mother. A variety of disorders leading to neonatal hypoglycemia are the result of fetal or neonatal hyperinsulinism. The prototype for this condition is the infant of a diabetic mother. These children are at risk for neonatal hypoglycemia caused by the persistence of fetal hyperinsulinism in the face of an interrupted supply of maternal glucose. Other maternal metabolic substrates (amino acids and lipids) may also play a role in maintaining the fetal hyperinsulinemic state. The fetal hyperinsulinemic state is induced by these abnormal quantities and types of metabolic fuels transplacentally acquired, resulting in fetal pancreatic beta-cell hypertrophy. Hypoglycemia in affected infants frequently occurs 4 to 6 hours after birth, although the coexistence of other complications may impact this timing. These infants also manifest augmented pancreatic beta-cell sensitivity to glucose, which persists for several days after birth, and thus continue to be at risk for hypoglycemia during this time.

The persistent fetal hyperinsulinemia leads to effects on all insulin sensitive tissues, giving rise to the myriad of clinical signs and symptoms seen in these infants. In addition to the disorders of carbohydrate metabolism, these infants are at significant risk for other types of perinatal morbidity. The observed increased incidence of respiratory distress in these infants is the result of many factors; the influences of glucose and insulin on surfactant and pulmonary function have been extensively studied. Affected infants may exhibit all of the manifestations of respiratory distress syndrome despite advanced gestational age or documented amniotic fluid lecithin-to-sphingomyelin ratios of more than 2:1.

The effects of chronic stimulation of insulin and insulin-like growth factor receptors in many fetal tissues including placenta, liver, heart, and adipose tissues may lead to large-for-gestational-age infants with their attendant difficulties during labor and delivery. The increased incidence of intrapartum fetal distress and third-trimester fetal demise may result from placental dysfunction caused by abnormal substrate accretion and decreased diffusion capacity. Perinatal stress may have an additive effect on the degree of hypoglycemia via effects of catecholamines, glucocorticoids, and glycogen depletion. Plethora and hyperviscosity resulting from increased red blood cell mass may further compromise these infants who are at risk of development of venous thromboses. Erythropoietin levels are elevated in the infants of diabetic mothers, but the relative contributions of placental insufficiency, perinatal stress, and insulin to increased red blood cell mass are not well characterized. Hyperbilirubinemia may be present as a result of the increased red cell mass or secondary to placental or hepatic dysfunction. These infants may also manifest hypocalcemia—again, reflecting reduced placental function; hypoxia and perinatal stress probably also contribute to neonatal hypocalcemia in affected infants. A subgroup of infants born to diabetic mothers have marked hypertrophy of the cardiac septum and present with congestive heart failure. The increased incidence of other structural heart lesions may complicate the differential diagnosis of these infants; specific diagnosis is usually confirmed by cardiac ultrasound.

The observed increase in congenital malformations in infants of diabetic mothers led to the hypothesis that alterations in maternal glucose metabolism in the first weeks of pregnancy may cause defects in organogenesis. Insulin does not seem to be teratogenic, but hyperglycemia, hyperketonemia, and hyperosmolality have all been shown to disrupt organogenesis in animal models. Increased attention to maternal glucose homeostasis later in pregnancy has dramatically improved perinatal mortality; the same may be true for early attention ameliorating associated congenital malformations. Transient hypoglycemia may also disrupt organogenesis as well as affect later fetal growth indices; both extremes of maternal hyperglycemia and hypoglycemia are therefore to be avoided.

In certain instances, the phenotype and clinical symptoms of hyperinsulinemic infants are so striking as to suggest the diagnosis of maternal diabetes mellitus. This diagnosis is supported by the finding of increased maternal levels of circulating glycosylated hemoglobin (Hgb A_{1c}). Although glucose homeostasis frequently returns toward normal in the days following delivery in women with gestational diabetes mellitus, Hgb A_{1c} levels remain elevated for weeks after delivery. Because of the impact of this condition on subsequent pregnancies, this diagnosis should be actively pursued in pregnancies complicated by inadequate prenatal care and large-for-gestational-age infants.

Mothers with severe long-standing diabetes associated with vasculopathy or retinopathy (White class F) may give birth to infants who are small for gestational age and prone to all the perinatal complications described.

Beckwith-Wiedemann Syndrome

Infants with the syndrome of exophthalmos, macroglossia, and gigantism often have associated omphaloceles, macrosomia, and neonatal hypoglycemia. This condition is associated with pancreatic beta-cell hypertrophy and hyperinsulinism; the metabolic defect is unknown. Most cases of Beckwith-Wiedemann syndrome are sporadic, but there is some evidence that it may be inherited as an autosomal dominant trait. Early recognition and treatment of the attendant hypoglycemia is likely to improve the intellectual outcome of these infants.

Erythroblastosis Fetalis

Infants with erythroblastosis fetalis complicating Rh incompatibility may also manifest hypoglycemia secondary to hyperinsulinism. Pancreatic beta-cell hyperplasia is demonstrable, but the underlying biochemical defect is unknown. Although unrelated, infants undergoing exchange transfusion for any cause are at risk for hypoglycemia afterward because of the transient stimulation of endogenous insulin by the added dextrose in citrated stored blood products. The insulin response then leads to rebound hypoglycemia as the infused glucose is metabolized. Heparinized blood contains no added glucose, but may lead to hypoglycemia owing to limited substrate availability during a double-volume exchange procedure.

Maternal Drug Effects on Neonatal Glucose Metabolism

Maternal chlorpropamide and benzothiazides increase fetal insulin secretion and predispose the newborn to hypoglycemia. The teratogenicity of chlorpropamide precludes most fetal exposure. Propranolol may also induce neonatal hypoglycemia via inhibition of catecholamine-induced glycogenolysis. Beta-sympathomimetics, commonly used in the prophylaxis of preterm labor, have been occasionally associated with neonatal hypoglycemia. This may result from both direct effects on fetal insulin secretion as well as effects mediated via abnormal maternal glucose concentrations. Inappropriate intrapartum maternal glucose administration may also lead to transient fetal hyperinsulinism and attendant neonatal hypoglycemia.

Diminished Glucose Production

Small for Gestational Age. Infants born small for gestational age not only have decreased glycogen stores but impaired gluconeogenesis. Elevated levels of gluconeogenic precursors (particularly alanine) have been reported in the blood of these infants. While insulin and glucagon secretion are similar in appropriate and small-for-gestational-age infants, the plasma amino acid response to glucagon may be altered in hypoglycemic small-for-gestational-age infants. Commonly, several days are required for these infants to maintain normal glucose homeostasis.

HYPERGLYCEMIA

Hyperglycemia, defined as a blood glucose greater than 125 mg/dL, is most commonly encountered in the very-low-birth-weight (less than 1500 g) infant receiving intravenous glucose infusions. The glucose infusion rate may inadvertently exceed 6 to 8 mg/kg per minute as the fluids are advanced if the concentration of glucose is not adjusted accordingly. The osmotic diuresis and resultant dehydration can be marked in these cases; the resultant hyperosmolar state has been associated with intraventricular hemorrhage.

Sepsis and stress have also been associated with hyperglycemia in any infant. Endotoxins have been proposed to have direct effects on insulin actions in septic infants.

A transient state of neonatal diabetes mellitus has also been described. In approximately one third of the cases there is a positive family history of diabetes mellitus. Some of these infants are thought to have a deficiency in pancreatic beta-cell adenylcyclase activity, which improves with time. The defect in the remaining infants is unknown. Many of these infants are small for gestational age and present with polyuria, glucosuria, and hyperglycemia. They may progress to severe dehydration, acidosis, and ketonemia. The syndrome is usually self-limiting, and normal glucose homeostasis after the neonatal period is common.

CHAPTER 14

The Eye

RETINOPATHY OF PREMATURITY

Retinopathy of prematurity (ROP), recognized since the early 1940s, continues to be a cause of serious visual morbidity in very-low-birth-weight children, despite the fact that the condition had been declared "eliminated" in the 1960s and 1970s. Rather than disappearing, this disorder of the developing retinal vasculature has been the focus of intense clinical and basic science research over the past 15 years. This time period has also been characterized by changes in terminology, classification, treatment options, and even the role of the ophthalmologist in the nursery. There is currently an internationally accepted classification of ROP and a treatment proven effective in a large, randomized multicenter trial, that is, cryotherapy for serious ROP as defined by the Cryotherapy for Retinopathy of Prematurity (CRYO-ROP) Cooperative Group.

The original term of retrolental fibroplasia, indicating an end stage of fibrosis and scarring in the space behind the lens, no longer adequately describes the retinal vasoproliferative process seen in the eyes of premature infants. Therefore, retrolental fibroplasia has been replaced by the term, retinopathy of prematurity.

CLASSIFICATION

A unified classification system has allowed for major strides forward in clinical research and collaborative efforts among investigators. The impetus for the development of an international classification came at a Ross Laboratory–sponsored conference on ROP in December 1981 when a group of 23 ophthalmologists and ophthalmic pathologists from 11 countries formed a working group to develop a common classification of ROP. Before that time, several classifications were in common use and each differed in emphasis, particularly in describing more severe retinopathy. Over the next few years, the group refined the protocol and put the developing system to use before recommending its broad use in the ophthalmic community.

The basic premise of the classification is that more extensive and more posterior retinopathy is a more serious disease. The classification is based on four observations: (1) stage (or description in a 1 to 5 grading system) of the retinopathy occurring at the junction between the vascularized and unvascularized peripheral retina; (2) extent in 30-degree sectors of involvement of the retinopathy along the circumferential junction of the vascularized and unvascularized retina; (3) anterior-posterior location of the retinopathy within the retina; and (4) the presence or absence of plus disease, defined as engorged and tortuous posterior pole vessels.

The acute phases of retinopathy occur along the junction of vascularized and unvascularized peripheral retina and are divided into five stages. The working group agreed that an eye should be staged according to the worst disease observed in any area of the retina. Stage 1 ROP is a distinct white line or demarcation line between vascular and avascular retina, often with abnormal branching of vessels leading to it. This was the earliest sign of ROP that the committee could agree on that would be clearly recognizable to ophthalmologists screening for ROP in the neonatal intensive care unit. The committee, however, recognized that earlier changes were observable, such as abnormal branching and equatorial turns of the vessels at the vascular-avascular junction. Stage 2 ROP consists of a heaping up of abnormal pink to salmon colored tissue in the region of the demarcation line that appeared to have depth when compared with the smooth surface of the retina. In stage 3 ROP, fine vessels appear along the surface of the ridge to just posterior to it and the fibrovascular proliferation invades the vitreous.

Stage 4 is a partial retinal detachment and is further subdivided into stage 4A for partial detachment not involving the macular region and stage 4B for partial detachment that involves the macula. Stage 5 is a total retinal detachment, although this may be difficult to distinguish on clinical grounds if a partial detachment obscures the view of the retina.

Extent of retinal involvement along the vascular-avascular junction was determined in 30-degree segments along the circumference of this line. Therefore, up to 12 sectors of involvement were possible, even though the retinopathy of various stages may occur in the various sectors.

The major breakthrough that led to widespread use of the international classification was the adoption of a method to determine the anterior-posterior location of retinopathy. Because it was thought that more posterior disease was more ominous for the eye, being able to locate the retinopathy with certainty became important. The committee recommended using the optic nerve as the central reference point, taking into account that the retinal vessels emerge from the optic nerve and grow out over the retina in a centrifugal fashion. Three concentric areas of retina were described as potential "zones" of retinal involvement. Zone 1 is the most posterior zone and is a circle centered on the optic nerve and with a radius of twice the distance from the optic nerve to the macula. Zone 2 is defined as that area outside zone 1 but within a circle defined by a radius of the distance from the optic nerve to the nasal ora serrata (where the peripheral retina ends just behind a flat area near the iris base). Zone 3 is that area of the retina that is peripheral to zones 1 and 2, and is not present at the nasal meridian. Zone 3 enlarges in anterior-posterior extent toward the superior and inferior retina and reaches its broadest extent at the temporal meridian.

One final aspect of ocular findings included in the classification was the notation of the appearance of the posterior pole vessels. Abnormally dilated veins and tortuous arterioles in the posterior pole were thought to be ominous signs suggesting more serious and rapidly progressive ROP, and the presence of these findings was noted by appending a plus sign (+) to the stage designation. Abnormal posterior pole vessels are usually seen with iris vessel engorgement, poor dilation of the pupil, and vitreous haze.

The usual course of acute phase retinopathy is to regress with few, if any, retinal sequelae. However, the long-term consequences for the child and family are extremely important because of the effect of retinal scarring on visual function and because of the increased likelihood of later retinal problems such as retinal detachment. The ophthalmologists who developed the classifications in 1984 and 1987 recommended recording the retinal findings in terms of retinal location, posterior or peripheral, and whether the findings were more vascular or retinal. The task of ordering the findings in terms of severity awaits more information about the impact of these findings on visual function and refractive error development. In the past decade, several investigators have added to the knowledge of the effect of retinal residua of ROP on visual function.

INCIDENCE

At Pennsylvania Hospital in Philadelphia, the incidence of ROP has been documented using a classification for acute phases of ROP since the early 1970s. Over this period, the number of low-birth-weight infants who survive has increased, but it appears that the incidence of ROP has only decreased in the larger birth-weight infants.

At this time, the report involving the largest number of serial eye examinations undertaken to document the incidence of acute phase ROP is from the CRYO-ROP study of infants with birth weights of less than 1251 g who were born during the 2 year period from 1986 to 1987. Eye examinations were undertaken from 4 to 6 weeks after birth in 4099 low-birth-weight infants to monitor the onset and course of the acute phase of ROP. The overall incidence of ROP observed was 65.8%, with the highest incidence (90%) being in the children with birth weights of less than 750 g, and lower incidences of 78% in the 751 to 1000 g birth-weight group and 47% in the largest 1000 to 1250 g birth-weight group. Stages 1, 2, or 3 ROP were the highest stage of ROP seen in 25%, 22%, and 18%, respectively, of the infants examined. The proportion of eyes in which more severe ROP develops is inversely related to the birth weight group of the child.

NATURAL HISTORY

In general, the natural course of ROP is an acute phase retinopathy to (1) develop in the weeks before term, (2) reach a peak severity around term, and then, (3) begin to regress with remodeling of the retinal vasculature or with cicatrization that sometimes leads to retinal detachment.

The data from the CRYO-ROP study argue for a simple relation between postconceptional age (as an indicator of retinal development) and age at onset of ROP, at least for infants with birth weights of less than 1251 g. The situation is more complex than this and it is undoubtedly perturbed by perinatal events that result in various degrees of insults.

Most ROP regresses, but the natural history of regressing ROP is not well documented. Children in whom mild ROP developed in peripheral zone 2 or zone 3 had vascularization into zone 3 by around term and had completed vascularization, and thus had complete regression, by 45 weeks' postconceptional age. Children in whom stage 3 ROP or ROP in zone 1 or posterior zone 2 developed had delay of retinal vascularization to an average of 51.7 to 55.4 weeks' postconceptional age. Therefore, more severe or more posterior ROP regresses more slowly and often lasts well into the time period after term due date.

TREATMENT
Retinal Ablation

By the late 1960s and early 1970s, it was apparent that ROP was not a preventable condition in the neonatal nursery and attention was directed to surgical treatment of already established retinopathy. Two modalities were initially considered and attempted: laser photocoagulation and cryotherapy.

Cryotherapy, rather than laser photocoagulation, emerged as the treatment modality of choice in the 1980s. This was largely based on the ease of administration of cryotherapy, because cryotherapy could be performed in the intensive care nursery with a neonatologist in attendance and using topical and subconjunctival anesthesia. Laser photocoagulation, on the other hand, required use of a cumbersome, nonportable instrument, usually required general anesthesia in the operating room, and was technically difficult in the sick, tiny premature infant.

Multicenter Trial of Cryotherapy

The multicenter trial of CRYO-ROP is a randomized study carried out at 23 centers in the United States and sponsored by the National Eye Institute that enrolled infants with birth weights of less than 1251 g who were born between January 1, 1986, and November 30, 1987.

The 3-month outcome report from the CRYO-ROP randomized trial documented a 98% followup rate with 273 of the eligible 279 infants returning for the examination (12 had died). Based on assessment by masked observers at the CRYO-ROP reading center in Portland, fundus photographs of 222 treated eyes and 216 control eyes could be assigned to the favorable or unfavorable categories. There was a 39.5% reduction of unfavorable outcome in treated eyes compared with control eyes ($\chi^2 = 25.4$, $P < 0.00001$). Among treated eyes, 31.1% had an unfavorable outcome and 51% of control eyes had an unfavorable outcome. When more severe ROP residua are considered, there was a 44.4% reduction in the occurrence of total retinal detachment or total retrolental and a 53.6% reduction in the occurrence of posterior retinal fold in treated eyes compared with control eyes.

Of particular importance in determining the cost benefit ratio of surgical intervention for threshold ROP, the cryotherapy procedure itself was relatively free of serious complications. The most common ocular complications were subconjunctival hematoma (11.7%) and conjunctival laceration (5.3%), and the most common systemic complications were bradycardia (9.4%) and acquired or increased cyanosis (1.1%).

Laser Photocoagulation for Retinopathy of Prematurity

Over the past few years, laser photocoagulation for ROP has become feasible with the advent of a laser instrument mounted on an indirect ophthalmoscope, allowing easier administration of laser photocoagulation than was possible previously with floor-mounted instruments. The use of this modality in the treatment of threshold ROP continues to be promising and outcomes after laser photocoagulation are similar to those obtained using cryotherapy at threshold ROP. The procedure appears to be less traumatic for the systemic and ocular condition of the infant. In addition, because the laser is applied directly to the retina and retinal pigment epithelium and not trans-sclerally as in cryotherapy, no conjunctival incision is needed. Laser photocoagulation may be of particular use in eyes with zone 1 ROP, because such eyes are difficult to treat with cryotherapy and the outcome of such eyes is still likely to be dismal despite timely administration of cryotherapy. Three of four eyes that received cryotherapy in the CRYO-ROP study had unfavorable structural outcomes at the 1-year study examination compared with more than nine of 10 eyes that were not randomized to receive cryotherapy. In the intensive care nursery of the 1990s, it appears that laser photocoagulation for threshold ROP in zone 1 has a much better outcome than the historical control or treated eyes in the CRYO-ROP study that admitted infants from January 1986 to November 1987.

INDEX

Note: Page numbers followed by the letter t refer to tables

A

Aa-Do$_2$, in hyaline membrane disease, 250
  measurement of, 251
Aagenaes syndrome, 448
Abdomen, distension of, obstruction causing, 436
  palpation of, 319
Abdominal wall defects, in Beckwith-Wiedemann syndrome, 65
Ablation, retinal, for retinopathy of prematurity, 548–549
ABO blood groups, incompatibility of, 472
Abscess, brain, 431
  breast, 210–211
Abstinence syndrome, in infant of substance abusing mother, 4
Abuse, substance. See *Substance abuse.*
Acetylcysteine, for meconium ileus, 439
N-Acetylglutamate synthetase (NAGS), 83
Acid-base balance, disturbances of. See also *Acidosis; Alkalosis.*
  in newborn, 155–163
Acidemia, glutaric, type 1, 96–97
  type 2, 97–98
  isovaleric, 95
  methylmalonic, 92–94
  propionic, 94–95

Acidosis, lactic, early lethal, 105–106
  metabolic, 155–159
    anion gap in, 156
      normal, 157
    correction of, resuscitation and, 128
    morbidity and mortality of, 158
    of prematurity, 156–157
    sodium bicarbonate for, 158–159
    tromethamine for, 159
  renal tubular, neonatal hypocalcemia associated with, 513
  respiratory, management of, 160
Acquired hemostatic disorder(s), 482–486
  disseminated intravascular coagulation as, 482–484
  periventricular-intraventricular hemorrhage as, 484
  vitamin K deficiency as, 484–486
Acquired immunodeficiency syndrome (AIDS). See *Human immunodeficiency virus (HIV) infection.*
Acrocyanosis, 314
Activated partial thromboplastin time (APTT), in hemorrhagic disorders, 480

Acute life-threatening event (ALTE), associated with apnea of infancy, 245
  increased risk of SIDS with, 245–246
Acute lymphoblastic leukemia (ALL), associated with Down syndrome, 52
Acute renal failure (ARF). See *Renal failure, acute.*
Acute tubular necrosis, 502
Acyclovir, for herpes simplex virus infection, 179
Acylcarnitine translocase deficiency, 101–102
Adenosine, for paroxysmal supraventricular tachycardia, 396
Adenosine arabinoside, for herpes simplex virus infection, 179
Adrenal hemorrhage, 518–520
Adrenal hyperplasia, congenital, 521–523
  21-hydroxylase deficiency in, 522–523
  clinical manifestations of, 522
  newborn screening for, 112
  screening for, 112
Adrenal hypoplasia, 521
Adrenal insufficiency, causes of, 518t
  transient, 520–521
Adrenaline, 147
Age, gestational, meconium staining of amniotic fluid and, 272
  small for, diminished glucose production in, 542–543
Agenesis, anal, 440
  of corpus callosum, 403
  rectal, 440
AHA-AAP (American Heart Association–American Academy of Pediatrics) approach, to meconium staining of amniotic fluid, 275–276
  to resuscitation, 123–131

AIDS (acquired immunodeficiency syndrome). See *Human immunodeficiency virus (HIV) infection.*
Airway resistance, in meconium aspiration syndrome, 273
Albuterol, for bronchopulmonary dysplasia, 293
Alcohol abuse, during pregnancy, 13–14
  enhanced risk for events after, 2t
  issues of, in child-bearing women, 3t
Alkalosis, metabolic, 160–163
  persistence of, factors in, 161
  respiratory, 163
ALL (acute lymphoblastic leukemia), associated with Down syndrome, 52
Alpha$_1$-antitrypsin deficiency, 446–447
  newborn screening for, 118
Alpha$_2$-antiplasmin, in hemorrhagic disorders, 480
Alpha-fetoprotein, maternal serum, in anencephaly, 400
  in Arnold-Chiari syndrome, 402
17-Alpha-hydroxyprogesterone (17-OHP), in congenital adrenal hyperplasia, 112
ALTE (acute life-threatening event), associated with apnea of infancy, 245
  increased risk of SIDS with, 245–246
Alveolar proteinosis, congenital, 70
Amegakaryocytic thrombocytopenia, 494
American Heart Association–American Academy of Pediatrics (AHA-AAP) approach, to meconium staining of amniotic fluid, 275–276
  to resuscitation, 123–131

Amino acid metabolism, inborn error(s) of, 75t, 87–92
　hereditary tyrosinemia type 1 as, 89–90
　maple syrup urine disease as, 87–89
　methionine synthetase deficiency as, 91
　nonketonic hyperglycinemia as, 90–91
　phenylketonuria as, 91–92
Ammonia metabolism, inborn error(s) of, 74t, 82–87
　argininosuccinate lyase (ASAL) deficiency as, 82, 85
　argininosuccinate synthetase (ASAS) deficiency as, 82, 85
　carbamylphosphate synthetase I (CPS-I) deficiency as, 82–85
　ornithine transcarbamylase (OTC) deficiency as, 82–85
　transient hyperammonemia of newborn as, 86–87
Amniotic fluid, meconium staining of, 271
　AHA-AAP approach to, 275–276
　cause of, 271–272
　procoagulant activity of, 500
Amniotic fluid volume, abnormalities of, 25, 26t
Amphetamine abuse, during pregnancy, 11–12
　enhanced risk for events after, 2t
Amphotericin B, causing ischemic and nephrotoxic renal injury, 504
Ampicillin, for bacterial meningitis, 197
　for infectious diarrhea, 201
Amyoplasia, arthrogryposis due to, 46, 46t
Anal agenesis, 440
Anal membrane, imperforate, 439
Anal stenosis, 439

Androgens, maternal overproduction of, virilization of female fetus by, 530–531
Anemia, hemolytic, nonspherocytic, 472–473
Anencephaly, 399–400
　diagnosis of, 400
Anion gap, in metabolic acidosis, 156
　normal, 157
Aniridia, 62
Annular pancreas, 441
Anorectal malformations, 439–440
Anterior horn cell disease, 434–435
Antibiotics. See also specific agent.
　for meconium aspiration syndrome, 274
　for septic arthritis, 205–206
　for urinary tract infections, 202
Antidiuretic hormone (vasopressin), 146
Antiepileptic drugs, 433
Antimicrobials. See Antibiotics; specific agent.
Aorta, coarctation of, 361–364
　juxtaductal, 362
　management of, 364
　signs and symptoms of, 362–363
Aortic arch, interruption of, 364–366
　clinical presentations of, 365
　treatment of, 366
Aortic stenosis, 366–369
　chest radiographs of, 368
　electrocardiographic patterns in, 368
　management of, 369
　murmur in, 367
Apert disease, 430
Apgar score(s), assignment of, intervals between, 121
　of 0, resuscitation of infants with, 124–125, 126t–127t
　of 1–3, resuscitation of infants with, 124
　of 4–6, resuscitation of infants with, 124

Apgar score(s) *(Continued)*
  of 7 or more, resuscitation of infants with, 123–124
Apgar scoring system, 122t
Apnea, bradycardia preceded by, 238–239
  central, 238
  hypocalcemic crisis with, treatment of, 514
  in chronic pulmonary insufficiency of prematurity, 297
  in relation to sleep state, 240
  obstructive, 239
  of infancy, 244–245
  of prematurity, 238–243
  symptomatic recurrent, 243
  treatment of, 240–242
    continuous positive airway pressure in, 242
    cutaneous stimulation in, 240–241
    heart rate monitors in, 240
    methylxanthines in, 241–242
    oxygen supplementation in, 241
Apnea monitoring programs, home, 246–247
Apneic spells, incidence of, 238
APTT (activated partial thromboplastin time), in hemorrhagic disorders, 480
Aqueductal stenosis, in utero, 408
ARF. See *Renal failure, acute.*
Argininosuccinate lyase (ASAL) deficiency, 82, 85
Argininosuccinate synthetase (ASAS) deficiency, 82, 85
Arnold-Chiari malformation, 401–402
Arrhythmia(s). See *Dysrhythmia(s).*
Arterial blood gas(es), measurement of, determinations from, 319–320
Arterial catheter–related thrombosis, 488–489
Arterial pulses, of extremities, measurement of, 319
Arteriovenous fistula(s), 379–381
Arteriovenous malformation, of vein of Galen, 407–408
Arthritis, septic, 203–206
  management of, 205–206
  signs and symptoms of, 204
Arthrogryposis, 45–46
  causes of, 46t
Asphyxia, 417–420
  assessment of, resuscitation and, 121, 122t
  birth, and hyaline membrane disease, 249
  definition of, 121
Aspiration, meconium. See also *Meconium aspiration pneumonia.*
  attention to, during resuscitation, 134
Asplenia, 359–361
  bilateral right-sidedness in, 359
  Heinz bodies in, 360
  Howell-Jolly bodies in, 360
  management of, 361
  vs. polysplenia, 360–361
Atlantoaxial subluxation, associated with Down syndrome, 51
Atresia, bowel, obstruction due to, 436–437
  pulmonary, tetralogy of Fallot with, 341–343
    with intact ventricular septum, 343–346
  tricuspid, 335, 348–350
Atrial flutter, 396–397
Atrial natriuretic peptide, 146–147
Atrioventricular block, first-degree, 397
  second-degree, 397–398
  third-degree, 398
Atrioventricular septal defect(s), 376–379
  electrocardiographic patterns in, 378
  in trisomy 21 (Down syndrome), 376–377
  surgical repair of, 379

Atrium (atria), enlargement of, 327
Auricular sinuses, 47–49
Auricular tags, 47–49
Auscultation, of chest, 316
   of heart, 317–318

B

Bacterial infection(s), 184–222
   botulism as, 221–222
   diarrhea in, 199–201
   diphtheria as, 218–219
   meningitis as, 194–198
   nosocomial, 211–215
      diarrhea in, 213
      gram-negative, 214–215
      staphylococcal, 211–213
      streptococcal group A, 213–214
   of skin, 208–211
   of urinary tract, 201–203
   ophthalmia neonatorum as, 206–208
   otitis media as, 198–199
   septic arthritis and osteomyelitis as, 203–206
   septicemia due to, 184–194
   tetanus neonatorum as, 219–221
   tuberculosis as, 215–218
Barbiturate abuse, during pregnancy, enhanced risk for events after, 2t
Barotrauma, in lung injury, 286
Barrel chest, in bronchopulmonary dysplasia, 289
Barth syndrome, 104
Basal encephalocele, 400
Beckwith Wiedemann syndrome, 64–65, 541
Bed rest, for premature labor, 31
Benign infantile mitochondrial myopathy/cardiomyopathy, 103–104
Benzathine penicillin G, for syphilis, in neonate, 236t
   in pregnant patient, 234t, 235t
Beta agonists, to suppress uterine contractions, in premature labor, 32
Beta-adrenergic agents, for bronchopulmonary dysplasia, 292–293
Betamethasone, for premature labor, 32
Bicarbonate. See *Sodium bicarbonate*.
Bilirubin, binding and transportation of, 464
   conjugation and excretion of, 464–465
   enterohepatic circulation of, 465
   excessive production of, 471–478. See also *Hyperbilirubinemia*.
   levels of, epidemiology of, 465–466
   synthesis of, increased, 464
   toxicity of, 467–470
Bilirubin encephalopathy, 415–416, 468
Biophysical profile, in fetal surveillance, 25–27
   elements of, 27t
   interpretation and management of, 28t
Biotin therapy, for biotinidase deficiency, 113
Biotinidase deficiency, newborn screening for, 112–113
Birth asphyxia, and hyaline membrane disease, 249
Birth defects, associated with Down syndrome, 50–51
Bleeding. See *Hemorrhage*.
Blennorrhea, inclusion, management of, 208
Blood, extravascular, hyperbilirubinemia due to, 477
Blood gas(es), arterial, measurement of, determinations from, 319–320
Blood group(s), ABO, incompatibility of, 472
   minor, incompatibility of, 472
Blood transfusion. See *Transfusion*.
"Blueberry muffin" lesions, rubella-associated, 169

Body composition,
    developmental changes
    in, 139–142
  during labor and delivery, 140–141
  regulation of, physiology of,
    142–145
Botulinal antitoxin, 222
Botulism, infant, 221–222
Bovine milk, human milk vs.,
    phosphorus content of,
    511
  neonatal hypocalcemia associated with, 510–511
BPD. See *Bronchopulmonary dysplasia (BPD)*.
Brachial plexus injury,
    426–427
Bradycardia, in chronic
    pulmonary insufficiency
    of prematurity, 297
  preceded by apnea, 238–239
  sinus, 393
Brain abscess, 431
Brain hemorrhage, in utero,
    410–411
Brain injury, traumatic,
    424–425
Brain lesion(s), in utero,
    408–411
  aqueductal stenosis as,
    408
  associated with metabolic
    disease, 411
  hemorrhagic, 410–411
  hydranencephaly as, 410
  hydrocephalus as, 409
  hypoxic-ischemic, 409–410
  infections causing, 411
Branched-chain 2-keto
    dehydrogenase
    (BCKAD) complex
    deficiency, 87–89
Breast abscess, 210–211
Breast milk. See *Human milk*.
Breast milk jaundice, 466
Breast-feeding, 450–452
  by HIV-positive mothers,
    WHO policy for, 452
  decreased morbidity associated with, 451–452
  jaundice in, 466–467
  substance abuse and, 16

Breast-feeding *(Continued)*
  vitamin supplementation in,
    452
Breathing. See also
    Respiratory entries.
  control of, 238–248
    home apnea monitoring
      programs in, 246–247
    in apnea of infancy, 244–245
    in apnea of prematurity,
      238–243
    in congenital hypoventilation syndrome, 243–244
    in sudden infant death
      syndrome, 245–246
    in symptomatic recurrent
      apnea, 243
    prone sleeping position
      in, 247–248
  diaphragmatic, in premature infants, 239
  labored, in infant with hyaline membrane disease, 252
Bronchopulmonary dysplasia
    (BPD), 284–296
  beta-adrenergic agents for,
    292–293
  bronchial lavage in, 287
  dexamethasone for, 293–294
    side effects of, 294
  factors predisposing to, 285
  incidence of, 284
  inhaled steroids for, 294
  lung compliance in, 290
  mortality rates in, 295
  nutritional support for,
    290–291
  organisms contributing to,
    288–289
  oxygen therapy for, 291
  patent ductus arteriosus associated with, 288
  selenium deficiency in, 289
  stage 4, 289–290
  vitamin A deficiency in,
    289

C

Café-au-lait lesions, in
    neurofibromatosis, 405

Caffeine abuse, during pregnancy, 15–16
Calcium, in total parenteral nutrition, 455
Calcium gluconate, for neonatal hypocalcemia, 513–515
  risks associated with, 513–514
Calcium metabolism, disorders of, 508–516. See also *Hypocalcemia.*
Campylobacter jejuni, in infectious diarrhea, 199
Candida albicans, 223. See also *Candidiasis.*
Candidiasis, disseminated, 222–224
  oral (thrush), in HIV-infected patient, ketoconazole for, 166
Cannabis, abuse of. See *Marijuana abuse.*
Capillary wall, water movement across, equation for, 143
Caput succedaneum, 424
Carbamylphosphate synthetase I (CPS-I) deficiency, 82–85
Carbimazole, for thyrotoxicosis, 536
Carbohydrate metabolism, disorders of, 536–543. See also *Hyperglycemia; Hypoglycemia.*
  inborn error(s) of, 74t, 76–82
    fructose-1,6-bisphosphatase deficiency as, 81–82
    glycogen storage diseases as, 78–80
    hereditary fructose intolerance as, 80–81
    hereditary galactosemia as, 76–78
Cardiac. See also *Heart.*
Cardiac catheterization, in evaluation of heart disorders, 332–333
Cardiac disorder(s), aortic stenosis as, 366–369
  asplenia and, 359–361
  atriovenous fistulas as, 379–381

Cardiac disorder(s) (*Continued*)
  atrioventricular septal defects as, 376–379
  cardiomyopathy in infant of diabetic mother as, 388–389
  coarctation of aorta as, 361–364
  cyanosis and, 308–309
  dysrhythmias as, 392–398
  early diagnosis of, 305–306
  Ebstein anomaly of tricuspid valve as, 350–353
  endocardial fibroelastosis as, 386–388
  evaluation of, 305–398
    arterial blood gas measurements in, 310–320
    auscultation of chest in, 316
    auscultation of heart in, 317–318
    cardiac catheterization in, 332–333
    chest radiographs in, 321–327
    differential cyanosis in, 314–315
    echocardiogram in, 330–332
    electrocardiographic patterns in, 329–330
    history of pregnancy in, 307–308
    in symptomatic newborn, 306
    laboratory tests in, 327–328
    localization of murmurs in, 317
    palpation of abdomen in, 319
    physical examination in, 310–312
  glycogen storage disease of heart as, 389–391
  hypoplastic left heart syndrome as, 369–372
  interrupted aortic arch as, 364–366
  myocarditis as, 382–386
  pulmonary stenosis with intact ventricular septum as, 346–348

Cardiac disorder(s) (*Continued*)
  tetralogy of Fallot as, 339–346
    with pulmonary atresia, 341–346
  total anomalous pulmonary venous connection as, 355–359
  transient myocardial ischemia as, 381–382
  transposition of great arteries as, 336–339
  tricuspid atresia as, 348–350
  truncus arteriosus as, 353–355
  tumors as, 391–392
  ventricular septal defects as, 372–376
  vs. pulmonary or systemic disease, 306–307
Cardiac lesions, rubella-associated, 169–170
Cardiac motion, precordial, visual assessment of, 316
Cardiac tumors, 391–392
Cardiomyopathy, in infant of diabetic mother, 388–389
  mitochondrial, infantile, benign, 103–104
Cardiovascular system, involvement of, in Marfan syndrome, 67
  in Noonan syndrome, 69
  support of, continuation of, after successful resuscitation, 130–131
  resuscitation and, 129–130
Cardioversion, for paroxysmal supraventricular tachycardia, 396
Carnitine palmitoyltransferase I deficiency, 101–102
Carnitine palmitoyltransferase II deficiency, 101–102
Carnitine transporter defect, 101–102
Cataracts, in GALT deficiency, 76–77
  rubella-associated, 168, 169
CATCH 22 acronym, in chromosome 22q11 deletion, 40

Catheterization, cardiac, in evaluation of cardiac disorders, 332–333
  of umbilical vessel, resuscitation and, 125, 128
Cefotaxime, for ophthalmia neonatorum, 207
Ceftriaxone, for ophthalmia neonatorum, 207
Central nervous system (CNS). See also *Brain* entries.
  anomalies of, in CHARGE association, 71
  asphyxial and hypoxic-ischemic injury involving, 417–420
  encephalopathies involving, 413–417
  intraventricular hemorrhage involving, 420–424
  involvement of, in congenital syphilis, 233
  in herpes simplex virus infection, 177
  malformation(s) of, 399–413
    destructive in utero lesions causing, 408–411
    drugs causing, 411–413
    neural tube defects causing, 399–408
  metabolic and degenerative diseases involving, 427–431
  neuromuscular disorders involving, 434–435
  seizures and paroxysmal disorders involving, 431–434
  superficial cranial injury involving, 424
  traumatic brain injury involving, 424–425
  traumatic nerve injury involving, 425–427
Cerebellum, malformations of, 405–407
Cerebrohepatorenal (Zellweger) syndrome, 448–449
Cerebrospinal fluid (CSF), excessive, in hydrocephalus, 409

Cerebrospinal fluid cell counts, in bacterial meningitis, interpretation of, 195–196
CHARGE association, 71–72
Chemical hyperbilirubinemia, definition of, 463
Chest, auscultation of, 316
Chest radiography, diagnostic, in lung disease vs. heart disease, 321–327
  evaluation of abdominal findings in, 322–324
  evaluation of lungs in, 324–326
  of aortic stenosis, 368
  of Ebstein anomaly, 352
  of meconium aspiration pneumonia, 273
  of myocarditis, 384
  of normal heart, 326–327
  of pulmonary atresia with intact ventricular septum, 344
  of pulmonary stenosis with intact ventricular septum, 347
  of transposition of great arteries, 338
  of ventricular septal defects, 375
  systematic review of, 326
Chest wall, compliant, in chronic pulmonary insufficiency of prematurity, 296
Chlamydia, in bronchopulmonary dysplasia, 288
Chloroquine, for transfusion-acquired malaria, 229
Choanal atresia, in CHARGE association, 71
Cholestasis, bacterial hepatitis causing, 446
  familial, 448
  in cystic fibrosis, 447
  TPN-associated, 449–450
  with lymphedema (Aagenaes syndrome), 448
Chromosome(s), marker, 64
Chromosome 22q11 deletion, conditions associated with, 40

Cigarette smoking, associated with premature delivery, 29
  during pregnancy, 14–15
  enhanced risk for events after, 2t
  issues of, in child-bearing women, 3t
Circulation, enterohepatic, of bilirubin, 465
  pulmonary and systemic, in transposition of great arteries, 336–337
Clamping, of umbilical cord, timing of, 141
Cleft lip and palate, 36–37
Clonic seizure(s), 432
Clostridium botulinum, 221. See also *Botulism*.
Clostridium difficile, in infectious diarrhea, 200
Clostridium tetani, 219. See also *Tetanus neonatorum*.
CMV. See *Cytomegalovirus (CMV)*.
CNS. See *Central nervous system (CNS)*.
Coarctation of aorta, 361–364
  juxtaductal, 362
  management of, 364
  signs and symptoms of, 362–363
Cocaine, pharmacologic actions of, 6–7
Cocaine abuse, during pregnancy, 6–11
  congenital abnormalities associated with, 8
  enhanced risk for events after, 2t
  fetal complications associated with, 7–8
  premature delivery and, 9–11, 29–30
Coeur-en-sabot appearance, of pulmonary artery, in tetralogy of Fallot, 341
Colistin sulfate, for infectious diarrhea, 201
Columba, in CHARGE association, 71
Communicating hydrocephalus, 409
Congenital dislocation of hip, 43

559

Congenital heart disease, 37–40
  cyanotic, 312–313
  syndromes associated with, 38t–39t
Conjunctivitis, neonatal, 206–208
  agents associated with, 206
  management of, 207–208
Conotruncal anomaly face syndrome, chromosome 22q11 deletion associated with, 40
Continuous positive airway pressure (CPAP), for apnea, 242
  for hyaline membrane disease, 260–261
Contraction stress test, in fetal surveillance, 24–25
Copper, in total parenteral nutrition, 455–456
Corpus callosum, agenesis of, 403
Corticosteroids, for hyaline membrane disease, 260
  for meconium aspiration syndrome, 274
  for thyrotoxicosis, 536
Corynebacterium diphtheriae, 218, 219
Courvoisier sign, 319
Coxsackie virus infection, myocarditis and, 383
CPAP (continuous positive airway pressure), for apnea, 242
  for hyaline membrane disease, 260–261
Cranial injury, superficial, 424
Cranial suture(s), premature closure of (craniosynostosis), 430–431
Craniofacial appearance, in Rubinstein-Taybi syndrome, 70
Craniosynostosis, 430–431
Cri du chat syndrome, 59
Crouzon disease, 430
Cryoprecipitate, for disseminated intravascular coagulation, 483

Cryotherapy, for retinopathy of prematurity, 549–550
C/S protein deficiency, homozygous, 487–488
CSF (cerebrospinal fluid), excessive, in hydrocephalus, 409
Cyanosis, associated with cardiac disorders, 308–309
  differential, 314–315
  definition of, 314
Cyanotic spells, without apnea, in premature infants, 242–243
Cystic fibrosis, 65–67, 443
  clinical manifestations of, 66
  genotyping for, 66–67
  liver disease in, 447
  meconium ileus in, 437–438
  newborn screening for, 114–115
  prenatal screening for, 438
Cytomegalovirus (CMV), in bronchopulmonary dysplasia, 288
  infection with, 171–175
  management of, 174
  transmission of, 172

D

Dandy-Walker malformation, 407
Deafness, rubella-associated, 168–169
Degenerative disease(s), 427–431
Deletion gene syndrome(s), 59–62
  cri du chat syndrome as, 59
  DiGeorge syndrome as, 60–61
  Miller-Dieker syndrome as, 59–60
  velocardiofacial syndrome as, 61
  Wolf-Hirschhorn syndrome as, 61–62
Delivery room, resuscitation in. See *Neonatal resuscitation*.
DES (diethylstilbestrol), in utero exposure to, 30

Desoxycorticosterone acetate, for transient adrenal insufficiency, 520
Developmental variability, associated with Down syndrome, 52
Dexamethasone, for bacterial meningitis, 197
　for bronchopulmonary dysplasia, 293–294
　for premature labor, 32
Diabetes mellitus, maternal, enhanced platelet function in, 499
　neural tube defects associated with, 411
Diabetic mother, infant of, cardiomyopathy in, 388–389
　hypocalcemia in, 510
　hypoglycemia in, 539–541
Dialysis, for hyperammonemia, 85
Diaphragmatic breathing, in premature infants, 239
Diarrhea, infectious, 199–201
　management of, 200–201
　nosocomial, 213
　organisms causing, 199–200
Diazepam, for seizures, 433
　for tetanus, 221
DIC (disseminated intravascular coagulation), 482–484
　diagnosis of, 483
　management of, 483–484
Diet, effect of, on platelet function, 499–500
　lactose-free, for GALT deficiency, 77
Diethylstilbestrol (DES), in utero exposure to, 30
DiGeorge syndrome, 60–61
　chromosome 22q11 deletion associated with, 40
Digoxin, for paroxysmal supraventricular tachycardia, 396
Diphtheria, 218–219
Diphtheria antitoxin, 219
Diploid-triploid mosaicism (mixoploidy), 58

Dislocation of hip, congenital, 43
Disseminated intravascular coagulation (DIC), 482–484
　diagnosis of, 483
　management of, 483–484
Dizygotic twins, 34
Dobutamine, for cardiovascular support, during resuscitation, 130
Dopamine, 147
　for acute renal failure, 506
　for cardiovascular support, during resuscitation, 129, 130
　for hyaline membrane disease, 260
　used in resuscitation, 127t
　of extremely premature infant, 133
Down syndrome. See *Trisomy 21 (Down syndrome)*.
Drug(s). See also specific drug or drug group.
　abuse of. See *Substance abuse*.
　and developing nervous system, 412–413
　for premature labor, 31–33
　for resuscitation, 126t–127t
　maternal ingestion of, virilization of female fetus by, 530
　transplacental passage of, thrombocytopenia due to, 494
Duchenne muscular dystrophy, newborn screening for, 116–117
Ductus arteriosus, constriction of, oxygen in, 299–300
　patent. See *Patent ductus arteriosus (PDA)*.
　premature closure of, in persistent pulmonary hypertension of newborn, 260
Duodenal stenosis, 437
Duplication(s), enteral, 440
Dysencephalia splanchnocystica, 68
Dysplasia, bronchopulmonary. See *Bronchopulmonary dysplasia (BPD)*.

561

Dysraphisms, ocular, 402
Dysrhythmia(s), 392–398
  atrial flutter as, 396–397
  atrioventricular block as, 397–398
  ectopic beats in, 393–394
  paroxysmal supraventricular tachycardia as, 394–396
  sinus arrhythmia as, 392
  sinus bradycardia as, 393
  sinus tachycardia as, 392–393
  ventricular tachycardia as, 397

E

$E_1\alpha$ gene mutation, in maple syrup urine disease, 88
Ear sinuses, 47–49
Ear tags, 47–49
Ebstein anomaly, of tricuspid valve, 350–353
  treatment of, 352
ECG. See *Electrocardiography (ECG)*.
Echocardiography, in evaluation of cardiac disorders, 330–332
  of pulmonary atresia with intact ventricular septum, 344
ECMO (extracorporeal membrane oxygenation), for persistent pulmonary hypertension of newborn, 271
Edema, hemorrhagic, of scalp, 424
  pulmonary, in transient tachypnea of newborn, 263, 264
  postasphyxial, 277–278
Edrophonium, for paroxysmal supraventricular tachycardia, 396
Edwards syndrome (trisomy 18), 53–55
  physical findings in, 53–54
Electrocardiography (ECG), in evaluation of cardiac disorders, 329–330
  of aortic stenosis, 368

Electrocardiography (ECG) *(Continued)*
  of atrioventricular septal defects, 378
  of ectopic beats, 393–394
  of endocardial fibroelastosis, 387–388
  of glycogen storage disease of heart, 390
  of hypoplastic left heart syndrome, 370
  of paroxysmal supraventricular tachycardia, 394
  of pulmonary stenosis with intact ventricular septum, 347
  of sinus arrhythmia, 392
  of sinus bradycardia, 393
  of sinus tachycardia, 393
Electrolyte(s). See also *Fluid(s)*.
  for infectious diarrhea, 200
  management of, in neonates, 148–155
  replacement of, calculations used in, 149–150
Electron transfer flavoprotein (ETF), 97
Elliptocytosis, hereditary, 477
ELN gene, in Williams syndrome, 63
Emphysema, pulmonary interstitial, 279–281
  causes of, 280
Encephaloceles, 400–401
Encephalomyelopathy, subacute necrotizing, 104–105
Encephalopathy, 413–417
  bilirubin, 415–416, 468
  hepatic, 415
  hypoxic-ischemic, 418–420
  intrauterine, 409–410
  infectious, 416–417
  metabolic, 414–415
  mild, 417
  moderate, 417–418
  postasphyxial, 413–414
  severe, 418
Endocardial fibroelastosis, 386–388
  electrocardiographic patterns in, 387–388
  heart murmurs in, 386–387
Enema, hyperosmolar, for meconium ileus, 438

Energy needs, of low-birth-weight infant, 453
Enteral nutrition, 457–459, 460t–461t, 462
  fatty acids in, 458
  protein in, 457–458, 460t
Enteric duplications, 440
Enterovirus infection(s), 175–176
Environmental toxin(s), and developing nervous system, 413
Enzyme abnormality(ies), of red blood cells, 472–476
  glucose-6-phosphate-dehydrogenase deficiency as, 473–475
  pyruvate kinase deficiency as, 475–476
Epidural abscess, 431
Epinephrine, administration of, during resuscitation, 125, 126t
Erb palsy, 427
Erythroblastosis fetalis, 541–542
Erythrocytes. See *Red blood cells (RBCs)*.
Erythromycin, for syphilis, in pregnant patient, 234t, 235t
ESAC (extra structurally abnormal chromosome), 64
Escherichia coli infection, 193
  in GALT deficiency, 77
ETF (electron transfer flavoprotein), 97
Ethambutol, for tuberculosis, 217
Exchange transfusion, for disseminated intravascular coagulation, 483–484
  for kernicterus, 468–469
Exencephaly, 400
Extra structurally abnormal chromosome (ESAC), 64
Extracorporeal membrane oxygenation (ECMO), for persistent pulmonary hypertension of newborn, 271

Extremely low-birth-weight infant(s), intubation of, 136
  resuscitation of, 132–133
Extremity(ies), arterial pulses of, measurement of, 319
Eye, herpes simplex virus infection of, 178

F

Facial nerve injury, 425–426
Facies, characteristic, in Marfan syndrome, 67
  "Greek helmet," in Wolf-Hirschhorn syndrome, 62
Factor deficiency(ies), congenital, 481–482
Factor XIII deficiency, in hemorrhagic disorders, 480
FAS (fetal alcohol syndrome), 13–14
  Pierre Robin sequence in, 44
Feces (stools), water loss through, 151
Feeding difficulties, in Pierre Robin sequence, 45
Fetal alcohol effects, 14
Fetal alcohol syndrome (FAS), 13–14
  Pierre Robin sequence in, 44
Fetal hydantoin syndrome, 412
Fetal lung field, delayed clearance of. See *Transient tachypnea of newborn (TTN)*.
Fetal surveillance, 23–28
  biophysical profile in, 25–27
    elements of, 27t
    interpretation and management of, 28t
  contraction stress test in, 24–25
  indications for, 23t
  nonstress test in, 25
Fetus, female, virilization of, 529–531
  by maternal ingestion of drugs, 530

563

Fetus (Continued)
by maternal overproduction of androgens, 530–531
Fibroelastosis, endocardial, 386–388
Fibroma(s), cardiac, 391
Fistula(s), arteriovenous, 379–381
Fluid(s), for infectious diarrhea, 200
management of, in neonates, 148–155
replacement of, calculations used in, 149–150
restriction of, in bronchopulmonary dysplasia, 291–292
in hyaline membrane disease, 258–259
Fluid compartments, developmental changes in, 139–142
during labor and delivery, 140–141
extracellular, osmolality changes in, 143
Fluid homeostasis, hydrops and, 16–17
Flutter, atrial, 396–397
Football sign, on chest radiograph, 323
Formula(s), infant, nutrient composition of, 460t–461t
Fresh-frozen plasma, for disseminated intravascular coagulation, 483
Frontonasal encephalocele, 400
Fructose intolerance, hereditary, 80–81, 447
Fructose–1,6-bisphosphatase deficiency, 81–82
Fructose–1,6-bisphosphate aldolase B deficiency, 80–81
Fumarylacetoacetate hydrolase (FAH) deficiency, 89–90
Fungal infection(s), 222–224. See also specific infection, e.g., *Candidiasis*.

G

G6PD (glucose-6-phosphate-dehydrogenase deficiency), 473–475
genetic forms of, 474
Galactose-1-phosphate-uridyltransferase (GALT) deficiency, 76–78
Galactosemia, 447
hereditary, 76–78
newborn screening for, 109–110
GALT (galactose-1-phosphate-uridyltransferase) deficiency, 76–78
Gastroenteritis, *Salmonella*, 199, 201
Gastrointestinal tract, duplications of, 440
malformations of, associated with Down syndrome, 51
Gene syndrome(s), deletion, 59–62
Genotyping, for cystic fibrosis, 66–67
Gentamicin, for bacterial meningitis, 197
Gestational age, meconium staining of amniotic fluid and, 272
small for, diminished glucose production in, 542–543
Glomerular filtration rate (GFR), in acute renal failure, 502
Glossoptosis, 43
Glucocorticoids, for premature labor, 31–32
Glucose, diminished production of, hypoglycemia and, 542–543
Glucose metabolism, neonatal, maternal drug effects on, 542
Glucose-6-phosphate deficiency, 78–79
Glucose-6-phosphate-dehydrogenase deficiency (G6PD), 473–475
genetic forms of, 474

Glutaric acidemia, type 1, 96–97
type 2, 97–98
Glutaryl-CoA dehydrogenase (GCDH) deficiency, 96–97
Glycine, for isovaleric acidemia, 95
Glycine cleavage complex (GCC) deficiency, 90–91
Glycogen metabolism, disorders of, associated with hypoglycemia, 538–539
Glycogen storage disease(s), 78–80
glucose-6-phosphate deficiency as, 78–79
lysosomal α-glucosidase deficiency as, 79–80
of heart, 389–391
electrocardiographic patterns in, 390
types of, 78
Glycogen stores, limited, associated with hypoglycemia, 538
Goldenhar syndrome, 73–74
Gonadal differentiation, disorder(s) of, 524–529
Klinefelter syndrome as, 57–58, 524
pure gonadal dysgenesis as, 527–528
true hermaphroditism as, 528–529
Turner syndrome as, 56–57, 524, 526–527
Gonadal dysgenesis, in Turner syndrome, 524, 526–527
pure (46,XX karyotype, 46,XY karyotype), 525t, 527–528
Granulomatosis infantisepticum, 192
Graves disease, neonatal, 535–536
Gray matter lesions, in utero, 410
Great arteries, transposition of, 336–339
chest radiographs of, 338
malformations associated with, 336
management of, 338–339

Great arteries *(Continued)*
murmurs in, 337
pulmonary and systemic circulations in, 336–337
"Greek helmet facies," in Wolf-Hirschhorn syndrome, 62
Growth deficiency, in CHARGE association, 71
Growth hormone therapy, for Turner syndrome, 57
Growth retardation, associated with Down syndrome, 51–52

H

Haemophilus influenzae infection, 194
Hashimoto's thyroiditis, 535
HBeAg (hepatitis B e antigen), 181, 182, 444, 445
HBsAg (hepatitis B surface antigen), 181, 182, 444, 445
HBV (hepatitis B virus), 444, 445
Health care workers, HIV infection in, 166–167
Hearing loss, associated with auricular tags and sinuses, 48–49
associated with Down syndrome, 51
Heart. See also *Cardiac; Cardio-* entries.
auscultation of, 317–318
congenital disease of, 37–40
cyanotic, 312–313
syndromes associated with, 38t–39t
glycogen storage disease of, 389–391
Heart beats, ectopic, 393–394
Heart block, atrioventricular, 397–398
Heart murmurs, in aortic stenosis, 367
in endocardial fibroelastosis, 386–387
in transposition of great arteries, 337

565

Heart murmurs *(Continued)*
  in truncus arteriosus, 354–355
  systolic and diastolic, 317–318
    localization of, 317
Heart rate, in paroxysmal supraventricular tachycardia, 395
Heart rate monitors, for apnea, 240
Heinz bodies, in asplenia, 360
  in G6PD deficiency, 474
  in hyperbilirubinemia, in septic infants, 476
Hemangioma(s), giant, 493–494
Hemifacial microsomia, 73–74
Hemivertebrae, in VACTERL syndrome, 322
Hemoglobin S, in sickle cell disease, 114
Hemolytic anemia, nonspherocytic, 472–473
Hemolytic disease of newborn, ABO incompatibility in, 472
  hyperbilirubinemia and, 471
  minor blood group incompatibility in, 472
  Rh isoimmunization in, 471–472
Hemophilia A, 481
Hemophilia B, 481
Hemorrhage, adrenal, 518–520
  brain, in utero, 410–411
  intraventricular, 420–424
    diagnosis of, 421–422
    grading of, 422–423
    treatment of, 423–424
      prophylactic, 423
  periventricular-intraventricular, 484
  subdural, 424–425
  VK-dependent. See *VK-dependent bleeding (VKDB)*.
Hemorrhagic disease of newborn. See *VK-dependent bleeding (VKDB)*.
Hemorrhagic disorder(s), 479–482

Hemorrhagic disorder(s) *(Continued)*
  due to vitamin K deficiency, 479–480
  hemophilia as, 481
  laboratory evaluation of, 480
  management of, 480–481
Hemorrhagic edema, of scalp, 424
Hemostatic disorder(s), 479–500
  acquired, 482–486
  hemorrhagic, 479–482
  of platelets, qualitative, 498–500
    quantitative, 490, 491t, 492–498
  thrombotic, 486–490
Heparin therapy, for renal vein thrombosis, 490
Hepatic. See also *Liver disorder(s)*.
Hepatic encephalopathy, 415
Hepatitis, 444–446
  bacterial, 446
  from syphilis, 446
Hepatitis B, 181–183, 444–445
  vaccination schedule for, 183
Hepatitis B e antigen (HBeAg), 181, 182
Hepatitis B e antigen (HbeAg), 444, 445
Hepatitis B surface antigen (HBsAg), 181, 182, 444, 445
Hepatitis B virus (HBV), 444, 445
Hepatitis C, 183, 445–446
Hepatomegaly, in congenital syphilis, 233
Hereditary elliptocytosis, 477
Hereditary fructose intolerance, 80–81, 447
Hereditary galactosemia, 76–78
Hereditary spherocytosis, 476–477
Hereditary tumor syndromes, of nervous system, 403
Hereditary tyrosinemia, type 1, 89–90
Hermaphroditism, true, 525t, 528–529

Heroin abuse, during pregnancy, 1, 3, 3t
Herpes simplex virus (HSV) infection, 176–179
 central nervous system involvement in, 177
 disseminated disease in, 177
 localized disease in, 177–178
 management of, 179
 transmission of, 177
 type 1, 176
 type 2, 176
High-frequency jet ventilation, for persistent pulmonary hypertension of newborn, 269–270
High-frequency oscillation ventilation, for persistent pulmonary hypertension of newborn, 269–270
Hip, congenital dislocation of, 43
Hirschsprung disease, 404, 442
HIV (human immunodeficiency virus), newborn screening for, 118–119
HIV infection. See *Human immunodeficiency virus (HIV) infection.*
HLA (human leukocyte antigen) typing, in 21-hydroxylase deficiency, 522–523
HMD. See *Hyaline membrane disease (HMD).*
Home apnea monitoring programs, 246–247
Homeostasis, fluid, hydrops and, 16–17
Homocystinuria, newborn screening for, 110–111
Homovanillic acid (HVA), in neuroblastoma, 117
Homozygous prethrombotic disorder(s), 487–488
Hormone(s). See specific hormone, e.g., *Thyroid-stimulating hormone (TSH).*

Hormone regulator(s), 145–148
 atrial natriuretic peptide as, 146–147
 dopamine, noradrenaline, and adrenaline as, 147
 kallikrein-kinin system as, 147
 prolactin, 147–148
 prostaglandins as, 147
 renin-angiotensin-aldosterone system as, 145–146
 vasopressin as, 146
Hospital-acquired infection(s), bacterial. See *Nosocomial infection(s), bacterial.*
Howell-Jolly bodies, in asplenia, 360
HSV infection. See *Herpes simplex virus (HSV) infection.*
Human immunodeficiency virus (HIV), newborn screening for, 118–119
Human immunodeficiency virus (HIV) infection, 164–168
 among health care workers, 166–167
 clinical categorization of, 165
 encephalopathy in, 417
 malaria and, 229–230
 management of, immunizations in, 166
  ketoconazole in, 166
  perspective in, 165
  zidovudine in, 165–166
 toxoplasmosis and, 225
 transmission of, 164–165
Human leukocyte antigen (HLA) typing, in 21-hydroxylase deficiency, 522–523
Human milk, fat content of, 459
 lactose in, 451
 lipids in, 451
 nutrient composition of, 460t–461t
 protein content of, 457–458
 vs. bovine milk, 450
  phosphorus content of, 511

567

Human milk *(Continued)*
  whey fraction of, 450
Human papillomavirus (HPV) infection, 184
HVA (homovanillic acid), in neuroblastoma, 117
H-Y antigen, negative, in pure gonadal dysgenesis, 528
  positive, in pure gonadal dysgenesis, 528
  in true hermaphroditism, 529
Hyaline membrane disease (HMD), 248–262
  Aa-Do$_2$ in, 250
    measurement of, 251
    approaches to, 254–255
  birth asphyxia and, 249
  elevated respiratory rate in, 250
  incidence of, 248
  labored breathing in, 252
  L/S ratio in, 253, 255
  NIH recommendations for, 256–257
  prenatal glucocorticoids for, 257
  surfactant deficiency in, 254
  treatment of, 257–262
    corticosteroids in, 260
    CPAP in, 260–261
    dopamine in, 260
    fluid restriction in, 258–259
    mechanical ventilation in, 261–262
    oxygen therapy for, 258
    surfactant in, 258
  V/Q in, 251
Hydantoins, and developing nervous system, 412–413
Hydramnios, 25
  diagnoses associated with, 26t
Hydranencephaly, intrauterine, 410
Hydration, use of, for premature labor, 31
Hydrocephalus, 409
  associated with meningomyelocele, 401
Hydrops, attention to, during resuscitation, 134–135

Hydrops fetalis, 16–23
  alloimmune, 17
  causes of, 17–18
  conditions associated with, 19t–20t
  investigation of, 21t
  neonates with, evaluation of, 18, 22t, 22–23
  pathogenesis of, 16–17
  prenatal ultrasound diagnosis of, 18
Hydrostatic pressure, in newborn, 144
21-Hydroxylase deficiency, in congenital adrenal hyperplasia, 522–523
Hyperaeration of lungs, 264
Hyperammonemia, 84–85
  transient, of newborn, 86–87
  treatment of, 85
Hyperbilirubinemia, ABO incompatibility and, 472
  chemical, definition of, 463
  definition of, 470
  extravascular blood and, 477
  hypothyroidism and, 478
  minor blood group incompatibility and, 472
  polycythemia and, 477–478
  red blood cell enzyme abnormalities and, 472–476
  red blood cell membrane defects and, 476–477
  Rh isoimmunization and, 471–472
  sepsis and, 476
  unconjugated, 470–478
  vs. physiologic jaundice, 463–464
Hyperglycemia, 543
Hyperglycinemia, ketonic, 94
  nonketonic, 90–91
Hyperinsulinemia, associated with hypoglycemia, 539–541
Hyperlipidemia, newborn screening for, 119
Hypernatremia, 148–153
  replacement therapy for, calculations governing, 149–150
  sodium chloride supplementation for, 152

Hypernatremia *(Continued)*
  sources of water loss and, 150–152
Hyperphosphatemia, in late neonatal hypocalcemia, 511
Hypersplenism, 495
Hyperthyroidism, treatment of, 536
Hypocalcemia, 508–516
  associated with hypomagnesemia, 512–513
    treatment of, 515–516
  definition of, 508
  early, 508–510
  late, 510–512
  treatment of, 513–515
Hypoglycemia, 536–543
  Beckwith-Wiedemann syndrome associated with, 541
  definition of, 414–415, 537
  diagnosis of, 536–537
  diminished glucose production in, 542–543
  erythroblastosis fetalis associated with, 541–542
  glycogen metabolism disorders associated with, 538–539
  hyperinsulinemia associated with, 539–541
  in Beckwith-Wiedemann syndrome, 65
  limited glycogen stores in, 538
  neonatal glucose metabolism associated with, maternal drug effects on, 542
  perinatal distress associated with, 538
  severe, 443–444
Hypomagnesemia, neonatal hypocalcemia associated with, 512–513
Hyponatremia, management of, 148
Hypoparathyroidism, transient, in late neonatal hypocalcemia, 511
Hypoplastic left heart syndrome, 369–372
  electrocardiographic patterns in, 370

Hypoplastic left heart syndrome *(Continued)*
  management of, 372
  ventricles in, 369–370
Hypothalamic-pituitary defects, 533
Hypothyroidism, congenital, 531–534
  dysgenesis in, 532–533
  hyperbilirubinemia with, 478
  hypothalamic-pituitary defects in, 533
  newborn screening for, 107–109
  transient, 534
Hypotonia, 40–42
  central, 434
  heritable disorders associated with, 41t
Hypoventilation syndrome, congenital, 243–244
Hypoxic-ischemic encephalopathy, 418–420
  intrauterine, 409–410
  neurologic sequelae in, 418
  treatment of, 419–420

I

IgM-FTA-ABS test, for syphilis, at birth, 237
Ileus, meconium. See *Meconium ileus.*
Immunizations, in HIV infection, 166
Immunoglobulin(s), after exposure to varicella, 180–181
Immunoglobulin A (IgA), detection of, in toxoplasmosis, 226
Immunoglobulin G (IgG), HIV-specific, 118
  in Rh isoimmunization, 471
Immunoglobulin M (IgM), detection of, in syphilis, 233, 237
  in toxoplasmosis, 226
  in congenital viral infections, 168
Immunoreactive trypsinogen, in cystic fibrosis, 114
Imperforate anal membrane, 439

Inborn errors of metabolism, 74–106. See also under *Amino acid metabolism; Ammonia metabolism; Carbohydrate metabolism; Organic acid metabolism.*
Incontinentia pigmenti, 406–407
Incubators, 138–139
  temperature regulation of, 138
Indomethacin, causing ischemic and nephrotoxic renal injury, 504
  for patent ductus arteriosus, 303–305
  platelet function and, 499
Infant(s). See also *Neonate(s).*
  apnea in, 244–245
  extremely low-birth-weight, intubation of, 136
    resuscitation of, 132–133
  low-birth-weight, energy needs of, 453
    enteral nutrition for, 457–459, 460t–461t, 462
    total parenteral nutrition for, 454–457
  of diabetic mother, cardiomyopathy in. 388–389
  hypocalcemia in, 510
  hypoglycemia in, 539–541
  premature. See *Premature infant(s).*
  small for gestational age, diminished glucose production in, 542–543
  very-low-birth-weight, bronchopulmonary dysplasia in, 284. See also *Bronchopulmonary dysplasia (BPD).*
    hyperglycemia in, 543
    osteopenia in, 517
    patent ductus arteriosus in, 300–301
Infant formula(s), nutrient composition of, 460t–461t
Infantile mitochondrial disease, benign, 103–104
  lethal, 104

Infection(s), 164–237. See also specific infection, e.g., *Tuberculosis.*
  bacterial, 184–222. See also *Bacterial infection(s).*
  fungal, 222–224
  in utero, brain lesions caused by, 411
  protozoal, 224–230
  spirochetal, 230–237
  viral, 164–184. See also *Viral infection(s).*
Infectious encephalopathy, 416–417
Inositol supplementation, in total parenteral nutrition, 455
Insulin therapy, for maple syrup urine disease, 88
Interstitial emphysema, pulmonary, 279–281
  causes of, 280
Intestinal obstruction(s), 436–443
  anal agenesis in, 440
  anal stenosis in, 439
  annular pancreas in, 441
  anorectal malformations in, 439–440
  atresia in, 436–437
  duodenal stenosis in, 437
  enteric duplications in, 440
  Hirschsprung disease in, 442
  imperforate anal membrane in, 439
  intussusception in, 441–442
  malrotation with volvulus in, 441
  meconium ileus in, 437–439
  meconium plug syndrome in, 442–443
  pseudo-obstruction syndromes in, 443
  rectal agenesis in, 440
Intestinal rotation, with volvulus, 441
Intracranial abscess, 431
Intranasal encephalocele, 400
Intraventricular hemorrhage, 420–424
  diagnosis of, 421–422
  grading of, 422–423
  treatment of, 423–424

Intraventricular hemorrhage (*Continued*)
prophylactic, 423
Intubation, of extremely low-birth-weight infant, during resuscitation, 136
Intussusception, 441–442
Iodine, for thyrotoxicosis, 536
Ipodate, for thyrotoxicosis, 536
Ischemia, and nephrotoxic injury, in acute renal failure, 504–505
myocardial, transient, 381–382
Ischemic-hypoxic injury, in acute renal failure, 502–503
Isoimmunization, Rh, 471–472
Isoniazid (INH), for tuberculosis, 216, 217
Isotretinoin, and developing nervous system, 412
Isovaleric acidemia, 95
Isovaleryl CoA dehydrogenase (IVCD) deficiency, 95

J

Jaundice. See also *Kernicterus*.
in G6PD deficiency, 473, 475
in GALT deficiency, 76
in pyruvate kinase deficiency, 475
phototherapy for, 469–470
physiologic, 463
vs. hyperbilirubinemia, 463–464
Joint contractures, multiple, 45–46, 46t

K

Kallikrein kinin system, 147
Kanamycin, for bacterial meningitis, 197
Kasabach-Merritt syndrome, 493–494
Kernicterus, 467–470. See also *Jaundice*.
exchange transfusion for, 468–469

Ketoconazole, for thrush, in HIV-infected patient, 166
Ketonic hyperglycinemia, 94
Kidney. See *Renal* entries.
Klinefelter syndrome (47,XXY karyotype), 57–58, 524, 525t
Klumpke palsy, 427

L

Labor and delivery, body composition and fluid compartment changes during, 140–141
premature. See *Premature labor and delivery*.
timing of cord clamping after, 141
Lactase, in human milk, 451
Lactose-free diet, for GALT deficiency, 77
LAMB syndrome, 403
Laser photoregulation, for retinopathy of prematurity, 550
Latex agglutination assays, for bacterial meningitis, 196
Lecithin/sphingomyelin (L/S) ratio, in hyaline membrane disease, 253, 255
Left-to-right shunting, in cardiac disorders, 312–313
through ductus arteriosus, 300, 301
Leigh disease (subacute necrotizing encephalomyelopathy), 104–105
LEOPARD syndrome, 403
Lethal infantile mitochondrial disease, 104
Lethal lactic acidosis, early, 105–106
Leukemia, acute lymphoblastic, associated with Down syndrome, 52
Leukomalacia, periventricular, 418–419
Lidocaine, for ventricular tachycardia, 397
Lip(s), cleft, 36–37

Lipid(s), emulsion of, in total parenteral nutrition, 454
  in human milk, 451
Lipid storage diseases, 448
Lipomeningomyelocele, 401
LIS1 gene, 60
Lissencephaly, 59–60
  hypotonia due to, 40, 42
Listeria monocytogenes infection, 192–193
  management of, 193
Liver disorder(s), 444–450
  alpha$_1$-antitrypsin deficiency as, 446–447
  cerebrohepatorenal syndrome as, 448–449
  cholestasis as, familial, 448
    TPN-associated, 449–450
    with lymphedema as, 448
  galactosemia as, 447
  hepatitis as, 444–446. See also *Hepatitis* entries.
  hereditary fructose intolerance as, 447
  in cystic fibrosis, 447
  lipid storage diseases as, 448
  tyrosinemia as, 448
Long-chain 3-hydroxy acyl-CoA dehydrogenase (LCHAD) deficiency, 100–101
Lorazepam, for seizures, 433
Low-birth-weight (LBW) infant(s), energy needs of, 453
  enteral nutrition for, 457–459, 460t–461t, 462
  total parenteral nutrition for, 454–457
Lung(s). See also *Pulmonary*; *Respiratory* entries.
  antioxidant enzymes of, 285–286
  chronic disease(s) of, 284–298
    bronchopulmonary dysplasia as, 284–296
    pulmonary insufficiency of prematurity as, 296–297
    Wilson-Mikity syndrome as, 297–298
  expansion of, resuscitation and, 125

Lymphedema, cholestasis with, 448
Lysosomal α-glucosidase deficiency, 79–80

M

Macroencephaly, 405
Macroglossia, in Beckwith-Wiedemann syndrome, 65
Magnesium, in total parenteral nutrition, 455
Magnesium sulfate, for neonatal hypocalcemia associated with hypomagnesemia, 515–516
Magnetic resonance imaging (MRI), diagnostic, of Arnold-Chiari syndrome, 401–402
Malaria, 228–230
  and HIV infection, 229–230
  incidence of, 228
  transfusion-acquired, 229
Malformation(s), severe, attention to, during resuscitation, 135–136
Malrotation with volvulus, 441
Mantoux test, 218
Maple syrup urine disease, 87–89
  e$_1$α gene mutation in, 88
  newborn screening for, 111
  nutritional approach to, 88
Marfan syndrome, 67
Marijuana abuse, during pregnancy, 15
  enhanced risk for events after, 2t
Maternal ingestion, of drugs, virilization of female fetus by, 530
Maternal overproduction, of androgens, virilization of female fetus by, 530–531
Maternal serum alpha-fetoprotein, in anencephaly, 400
  in Arnold-Chiari syndrome, 402
Mean platelet volume (MPV), in thrombocytopenia, 492

Mechanical ventilation, for bronchopulmonary dysplasia, 286
  for hyaline membrane disease, 261–262
  pulmonary interstitial emphysema due to, 281
Meckel syndrome, 68
  postaxial polydactyly in, 47
Meconium, 271
  aspiration of, during resuscitation, 134
  passage of, 134
Meconium aspiration pneumonia, 271–276
  airway resistance in, 273
  antibiotics for, 274
  corticosteroids for, 274
  infant postmaturity and, 273
Meconium ileus, 437–439
  in cystic fibrosis, 66, 437–438
  simple, management of, 438–439
Meconium plug syndrome, 442–443
Meconium staining, of amniotic fluid, 271
  American Heart Association and American Academy of Pediatrics approach to, 275–276
  cause of, 271–272
Medium-chain acyl-coA dehydrogenase deficiency, newborn screening for, 115–116
Medium-chain acyl-CoA dehydrogenase (MCAD) deficiency, 98–99
Meningitis, bacterial, 194–198
  cerebrospinal fluid cell counts in, interpretation of, 195–196
  Escherichia coli in, 195
  group B streptococcus in, 194–195
  management of, 196–198
  mortality in, 198
  signs and symptoms of, 186t, 195
  tuberculous, prednisone for, 217

Meningocele, 401
Meningomyelocele, 401
  Arnold-Chiari syndrome with, 401–402
Mental retardation, in CHARGE association, 71
Mercury, exposure to, developing nervous system and, 413
Metabolic acidosis, 155–159
  anion gap in, 156
    normal, 157
  correction of, resuscitation and, 128
  morbidity and mortality of, 158
  of prematurity, 156–157
  sodium bicarbonate for, 158–159
  tromethamine for, 159
Metabolic alkalosis, 160–163
  persistence of, factors in, 161
Metabolic disease(s), 427–431
  in utero, brain lesions associated with, 411
  Type I, 427
  Type II, 427–428
  Type III, 428
  Type IVa, 428–429
  Type IVb, 429
  Type IVc, 429
  Type V, 429–430
Metabolic encephalopathy, 414–415
Metabolism, disorders of. See also specific disorder, e.g., *Hypocalcemia*.
  maternal, umbilical cord blood screening for, 119–120
  inborn errors of, 74–106. See also under *Amino acid metabolism; Ammonia metabolism; Carbohydrate metabolism; Organic acid metabolism*.
  associated with hypotonia, 42
Metered dose inhalers, for bronchopulmonary dysplasia, 294
Methadone maintenance, during pregnancy, 5

Methimazole, for thyrotoxicosis, 536
Methionine synthetase deficiency, 91
Methylmalonic acidemia, 92–94
L-Methylmalonyl-CoA mutase (MCM) deficiency, 92–94
Methylxanthines, for apnea, 241–242
Microencephaly, 404–405
Microencephaly vera, 404
Micrognathia, 43–45
Microsomia, hemifacial, 73–74
Miller-Dieker syndrome, 59–60
  hypotonia due to, 40, 42
Mitochondrial disease, infantile, benign, 103–104
  lethal, 104
Mitochondrial myopathy/cardiomyopathy, infantile, benign, 103–104
Mixoploidy, 58
Möbius syndrome, 404
Mohr syndrome, postaxial polydactyly in, 47
Monozygotic twins, 34
Morbidity and mortality, in acute renal failure, 507
  in bronchopulmonary dysplasia, 295
  in metabolic acidosis, 158
Motor neuron disease(s), 434–435
MPV (mean platelet volume), in thrombocytopenia, 492
MRI (magnetic resonance imaging), diagnostic, of Arnold-Chiari syndrome, 401–402
Multicenter trial of cryotherapy for retinopathy of prematurity (CRYO-ROP) study, 549–550
Multiple carboxylase deficiency, 96, 113
Multiple joint contractures, 45–46, 46t
Murmurs. See *Heart murmurs.*

Myasthenia gravis, maternal, neonatal hypotonia associated with, 42
Myocardial ischemia, transient, 381–382
Myocarditis, 382–386
  chest radiographs of, 384
  coxsackie virus infection and, 383
  diagnosis of, 384–385
Myoclonic seizure(s), 432
Myopathy, mitochondrial, infantile, benign, 103–104
MZ phenotype, in alpha$_1$-antitrypsin deficiency, 446

N

NAGS (*N*-acetylglutamate synthetase), 83
Naloxone hydrochloride, for resuscitation, 127t
NAME syndrome, 403
Necrotizing encephalomyelopathy, subacute, 104–105
Necrotizing fasciitis, 210
Neisseria gonorrhoeae, ophthalmia neonatorum associated with, 206, 207, 208
Neomycin, for infectious diarrhea, 201
Neonatal Abstinence Score, 4
Neonatal Narcotic Withdrawal Index, 4
Neonatal resuscitation, 121–137
  AHA-AAP approach to, 123–131
  assessment of asphyxia in, 121, 122t
  cardiovascular support in, 129–130
    continuation of, after successful resuscitation, 130–131
  condition(s) requiring attention during, 132–136
  extremely premature infant and, 132–133
  hydrops as, 134–135
  meconium aspiration as, 134

Neonatal resuscitation (*Continued*)
   severe malformations as, 135–136
  controversies in, 136–137
  duration of, 137
  epinephrine administration in, 125
  expansion of lungs in, 125
  intubation of extremely low-birth-weight infant and, 136
  medications for, 126t–127t
  metabolic acidosis correction in, 128
  of depressed infant, 123
  of infants with Apgar score of 0, 124–125, 126t–127t
  of infants with Apgar score of 1–3, 124
  of infants with Apgar score of 4–6, 124
  of infants with Apgar score of 7 or more, 123–124
  overview of, 123
  rules of, 131–132
  sodium bicarbonate administration in, 136
  umbilical vessel catheterization in, 125, 128
  with room air vs. 100% oxygen in, 137

Neonatal screening program(s), 106t, 106–120
  for alpha$_1$-antitrypsin deficiency, 118
  for biotinidase deficiency, 112–113
  for congenital adrenal hyperplasia, 112
  for congenital hypothyroidism, 107–109
  for congenital toxoplasmosis, 115
  for cystic fibrosis, 114–115
  for Duchenne muscular dystrophy, 116–117
  for galactosemia, 109–110
  for homocystinuria, 110–111
  for human immunodeficiency virus, 118–119
  for hyperlipidemia, 119

Neonatal screening program(s) (*Continued*)
  for maple syrup urine disease, 111
  for medium-chain acyl-CoA dehydrogenase deficiency, 115–116
  for neuroblastoma, 117
  for phenylketonuria, 106–107
  for sickle cell disease, 113–114
  of umbilical cord blood, for maternal metabolic disorders, 119–120

Neonate(s). See also *Infant(s)*.
  acid-base balance in, disturbances of, 155–163
  asphyxial and hypoxic-ischemic injury in, 417–420
  body composition of, developmental changes in, 139–142
    physiology of regulation of, 142–145
  cardiac disorders in, evaluation of, 305–398. See also *Cardiac disorder(s)*; specific disorder, e.g., *Tetralogy of Fallot*.
  encephalopathies in, 413–417
  endocrine disorders in. See specific disorder, e.g., *Hypocalcemia*.
  fluid and electrolyte management in, 148–155
  fluid compartments in, developmental changes of, 139–142
  hormone regulator(s) in, 145–148
    atrial natriuretic peptide as, 146–147
    dopamine, noradrenaline, and adrenaline as, 147
    kallikrein-kinin system as, 147
    prolactin as, 147–148
    prostaglandins as, 147
    renin-angiotensin-aldosterone system as, 145–146

Neonate(s) *(Continued)*
  vasopressin as, 146
  intraventricular hemorrhage in, 420–424
  metabolic and degenerative diseases in, 427–431
  neuromuscular disorders in, 434–435
  respiratory distress in. See *Hyaline membrane disease (HMD); Respiratory distress.*
  seizures in, 431–434
  superficial cranial injury in, 424
  thermal neutral zone in, 138–139
  transient hyperammonemia of, 86–87
  traumatic brain injury in, 424–425
  traumatic nerve injury in, 425–427
Nephropathy, uric acid, 505
Nerve injury(ies). See also specific nerve.
  traumatic, 425–427
Nervous system, central. See *Central nervous system (CNS).*
Nesidioblastosis, 443–444
Neural crest, migration, disorders of, 403–404
Neural tube defect(s), 399–408
  anencephaly as, 399–400
  Arnold-Chiari malformation as, 401–402
  arteriovenous malformation of vein of Galen as, 407–408
  cerebellar malformations as, 405–407
  corpus callosum agenesis as, 403
  encephaloceles as, 400–401
  lipmeningomyelocele as, 401
  macroencephaly as, 405
  meningocele as, 401
  meningomyelocele as, 401
  microencephaly as, 404–405
  Möbius syndrome as, 404
  neurocristopathies as, 403–404

Neural tube defect(s) *(Continued)*
  neurocutaneous syndromes as, 405–407
  ocular dysraphisms as, 402
Neuroblastoma, 404
  newborn screening for, 117
Neurocristopathy(ies), 403–404
Neurocutaneous syndrome(s), 405–407
Neurofibromatosis, *ras* proto-oncogene in, 405
Neuromuscular disorder(s), 434–435
Nitric oxide, and platelet adhesion, 500
  inhalation of, for persistent pulmonary hypertension of newborn, 270
  synthesis of, in persistent pulmonary hypertension of newborn, 266
Nitrogen, in total parenteral nutrition, 453–454
Noncommunicating hydrocephalus, 409
Nonimmune hydrops, 16–23. See also *Hydrops fetalis.*
Nonketotic hyperglycinemia, 90–91
Nonstress test, in fetal surveillance, 25
Noonan syndrome, 68–69
Noradrenaline, 147
Nosocomial infection(s), bacterial, 211–215
  diarrhea in, 213
  gram-negative, 214–215
  staphylococcal, 211–213
  streptococcal group A, 213–214
Nutrient(s), essential, in total parenteral nutrition, 454
Nutrient composition, of human milk, 460t–461t
  of infant formulas, 460t–461t
Nutrition, enteral, 457–459, 460t–461t, 462
  fatty acids in, 458
  protein in, 457–458, 460t
  parenteral, 453–457
  total. See *Total parenteral nutrition (TPN).*

Nutritional support, for bronchopulmonary dysplasia, 290–291

O

Obstruction, intestinal, 436–443. See also *Intestinal obstruction(s)*.
Ocular disorders, associated with Down syndrome, 51
Ocular dysraphisms, 402
Oculo-auriculo-vertebral spectrum, 73–74
Oligohydramnios, 25
  diagnoses associated with, 26t
Oncotic pressure, in newborn, 144
Ophthalmia neonatorum, 206–208
  agents associated with, 206
  management of, 207–208
  prevention of, 208
Opiate abuse, during pregnancy, 1, 3–6
  and sudden infant death syndrome, 5–6
  enhanced risk for events after, 2t
  obstetric complications and, 3–4
Oral candidiasis (thrush), in HIV-infected patient, ketoconazole for, 166
Organic acid metabolism, 414
  inborn error(s) of, 75t, 92–106
    acylcarnitine translocase deficiency as, 101–102
    Barth syndrome as, 104
    benign infantile mitochondrial myopathy/cardiomyopathy as, 103–104
    carnitine palmitoyltransferase I and II deficiencies as, 101–102
    carnitine transporter defect as, 101–102
    early lethal lactic acidosis as, 105–106
    glutaric acidemia type 1 as, 96–97

Organic acid metabolism (*Continued*)
    glutaric acidemia type 2 as, 97–98
    isovaleric acidemia as, 95
    lethal infantile mitochondrial disease as, 104
    long-chain 3-hydroxy acyl-CoA dehydrogenase (LCHAD) deficiency as, 100–101
    medium-chain acyl-CoA dehydrogenase (MCAD) deficiency as, 98–99
    methylmalonic acidemia as, 92–94
    multiple carboxylase deficiency as, 96
    phosphoenolpyruvate carboxykinase deficiency as, 103
    propionic acidemia as, 94–95
    pyruvate carboxylase (PC) deficiency as, 103
    pyruvate dehydrogenase deficiency as, 102
    short-chain acyl-CoA dehydrogenase (SCAD) deficiency as, 100
    subacute necrotizing encephalomyelopathy (Leigh disease) as, 104–105
    very-long-chain acyl-CoA dehydrogenase (LCAD) deficiency as, 99–100
Ornithine transcarbamylase (OTC) deficiency, 82–85
Orofacial clefting, 36–37
Osmolality, changes in, of extracellular fluid compartments, 143
Osseous lesions, rubella-associated, 169
Osteomalacia, 516
Osteomyelitis, 203–206
  management of, 205–206
Osteopenia, in premature infants, 516–518
Osteoporosis, 516–517

Osteoporosis (Continued)
definition of, 516
Otitis media, 198–199
Oxygen (100%), vs. room air, for resuscitation, 137
Oxygen tension, maintenance of, in persistent pulmonary hypertension of newborn, 268–269
Oxygen therapy, for apnea, 241
for bronchopulmonary dysplasia, 291
for hyaline membrane disease, 258
for persistent pulmonary hypertension of newborn, 269

P

Palate, cleft, 36–37
Pallister-Hall syndrome, postaxial polydactyly in, 47
Pancreas, annular, 441
disorders of, 443–444. See also specific disorder, e.g., *Cystic fibrosis*.
Pancuronium bromide, for tetanus, 221
Paralysis, facial, congenital, 425–426
Parathyroid hormone (PTH), in early neonatal hypocalcemia, 509
in late neonatal hypocalcemia, 511
secretion of, hypomagnesemia and, 512
Paroxysmal supraventricular tachycardia. See *Supraventricular tachycardia, paroxysmal*.
Patau syndrome (trisomy 13), 55–56
postaxial polydactyly in, 47
skin holes in, 313
Patent ductus arteriosus (PDA), 299–305
associated with bronchopulmonary dysplasia, 288
clinical signs of, 302
in very-low-birth-weight infants, 300–301

Patent ductus arteriosus (PDA) (Continued)
incidence of, surfactant therapy and, 302
indomethacin for, 303–305
left-to-right shunt in, 300, 301
positive end-expiratory pressure for, 302–303
PCBs (polychlorinated biphenyls), exposure to, developing nervous system and, 413
PDA. See *Patent ductus arteriosus (PDA)*.
PEEP. See *Positive end-expiratory pressure (PEEP)*.
Penicillin G, for ophthalmia neonatorum, 207
for syphilis, in newborn, 236t
in pregnant patient, 234t, 235t
Perinatal distress, associated with hypoglycemia, 538
Periventricular leukomalacia, 418–419
Periventricular-intraventricular hemorrhage, 484
Persistent pulmonary hypertension of newborn (PPHN), 265–271
nitric oxide synthesis in, 266
premature closure of ductus arteriosus in, 266
treatment of, 267–271
ECMO in, 271
high-frequency jet ventilation for, 269–270
high-frequency oscillation ventilation for, 269–270
inhalation of nitric oxide in, 270
oxygen tension in, maintenance of, 268–269
oxygen therapy for, 269
PEEP for, 269
tolazine in, 270
Peutz-Jeghers-Touraine syndrome, 403
Phencyclidine abuse, during pregnancy, 12–13

Phencyclidine abuse *(Continued)*
　enhanced risk for events after, 2t
Phenobarbital, for seizures, 433
Phenylalanine hydroxylase (PAH) deficiency, 91–92
Phenylephrine, for paroxysmal supraventricular tachycardia, 396
Phenylketonuria (PKU), 91–92
　newborn screening for, 106–107
Phenytoin, for seizures, 433
Phosphate deficiency rickets, risk of, 517–518
Phosphatidylglycerol, in hyaline membrane disease, 253, 255
Phosphoenolpyruvate carboxykinase deficiency, 103
Phosphorus, in human milk and bovine milk, 511
　in total parenteral nutrition, 455
Photoregulation, laser, for retinopathy of prematurity, 550
Phototherapy, for jaundice, 469–470
Pierre Robin sequence, 43–45
Pituitary hypoplasia, 521
PKU (phenylketonuria), 91–92
　newborn screening for, 106–107
Plasmodium species, in malaria, 228
Platelet(s), consumption of, disease states associated with, 493
　destruction of, increased, 492–494
　production of, decreased, 494
Platelet concentrates, for thrombocytopenia, 495
Platelet disorder(s), qualitative, 498–500
　quantitative, 490, 491t, 492–498

Platelet transfusion, for alloimmune thrombocytopenia, 497–498
Pneumomediastinum, 281–284
　spontaneous, incidence of, 281
Pneumonia, meconium aspiration, 271–276. See also *Meconium aspiration pneumonia.*
Pneumopericardium, 283
Pneumoperitoneum, 283–284
Pneumothorax, 282
Polychlorinated biphenyls (PCBs), exposure to, developing nervous system and, 413
Polycythemia, 477–478
Polydactyly, 47
Polysplenia, vs. asplenia, 360–361
Pompe disease, 380
Positive end-expiratory pressure (PEEP), for cyanotic spells without apnea, 242, 243
　for patent ductus arteriosus, 302–303
　for persistent pulmonary hypertension of newborn, 269
Postasphyxial encephalopathy, 413–414
Potassium, in total parenteral nutrition, 455
PPHN. See *Persistent pulmonary hypertension of newborn (PPHN).*
PPROM (preterm premature rupture of membranes), 29, 33
Prader-Willi syndrome, hypotonia due to, 40, 42
Preauricular pits, 48
Prednisone, for tuberculosis, 217
　for tuberculous meningitis, 217
Pregnancy, substance abuse in, 1–16. See also *Substance abuse, during pregnancy.*

579

Premature infant(s), apnea in, 238–243. See also *Apnea.*
  cyanotic spells without, 242–243
  chronic pulmonary insufficiency in, 296–297
  diaphragmatic breathing in, 239
  limited glycogen stores in, 538
  metabolic acidosis in, 156–157
  osteopenia in, 516–518
  patent ductus arteriosus in, 299–305. See also *Patent ductus arteriosus (PDA).*
  retinopathy in, 544–550. See also *Retinopathy of prematurity (ROP).*
  temperature regulation of, 138–139
Premature labor and delivery, 29–33
  cocaine abuse and, 9–11, 29–30
  defined, 29
  treatment for, 31–33
Premature rupture of membranes (PROM), 29
Preterm premature rupture of membranes (PPROM), 29, 33
Procaine penicillin G, for syphilis, in newborn, 236t
  in pregnant patient, 234t, 235t
Prolactin, 147–148
PROM (premature rupture of membranes), 29
Prone sleeping position, in control of breathing, 247–248
  SIDS associated with, 247
Propionic acidemia, 94–95
Propionyl CoA carboxylase (PCC) deficiency, 94–95
Propranolol, for paroxysmal supraventricular tachycardia, 396
Propylthiouracil, for thyrotoxicosis, 536

Prosencephalon, disorders of, 403
Prostaglandin(s), 147
  for asplenia, 361
  for coarctation of aortic arch, 364
  for interrupted aortic arch, 366
  for pulmonary atresia with intact ventricular septum, 345
Protein intake, for low-birth-weight infants, 457–458, 460t
Proteinosis, congenital alveolar, 70
Prothrombin time (PT), in hemorrhagic disorders, 480
Protozoal infection(s), 224–230
  malaria as, 228–230
  toxoplasmosis as, 224–228
Pseudomonas infection, 193
Pseudo-obstruction syndromes, 443
PT (prothrombin time), in hemorrhagic disorders, 480
PTH. See *Parathyroid hormone (PTH).*
Pulmonary. See also *Lung(s).*
Pulmonary artery, coeur-en-sabot appearance of, in tetralogy of Fallot, 341
Pulmonary atresia, tetralogy of Fallot with, 341–343
  with intact ventricular septum, 343–346
    chest radiographs of, 344
    echocardiography of, 344
    initial management of, 345
    QRS axis in, 345
    surgical management of, 345–346
Pulmonary compliance, in bronchopulmonary dysplasia, 290
Pulmonary edema, in transient tachypnea of newborn, 263, 264
  postasphyxial, 277–278
Pulmonary insufficiency of prematurity, 296–297

Pulmonary interstitial emphysema, 279–281
  causes of, 280
Pulmonary stenosis, with intact ventricular septum, 346–348
  chest radiographs of, 347
  electrocardiographic patterns in, 347
  management of, 348
  QRS axis in, 347
  right-to-left shunting in, 346–347
Pyrazinamide, for tuberculosis, 217
Pyrimethamine, for toxoplasmosis, 227
Pyruvate carboxylase (PC) deficiency, 103
Pyruvate dehydrogenase deficiency, 102
Pyruvate kinase deficiency, 475–476

Q

QRS axis, in pulmonary atresia with intact ventricular septum, 345
  in pulmonary stenosis with intact ventricular septum, 347

R

Radiant warmer beds, open, 139
Radiography, chest. See *Chest radiography.*
ras proto-oncogene, in neurofibromatosis 1, 405
Rash, rubella-associated, 170
Rectal agenesis, 440
Red blood cells (RBCs), detection of GALT enzyme deficiency in, 78
  enzyme abnormality(ies) of, 472–476
    glucose-6-phosphate-dehydrogenase deficiency as, 473–475
    pyruvate kinase deficiency as, 475–476

Red blood cells (RBCs) *(Continued)*
  life span of, 464
  membrane defect(s) of, hereditary elliptocytosis as, 477
    hereditary spherocytosis as, 476–477
Renal failure, acute, clinical course of, 506–507
  glomerular filtration rate in, 502
  intrinsic, 501–505
    course of, 502
    treatment of, 506
  ischemic-hypoxic injury in, 502–503
  nephrotoxic injury in, 503–504
    ischemia and, 504–505
  outcome of, 507
  treatment of, 505–506
Renal tubular acidosis, neonatal hypocalcemia associated with, 513
Renal vein thrombosis, 489–490
Renin-angiotensin-aldosterone system, 145–146
Respiration. See *Breathing.*
Respiratory acidosis, management of, 160
Respiratory alkalosis, 163
Respiratory distress, 248–278
  hyaline membrane disease causing, 248–262
  in Pierre Robin sequence, 45
  late-onset, 296–297
  meconium aspiration pneumonia causing, 271–276
  persistent pulmonary hypertension of newborn causing, 265–271
  postasphyxial pulmonary edema in, 277–278
  surfactant protein B deficiency in, 278
  transient tachypnea of newborn causing, 262–265
Respiratory distress syndrome. See *Hyaline membrane disease (HMD).*

Respiratory rate, elevated, in hyaline membrane disease, 250
Respiratory tract, water losses through, 151
Resuscitation, neonatal. See *Neonatal resuscitation.*
RET proto-oncogene, in Hirschsprung disease, 404
Retinal ablation, for retinopathy of prematurity, 548–549
Retinoic acid, and developing nervous system, 412
Retinopathy of prematurity (ROP), 544–550
  acute phase of, 545–546
  classification of, 544–547
    basic premise in, 545
    international, 456
  incidence of, 547–548
  long-term consequences of, 457
  natural history of, 548
  treatment of, cryotherapy in, 549–550
    laser photoregulation in, 550
    retinal ablation in, 548–549
  zones of retinal involvement in, 456
Retrolental fibroplasia. See *Retinopathy of prematurity (ROP).*
Rh isoimmunization, 471–472
Rhabdomyoma(s), 391
Rickets, 516
  phosphate deficiency, risk of, 517–518
  vitamin D deficiency, treatment of, 516
Rifampin, for staphylococcal infection, 192
  for tuberculosis, 217
Right-to-left shunting. See *Shunt (shunting), right-to-left.*
Rocker-bottom feet, in trisomy 18 (Edwards syndrome), 54
Room air, vs. 100% oxygen, for resuscitation, 137
ROP. See *Retinopathy of prematurity (ROP).*

Rubella, congenital, 168–171
  cardiac lesions in, 169–170
  classic findings in, 168–169
  consequences of, 171
  rash in, 170
  skin and osseous lesions in, 169
  maternal, 168–169
  management of, 171
Rubinstein-Taybi syndrome, 70–71
  preaxial polydactyly in, 47
"Rules" of resuscitation, 131–132

S

Salmonella, in infectious diarrhea, 199
Salt wasting, virilization with, in congenital adrenal hyperplasia, 523
Scalp, hemorrhagic edema of, 424
Screening program(s), neonatal, 106t, 106–120
  for alpha$_1$-antitrypsin deficiency, 118
  for biotinidase deficiency, 112–113
  for congenital adrenal hyperplasia, 112
  for congenital hypothyroidism, 107–109
  for congenital toxoplasmosis, 115
  for cystic fibrosis, 114–115
  for Duchenne muscular dystrophy, 116–117
  for galactosemia, 109–110
  for homocystinuria, 110–111
  for human immunodeficiency virus, 118–119
  for hyperlipidemia, 119
  for maple syrup urine disease, 111
  for medium-chain acyl-CoA dehydrogenase deficiency, 115–116

Screening program(s) (*Continued*)
  for neuroblastoma, 117
  for phenylketonuria, 106–107
  for sickle cell disease, 113–114
  of umbilical cord blood, for maternal metabolic disorders, 119–120
Seizure(s), 431–434
  hypocalcemic crisis with, treatment of, 514
  risk of, 431
  treatment of, maintenance schedules in, 433–434
  phases in, 433
  types of, 431–432
Selenium deficiency, in bronchopulmonary dysplasia, 289
Sepsis, associated with bilirubin overproduction, 476
  Escherichia coli, 193
  in GALT deficiency, 77
  neonatal. See *Septicemia*.
Septal defect(s), atrioventricular, 376–379
  ventricular, 372–376
Septic arthritis, 203–206
  management of, 205–206
  signs and symptoms of, 204
Septicemia, 184–194
  Escherichia coli infection causing, 193
  Haemophilus influenzae infection causing, 194
  incidence of, 184
  Listeria monocytogenes infection causing, 192–193
  Pseudomonas infection causing, 193
  risk of, antenatal treatment for, 185
  signs and symptoms of, 186, 186t
  staphylococcal disease causing, 190–192
  streptococcal disease causing, 188–190
  white blood count in, 187

Sexual differentiation, abnormalities of, 524–531. See also specific disorder, e.g., *Turner syndrome*.
  classification of, 525t
Sexually transmitted disease(s). See also specific disease, e.g., *Syphilis*.
  ophthalmia neonatorum associated with, 206–208
Shigellosis, 200
  ampicillin for, 201
Short-chain acyl-CoA dehydrogenase (SCAD) deficiency, 100
Shunt (shunting), left-to-right, in atrioventricular septal defects, 377
  in cardiac disorders, 312–313
  through ductus arteriosus, 300, 301
  right-to-left, causing differential cyanosis, 314
  in aortic stenosis, 367
  in cardiac disorders, propensity for, 320
  in Ebstein anomaly, 351–352
  in pulmonary stenosis with intact ventricular septum, 346–347
Sickle cell disease, newborn screening for, 113–114
SIDS. See *Sudden infant death syndrome (SIDS)*.
Sinus arrhythmia, 392
Sinus bradycardia, 393
Sinus tachycardia, 392–393
Sinuses, auricular, 47–49
Skin, lesions of, rubella-associated, 169
  stimulation of, for apnea, 240–241
  water losses through, 150–151
Skin infection(s). See also *Rash*.
  bacterial, 208–211
  streptococcus group A and B in, 209
Sleep state, apnea in relation to, 240

583

Sleeping position, lateral, 247
  prone, 247–248
    SIDS associated with, 247
  supine, 247
Small for gestational age (SGA) infant(s), diminished glucose production in, 542–543
Smoking. See *Cigarette smoking.*
Sodium, in total parenteral nutrition, 455
Sodium bicarbonate, administration of, during resuscitation, 126t, 136
  for correction of metabolic acidosis, 128
  for metabolic acidosis, 158–159
SP-B (surfactant protein B) deficiency, 69–70
  in respiratory distress syndrome, 278
Spherocytosis, hereditary, 476–477
Spina bifida cystica, 401
Spinal muscular atrophy, 434–435
  types of, 435
Spinal muscular atrophy (Werdnig-Hoffman disease), hypotonia due to, 42
Spiramycin, for toxoplasmosis, 227
Spirochetal infection(s), 230–237. See also *Syphilis.*
Splenomegaly, in congenital syphilis, 233
Staphylococcal infection(s), 190–192
  nosocomial, 211–213
  treatment of, 191–192
  types of, 190–191
Staphylococcus aureus, 190–191
Staphylococcus epidermidis, 190, 191
Starling equation, 17
Stenosis, anal, 439
  aortic, 366–369
  aqueductal, in utero, 408
  duodenal, 437

Stenosis *(Continued)*
  pulmonary, with intact ventricular septum, 346–348
Steroids, inhaled, for bronchopulmonary dysplasia, 294
Stickler syndrome, 44
Stimulation, cutaneous, for apnea, 240–241
Stools (feces), water loss through, 151
Storage diseases(s), glycogen, 389–391
  lipid, 448
Streptococcal infection(s), 188–190
  clinical manifestations of, 188–189
  group A, 189–190
    nosocomial, 213–214
  group B, 188–189, 190
    in meningitis, 194–195
  late-onset meningitic form of, 189
Streptomycin, for tuberculosis, 217
Sturge-Weber disease, 406
Subacute necrotizing encephalomyelopathy (Leigh disease), 104–105
Subdural hemorrhage, 424–425
Subluxation, atlantoaxial, associated with Down syndrome, 51
Substance abuse, breastfeeding and, 16
  during pregnancy, 1–16
    enhanced risk for events after, 2t
    methadone maintenance for, 5
  of alcohol, 13–14
  of amphetamines, 11–12
  of caffeine, 15–16
  of cocaine, 6–11
    premature delivery associated with, 9–11, 29–30
  of opiates, 1, 2t, 3–6
    and sudden infant death syndrome, 5–6
    obstetric complications and, 3–4

Substance abuse *(Continued)*
   of phencyclidine, 12–13
   of tobacco, 14–15
   issues of, in child-bearing women, 3t
Sudden infant death syndrome (SIDS), 245–246
   near-miss, 245
   opiates and, 5–6
   prone sleeping position associated with, 247
Sulfadiazine, for toxoplasmosis, 227
Supraventricular tachycardia, paroxysmal, 394–396
   electrocardiographic patterns in, 394
   heart rates in, 395
   medical management of, 396
Surfactant metabolism, inborn error of, 70
Surfactant protein B (SP-B) deficiency, 69–70
   in respiratory distress syndrome, 278
Surfactant therapy, for hyaline membrane disease, 258
   for patent ductus arteriosus, 302
Symptomatic recurrent apnea, 243
Syphilis, congenital, 230–237
   diagnosis of, 233, 237
   IgM-FTA-ABS test for, 237
   radiographic studies of, 232–233
   signs of, 237–238
   transplacental transmission of, 230–231
   visceral involvement in, 233
   hepatitis from, 446
   treatment of, in newborn, 236t
   in pregnant patient, 234t–235t

T

Tachycardia, sinus, 392–393
   supraventricular, paroxysmal, 394–396

Tachycardia *(Continued)*
   electrocardiographic patterns in, 394
   heart rates in, 395
   medical management of, 396
   ventricular, 397
Tags, auricular, 47–49
TAPVC. See *Total anomalous pulmonary venous connection (TAPVC)*.
TAPVD. See *Total anomalous pulmonary venous drainage (TAPVD)*.
TAR (thrombocytopenia absent radius) syndrome, 494
Temperature, regulation of, in premature infant, 138–139
Terbutaline, for bronchopulmonary dysplasia, 293
Tetanus antitoxin, 220
Tetanus neonatorum, 219–221
   agent causing, 219
   management of, 220–221
   vs. tetany, 220
Tetany, hypocalcemic crisis with, treatment of, 514
   late infantile, 510
   neonatal, treatment of, 515
   vs. tetanus neonatorum, 220
Tetracycline, for tetanus neonatorum, 221
Tetralogy of Fallot, 333–334, 339–343
   anomalies associated with, 339
   coeur-en-sabot appearance of pulmonary artery in, 341
   surgical management of, 341
   with pulmonary atresia, 341–343
THAN (transient hyperammonemia of newborn), 86–87
Thermal neutral zone, 138–139
Thrombin clotting time (TCT), in hemorrhagic disorders, 480

Thrombocytopenia, 490, 492
  alloimmune, 496–498
    clinical presentation of, 497
    management of, 497–498
  amegakaryocytic, 494
  autoimmune, 498
  clinical impact of, 495
  decreased production of platelets causing, 494
  definition of, 490
  disease states associated with, 491t, 493
  drug-induced, 494
  increased destruction of platelets causing, 492–494
  mean platelet volume in, 492
  with giant hemangiomas, 493–494
Thrombocytopenia absent radius (TAR) syndrome, 494
Thrombotic disorder(s), 486–490
  arterial catheter–related, 488–489
  homozygous prethrombotic, 487–488
  renal vein thrombosis as, 489–490
  venous catheter–related, 488
Thrush (oral candidiasis), in HIV-infected patient, ketoconazole for, 166
Thumb polydactyly, 47
Thyroid dysgenesis, 532–533
Thyroid gland, disorder(s) of, 531–536
  associated with Down syndrome, 52
  congenital hypothyroidism as, 531–534
  dysgenesis in, 532–533
  hypothalamic-pituitary defects in, 533
  transient, 534
  thyrotoxicosis as, 535–536
Thyroiditis, Hashimoto's, 535
Thyroid-stimulating antibody (TSA), in thyrotoxicosis, 535

Thyroid-stimulating hormone (TSH), in congenital hypothyroidism, 531–532
  screening for, 108–109
  in hypothalamic-pituitary defects, 533
  in thyroid dysgenesis, 533
Thyrotoxicosis, 535–536
Thyrotropin-releasing hormone (TRH), in hypothalamic-pituitary defects, 533
Thyroxine (T_4), in congenital hypothyroidism, 532
  screening for, 108–109
  in thyroid dysgenesis, 532, 533
Tincture of opium, for neonatal opiate withdrawal, 4
Tolazine, for persistent pulmonary hypertension of newborn, 270
Tonic seizure(s), 432
TORCH infections, 167
Total anomalous pulmonary venous connection (TAPVC), 355–359
  postnatal presentation of, 356
  treatment of, 358–359
Total anomalous pulmonary venous drainage (TAPVD), 312–313, 334–335
  infradiaphragmatic, 322
  supracardiac, 315
Total parenteral nutrition (TPN), 453–457
  calcium, phosphorus, and magnesium in, 455
  cholestasis associated with, 449–450
  copper and zinc in, 455–456
  essential nutrients included in, 454
  inositol supplementation in, 455
  lipid emulsions in, 454
  nitrogen in, 453
    retention of, 453–454
  sodium and potassium in, 455

Total parenteral nutrition (TPN) *(Continued)*
  vitamin A in, 456
  vitamin E in, 456
  water-soluble vitamins in, 456–457
Toxicity, bilirubin, 467–470
Toxoplasma gondii, 224
Toxoplasmosis, 224–228
  and co-infection with HIV, 225
  classic triad of, 225
  congenital, newborn screening for, 115
  diagnosis of, 226
  immunoglobulin antibodies in, detection of, 226
  maternal, therapeutic abortion option in, 227–228
  treatment of, 227
TPN. See *Total parenteral nutrition (TPN).*
Transepidermal water losses, 150–151
Transfusion, exchange, for disseminated intravascular coagulation, 483–484
  for kernicterus, 468–469
  platelet, for alloimmune thrombocytopenia, 497–498
Transfusions, blood, for bronchopulmonary dysplasia, 291
Transient hyperammonemia of newborn (THAN), 86–87
Transient tachypnea of newborn (TTN), 262–265
  hyperaeration of lungs in, 264
  pulmonary edema in, 263, 264
  symptoms of, 263–264
Transposition of great arteries, 336–339
  chest radiographs of, 338
  malformations associated with, 336
  management of, 338–339
  murmurs in, 337
  pulmonary and systemic circulations in, 336–337

Treponema pallidum, 230. See also *Syphilis.*
Treponema pertenue, 230
TRH (thyrotropin-releasing hormone), in hypothalamic-pituitary defects, 533
Trichorrhexis nodosa, 84
Tricuspid atresia, 335, 348–350
Tricuspid valve, Ebstein anomaly of, 350–353
  treatment of, 352
Triploidy, 58–59
Trisomy 13 (Patau syndrome), 55–56
  postaxial polydactyly in, 47
  skin holes in, 313
Trisomy 18 (Edwards syndrome), 53–55
  physical findings in, 53–54
Trisomy 21 (Down syndrome), 49–52, 321–322
  acute lymphoblastic leukemia associated with, 52
  atlantoaxial subluxation associated with, 51
  atrioventricular septal defects in, 376–377
  birth defects associated with, 50–51
  cardinal signs of, in newborn, 49–50, 50t
  developmental variability associated with, 52
  gastrointestinal malformations associated with, 51
  growth problems associated with, 51–52
  hearing loss associated with, 51
  hypotonia due to, 40, 42
  long-term survival and prognosis for, 52
  ocular disorders associated with, 51
  prenatal diagnosis of, 49
  thyroid dysfunction associated with, 52
Tromethamine, for metabolic acidosis, 159
Truncus arteriosus, 335, 353–355

587

Truncus arteriosus (*Continued*)
  definition of, 353
  management of, 355
  murmurs in, 354–355
TSA (thyroid-stimulating antibody), in thyrotoxicosis, 535
TSH. See *Thyroid-stimulating hormone (TSH)*.
TTN. See *Transient tachypnea of newborn (TTN)*.
Tuberculin skin test, 218
Tuberculosis, 215–218
  management of, 217
  maternal, management of, 216
  miliary, 217
  sputum-positive, 217
  risk of, AIDS/HIV epidemic and, 215
Tuberous sclerosis, 406
Tumor(s), cardiac, 391–392
Turner syndrome (45,X karyotype), 56–57, 524, 525t, 526–527
  definition of, 524
  variants of, 527
Twins, 34–36
  congenital anomalies associated with, 35–36
  dizygotic (fraternal), 34
  monozygotic (identical), 34–35
  zygosity determination in, 36
Tyrosinemia, 448
  hereditary, type 1, 89–90

U

UCEDs (urea cycle enzyme defects), laboratory findings in, 84
Ultrasonography, diagnostic, of Arnold-Chiari syndrome, 401–402
  of renal vein thrombosis, 489–490
Umbilical cord, clamping of, timing of, 141
Umbilical cord blood, screening of, for maternal metabolic disorders, 119–120
Umbilical vessel, catheterization of, resuscitation and, 125, 128
Urea cycle enzyme defects (UCEDs), laboratory findings in, 84
Ureaplasma, in bronchopulmonary dysplasia, 288–289
Uric acid nephropathy, 505
Urinary tract infection(s), 201–203
Urine, water loss through, 151

V

Vaccination schedule, for hepatitis B, 183
VACTERL association, 72–73, 307
  hemivertebrae in, 322
Van der Woude syndrome, 37
Vancomycin, for staphylococcal infection, 192
Vanillylmandelic acid (VMA), in neuroblastoma, 117
Varicella zoster immune globulin (VZIG), 181
Varicella zoster virus infection, 179–181
  management of, 180–181
Vasopressin (antidiuretic hormone), 146
Vein of Galen, arteriovenous malformation of, 407–408
Velocardiofacial (Sprintzen) syndrome, 44, 61
  chromosome 22q11 deletion associated with, 40
Venous catheter–related thrombosis, 488
Ventilation, high-frequency, for persistent pulmonary hypertension of newborn, 269–270
  mechanical, for bronchopulmonary dysplasia, 286
  for hyaline membrane disease, 261–262
  pulmonary interstitial emphysema due to, 281

Ventricle(s), in hypoplastic left heart syndrome, 369–370
Ventricular septum, defects of, 372–376
  chest radiographs of, 375
  intact, pulmonary atresia with, 343–346
  pulmonary stenosis with, 346–348
Ventricular tachycardia, 397
Very-long-chain acyl-CoA dehydrogenase (LCAD) deficiency, 99–100
Very-low-birth-weight (VLBW) infant(s), bronchopulmonary dysplasia in, 284. See also *Bronchopulmonary dysplasia (BPD)*.
  hyperglycemia in, 543
  osteopenia in, 517
  patent ductus arteriosus in, 300–301
Viral infection(s), 164–184
  congenital, 167–168
  cytomegaloviral, 171–175
  enteroviral, 175–176
  hepatitis B as, 181–183
  hepatitis C as, 183
  herpes simplex, 176–179
  human immunodeficiency, 164–168
  human papillomavirus, 184
  rubella as, 168–171
  varicella, 179–181
Virilization, associated with congenital adrenal hyperplasia, 523
  of female fetus, 529–531
    by maternal ingestion of drugs, 530
    by maternal overproduction of androgens, 530–531
Vitamin(s), water-soluble, in total parenteral nutrition, 456–457
Vitamin A, in total parenteral nutrition, 456
Vitamin A deficiency, in bronchopulmonary dysplasia, 289
Vitamin B$_{12}$, for methylmalonic acidemia, 93–94

Vitamin D, for breast-fed infant, 452
  for vitamin D deficiency rickets, 516
Vitamin D deficiency, early neonatal hypocalcemia and, 509
  late neonatal hypocalcemia and, 511
Vitamin E, in total parenteral nutrition, 456
Vitamin K, daily requirements of, for VK-dependent bleeding, 486
  for breast-fed infant, 452
  prophylactic, for intraventricular hemorrhage, 423
Vitamin K deficiency, 484–486
  hemorrhagic disorders due to, 479–480
VK-dependent bleeding (VKDB), 484–486
  classic form of, 485
  daily requirements of vitamin K for, 486
  early form of, 485
  late form of, 485
  vitamin K prophylaxis in, 485–486
VMA (vanillylmandelic acid), in neuroblastoma, 117
Volume expanders, for resuscitation, 126t
Volutrauma, 286
Volvulus, malrotation with, 441
Vomiting, intestinal obstruction causing, 436
V/Q, in hyaline membrane disease, 251
V/Q spells, in premature infants, 242–243
VZIG (varicella zoster immune globulin), 181

W

Water losses, insensible, 150–151
  sensible, 151
  surgical, 151–152
Water requirements, for sick newborn, estimation of, 150

589

Water-soluble vitamins, in total parenteral nutrition, 456–457
Werdnig-Hoffman disease (spinal muscular atrophy), hypotonia due to, 42
Werdnig-Hoffmann disease, 435
Whey fraction, constituents of, 450–451
  in human milk vs. bovine milk, 450
White blood cell (WBC) count, in septicemia, 187
White matter injury, 418–419
Williams syndrome, 62–63
Wilms tumor, 62
Wilson-Mikity syndrome, 297–298
Withdrawal syndrome, in infant of substance abusing mother, 4
Wolf-Hirschhorn syndrome, 61–62
World Health Organization (WHO) policy, for breast-feeding by HIV-positive mothers, 452

X

45,X karyotype (Turner syndrome), 56–57, 524, 525t, 526–527
  definition of, 524
  variants of, 527
47,XXX karyotype, 57
46,XX/XY karyotype (pure gonadal dysgenesis), 525t, 527–528
47,XXY karyotype (Klinefelter syndrome), 57–58, 524, 525t
47,XYY karyotype, 58

Z

Zellweger (cerebrohepatorenal) syndrome, 448–449
Zidovudine, for HIV infection, 165–166
Zinc, in total parenteral nutrition, 455–456
Zygosity determination, in twinning, 36
ZZ phenotype, in alpha$_1$-antitrypsin deficiency, 446